Essentials in Ophthalmology

Cornea and External Eye Disease

T. Reinhard   F. Larkin
Editors

Essentials in Ophthalmology

G. K. Krieglstein   R. N. Weinreb
Series Editors

Glaucoma

Cataract and Refractive Surgery

Uveitis and Immunological Disorders

Vitreo-retinal Surgery

Medical Retina

Oculoplastics and Orbit

**Pediatric Ophthalmology,
Neuro-Ophthalmology, Genetics**

Cornea and External Eye Disease

Editors Thomas Reinhard
Frank Larkin

Cornea and External Eye Disease

Corneal Allotransplantation,
Allergic Disease and Trachoma

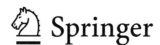

Series Editors

Günter K. Krieglstein, MD
Professor and Chairman
Department of Ophthalmology
University of Cologne
Joseph-Stelzmann-Straße 9
50931 Köln
Germany

Robert N. Weinreb, MD
Professor and Director
Hamilton Glaucoma Center
Department of Ophthalmology – 0946
University of California at San Diego
9500 Gilman Drive
La Jolla, CA 92093-0946
USA

Volume Editors

Thomas Reinhard
Professor and Chairman
University Eye Hospital
Killianstraße 5
79106 Freiburg
Germany

Frank Larkin
Moorfields Eye Hospital
162 City Road
London EC1V 2PD
United Kingdom

ISBN: 978-3-540-85543-9   e-ISBN: 978-3-540-85544-6

DOI: 10.1007/978-3-540-85544-6

Library of Congress Control Number: 2009931341

© Springer-Verlag Berlin Heidelberg 2010

This work is subject to copyright. All rights are reserved, whether the whole or part of the material is concerned, specifically the rights of translation, reprinting, reuse of illustrations, recitation, broadcasting, reproduction on microfilm or in any other way, and storage in data banks. Duplication of this publication or parts thereof is permitted only under the provisions of the German Copyright Law of September 9, 1965, in its current version, and permission for use must always be obtained from Springer. Violations are liable to prosecution under the German Copyright Law.

The use of general descriptive names, registered names, trademarks, etc. in this publication does not imply, even in the absence of a specific statement, that such names are exempt from the relevant protective laws and regulations and therefore free for general use.

Product liability: The publishers cannot guarantee the accuracy of any information about dosage and application contained in this book. In every individual case the user must check such information by consulting the relevant literature.

Cover design: wmx Design, Heidelberg, Germany

Printed on acid-free paper

9 8 7 6 5 4 3 2 1

(www.springer.com)

Foreword

The Essentials in Ophthalmology series represents an unique updating publication on the progress in all subspecialties of ophthalmology.

In a quarterly rhythm, eight issues are published covering clinically relevant achievements in the whole field of ophthalmology. This timely transfer of advancements for the best possible care of our eye patients has proven to be effective. The initial working hypothesis of providing new knowledge immediately following publication in the peer-reviewed journal and not waiting for the textbook appears to be highly workable.

We are now in the third cycle of the Essentials in Ophthalmology series, having been encouraged by readership acceptance of the first two series, each of eight volumes. This is a success that was made possible predominantly by the numerous opinion-leading authors and the outstanding section editors, as well as with the constructive support of the publisher. There are many good reasons to continue and still improve the dissemination of this didactic and clinically relevant information.

G.K. Krieglstein
R.N. Weinreb
Series Editors

Preface

This third *Cornea and External Eye Disease* volume comprises eleven reviews of moving points in corneal biology, disease pathogenesis and management.

In this volume we have gathered a number of chapters on and around the topic of cornea and limbus transplantation. Jerry Niederkorn reviews our increasing understanding of the components of immune privilege enjoyed by corneal transplants, a privilege unrivalled in the field of transplantation. This privilege is relative and is neither universal nor immutable. Rejection remains the major threat for corneal transplants, in the settings of conventional penetrating keratoplasty, of newer lamellar surgical techniques and of course especially in patients at high rejection risk.

Strategy on how to prevent immune rejection is controversial; differing analyses being described in the chapters by Douglas Coster and Alex Reis. Some benefit of HLA matching has been found in high rejection risk corneal transplantation, but transplantation antigen matching is undertaken only in European centres. Is use of systemic immunosuppressive drugs justified in corneal graft recipients, among whom are some in whom blindness would result from loss of donor corneal transparency? Risks of drug adverse effects vs. benefits of maintaining a functioning transplant should be considered in any candidate for a corneal transplant at high rejection risk. It is noteworthy that quality of life in blind patients is significantly more compromised than in those renal failure patients requiring dialysis [1, 2]. We hope you enjoy reading this volume.

Thomas Reinhard
Frank Larkin

References

1. Brown MM, Brown GC, Sharma S, Kistler J, Brown H (2001) Utility values associated with blindness in an adult population. Br J Ophthalmol 85:327–331
2. Liem YS, Bosch JL, Hunink MG (2008) Preference-based quality of life of patients on renal replacement therapy: a systemic review and meta-analysis. Value Health 11:733–741

Contents

Chapter 1
Immune Privilege of Corneal Allografts
Jerry Y. Niederkorn

1.1	History of Corneal Transplantation and Immune Privilege	1
1.2	How Successful Is Corneal Transplantation?	2
1.3	Immune Rejection of Corneal Allografts	3
1.3.1	Role of CD4+ T Lymphocytes in Corneal Allograft Rejection	3
1.3.2	Role of CD8+ T Lymphocytes in Corneal Allograft Rejection	3
1.3.3	Role of Antibodies in Corneal Allograft Rejection	4
1.3.4	Role of Macrophages and NK Cells in Corneal Allograft Rejection	4
1.3.5	What are the Effectors of Corneal Allograft Rejection?	5
1.4	Role of Atopic Diseases in Corneal Allograft Rejection	5
1.5	Immune Privilege of Corneal Allografts Is a Tripartite Phenomenon	5
1.5.1	Afferent Blockade of the Immune Response to Corneal Allografts	6
1.5.2	Immune Deviation in the Central Processing Component of the Immune Reflex Arc	8
1.5.3	Efferent Blockade of the Immune Response to Corneal Allografts	9
	References	10

Chapter 2
Mechanisms of Corneal Allograft Rejection and the Development of New Therapies
Douglas J. Coster, Claire F. Jessup, and Keryn A. Williams

2.1	Status of Corneal Transplantation	13
2.2	Success Rate of Corneal Transplantation	13
2.3	Maintenance and Erosion of Corneal Privilege	14
2.4	The Corneal Allograft Response	15
2.5	Antigen Uptake in the Eye	15
2.6	Antigen Processing	16
2.7	Antigen Presentation	16
2.8	T Cell Activation, Proliferation, and Clonal Expansion	17
2.9	Effector Arm of the Allograft Response	17
2.10	Current Management of Corneal Transplants	17
2.11	Prevention of Allograft Rejection	17
2.12	Stratification of Risk	18
2.13	Protecting Immune Privilege	18
2.14	Minimizing Antigenic Differences Between Donor and Recipient	18
2.15	Systemic Immunosuppression	18
2.16	Surgical Techniques and Postoperative Management	18
2.17	Management of Acute Rejection Episodes	19
2.18	New Therapies with Novel Mechanisms	19
2.19	Antibody-based Immunosuppressive Agents in Transplantation	19
2.20	Engineered Antibodies for Eye Disease	19
2.21	Gene Therapy of the Donor Cornea	20
2.22	Vectors for Gene Therapy of the Cornea	20
2.23	Transgenes for Prolonging Corneal Graft Survival	20
2.24	Future Prospects	20
	References	22

Chapter 3
New Developments in Topical and Systemic Immunomodulation Following Penetrating Keratoplasty
Alexander Reis and Thomas Reinhard

3.1	Introduction	25
3.2	Immunology	26
3.2.1	Acute Rejection	26
3.2.2	Major Histocompatibility Complex (MHC)	26

3.2.2.1	Direct Pathway of Allorecognition	26	4.1.1	Anterior Chamber-Associated Immune Deviation (ACAID)	38
3.2.2.2	Indirect Pathway of Allorecognition	26	4.1.2	The Th1/Th2 Paradigm	38
3.2.3	Chronic Rejection	26	4.2	Pitfalls in the Determination of Cytokine Levels from Aqueous Humor	38
3.3	Normal-risk vs. High-risk Transplantation	27			
3.3.1	Normal-risk Transplantation	27			
3.3.2	High-risk Transplantation	27	4.3	Relevance of Individual Cytokines in Corneal Transplantation	40
3.3.3	Rationale for Systemic Immunosuppression	27	4.3.1	Interleukin 1b	40
3.3.4	Why Is Immunomodulation with Topical Steroids Not Sufficient to Prevent Immunologic Graft Rejection in High-Risk Patients?	27	4.3.1.1	General Functions from In Vitro Experiments	40
			4.3.1.2	Effects in Animal Models of Corneal Transplantation	40
3.3.5	Rationale for Topical Immunomodulation	27	4.3.1.3	Interleukin 1b Levels in Human Aqueous Humor	40
3.4	Immunosuppressive Agents	28	4.3.2	Interleukin 2	40
3.4.1	History	28	4.3.2.1	General Functions from In Vitro Experiments	40
3.4.2	Corticosteroids	28			
3.4.3	Cyclosporine A	28	4.3.2.2	Effects in Animal Models of Corneal Transplantation	40
3.4.3.1	CSA in Corneal Transplantation	29			
3.4.4	Tacrolimus (fk506)	29	4.3.2.3	Interleukin 2 Levels in Human Aqueous Humor	40
3.4.4.1	Tacrolimus in Corneal Transplantation	29			
3.4.5	Mycophenolate Mofetil (MMF)	29	4.3.3	Interleukin 6	41
3.4.6	Rapamycin (Sirolimus)	30	4.3.3.1	General Functions from In Vitro Experiments	41
3.4.7	RAD (Everolimus)	30			
3.4.8	FTY 720	31	4.3.3.2	Effects in Animal Models of Corneal Transplantatoin	41
3.4.9	FK788	31			
3.5	Pimecrolimus	31	4.3.3.3	Interleukin 6 Levels in Human Aqueous Humor	41
3.5.1	Pimecrolimus in Corneal Transplantation	31			
			4.3.4	Interleukin 10	41
3.5.2	Biologic Agents	31	4.3.4.1	General Functions from In Vitro Experiments	41
3.5.2.1	Basiliximab and Daclizumab	31			
3.6	Guidelines for Practitioners	32	4.3.4.2	Effects in Animal Models of Corneal Transplantation	41
3.6.1	Systemic Immunosuppression with Drugs with Proven Efficacy in Corneal Transplantation	32			
			4.3.4.3	Interleukin10 Levels in Human Aqueous Humor	41
3.6.1.1	Preoperative Evaluation	32	4.3.5	Interferon Gamma (IFN-γ)	42
3.6.1.2	How to Use Cyclosporine in High-risk Corneal Transplantation	32	4.3.5.1	General Functions from In Vitro Experiments	42
3.6.1.3	How to Use MMF in High-risk Corneal Transplantation	32	4.3.5.2	Effects in Animal Models of Corneal Transplantation	42
			4.3.5.3	INF-γ Levels in the Aqueous Humor	42
3.6.2	Topical Immunosuppression	33	4.3.6	Tumor Necrosis Factor Alpha (TNF-α)	42
3.7	Conclusion	33	4.3.6.1	General Functions from In Vitro Experiments	42
	References	33			
			4.3.6.2	Effects in Animal Models of Corneal Transplantation	42

Chapter 4
Cytokines Analysis of the Aqueous Humor in the Context of Penetrating Keratoplasty

Philip Maier and Thomas Reinhard

4.1	Immune Privilege of the Anterior Ocular Segment	38	4.3.6.3	TNF-α Levels in Human Aqueous Humor	42
			4.3.7	Transforming Growth Factor Beta (TGF-β)	43
			4.3.7.1	General Functions from In Vitro	

	Experiment	43
4.3.7.2	Effects in Animal Models of Corneal Transplantation	44
4.3.7.3	TGF-β2 Levels in Human Aqueous Humor.................................	44
4.3.8	Fas, Fas Ligand and Soluble Fas Ligand	44
4.3.8.1	General Functions from In Vitro Experiments	44
4.3.8.2	Effects in Animal Models of Corneal Transplantation	45
4.3.8.3	sFasL Levels in Human Aqueous Humor.................................	45
4.3.9	Further Cytokines and Immunomodulative Factors	45
4.3.9.1	Interleukin 1 Receptor Antagonist	45
4.3.9.2	Interleukin 4	46
4.3.9.3	Interleukin 5	46
4.3.9.4	Interleukin 8	46
4.3.9.5	Interleukin 12.........................	46
4.3.9.6	Alpha-Melanocyte-Stimulating Hormone/Calcitonin Gene-Realted Peptide/Thrombospondin/Somatostatin	46
4.4	Cytokine Profiles in the Context of Corneal Transplantation.............	49
4.4.1	Cytokine Profiles in Animal Models	49
4.4.2	Cytokine Profiles in Humans	49
4.4.2.1	Cytokines in the Serum of Patients Following PK..........................	49
4.4.2.2	Cytokines in Human Corneas	49
4.4.2.3	Cytokines in Human Aqueous Humor ...	49
	References.............................	50

Chapter 5
Limbal Stem Cell Transplantation: Surgical Techniques and Results
Alex J. Shortt, Stephen J. Tuft, and Julie T. Daniels

5.1	Introduction	53
5.1.1	The Corneal Epithelium................	53
5.1.2	The Limbus and Corneal Epithelial Homeostasis	53
5.2	Corneal LESC Deficiency...............	55
5.2.1	Diagnosis and Classification of Corneal LESC Deficiency	55
5.3	Management of Patients with Limbal Stem Cell Deficiency	57
5.3.1	Conservative Options	57
5.3.2	Surgical Options for Partial Limbal Stem Cell Deficiency	57

5.3.3	Surgical Options for Total Limbal Stem Cell Deficiency	57
5.4	Surgical Techniques for Transplanting Corneal Limbal Stem Cells	58
5.4.1	Conjunctival Limbal Autograft (CLAU)...	58
5.4.2	Living-Related Conjunctival Limbal Allograft Transplant (lr-CLAL)	58
5.4.2.1	Clinical Outcomes of CLAU and lr-CLAL...	59
5.4.3	Keratolimbal Allograft Transplant	59
5.4.4	Ex Vivo Expansion and Transplantation of Cultured Limbal Stem Cells...........	60
5.4.5	Regulations Governing the Clinical Use of Ex vivo Cultured Tissue	60
5.4.6	Evidence of the Presence of Stem Cells in Ex vivo Cultures and Grafts......	61
5.4.7	Assessing Outcomes Following LESC Transplantation	61
5.4.8	Evidence for Donor Cell Survival Following Ex Vivo Cultured LESC Transplantation	61
5.4.9	Role of Tissue Matching in Transplantation of Allogeneic Tissue or Cells...........................	62
5.4.10	Alternative Sources of Autologous Stem Cells	62
5.4.11	Issues Surrounding Ex Vivo Cultured LESC Transplantation that Require Further Investigation...................	62
5.5	Conclusion............................	63
	References.............................	63

Chapter 6
Cell Cycle Control and Replication in Corneal Endothelium
Nancy C. Joyce

6.1	Relationship of Endothelial Barrier Function to Corneal Transparency	70
6.2	Corneal Endothelial Cell Loss and Repair Mechanisms	71
6.2.1	Causes of Cell Loss	71
6.2.2	Repair of the Endothelial Monolayer	71
6.3	Are Human Corneal Endothelial Cells Able to Divide?.....................	71
6.3.1	Proliferative Status In Vivo	71
6.3.2	Evidence that HCEC Retain Proliferative Capacity....................	71
6.4	The Cell Cycle	72
6.4.1	Positive Regulation of the Cell Cycle	72
6.4.2	Negative Regulation of G1-Phase of the Cell Cycle	73

6.5	Potential Causes for Inhibition of HCEC Proliferation In Vivo	74		7.3.2.4	Hybrid Lenses	89
6.5.1	Cell–Cell Contacts Inhibit Division	74		7.3.3	Fitting Techniques	89
6.5.2	Endothelium In Vivo Lacks Effective Paracrine or Autocrine Growth Factor Stimulation	75		7.3.3.1	The Reshape and Splint Method	89
				7.3.3.2	The Three-Point Touch Method	89
				7.3.3.3	The Apical Clearance Method	90
				7.3.3.4	Scleral Fitting Method	90
6.5.3	TGF-Beta2 Has a Suppressive Effect on S-phase Entry	75		7.3.4	GP Fitting Following Cross Linking	90
				7.4	CL Fitting Following Penetrating Keratoplasty	91
6.6	Proliferative Capacity of HCEC Differs with Donor Age	76		7.4.1	Indications for CLs Following PK	91
6.6.1	Analysis of pRb Hyperphosphorylation	77		7.4.2	Indications for CLs Following PK in Comparison with Newer Techniques	91
6.6.2	Analysis of Replication Competence	77				
6.6.3	Analysis of CKI Protein Expression	77		7.4.3	PK Peculiarities in Conjunction with CLs	92
6.7	Efforts to Stimulate Corneal Endothelial Proliferation by Interfering with G1-phase Inhibition	78		7.4.3.1	Corneal Sensitivity, Fitting Quality, and Frequent Follow-Ups	92
				7.4.3.2	The Endothelium and Choice of GP Materials	92
6.7.1	Overcoming G1-phase Inhibition	79				
6.7.2	Bypassing G1-phase Inhibition	79		7.4.3.3	Immune Reactions	92
6.8	Endothelial Topography Affects the Proliferative Capacity of HCEC	79		7.4.4	When to Fit?	92
				7.4.5	Fitting Techniques	93
6.8.1	Differences in Proliferative Capacity	79		7.4.5.1	PK with One or Two Sutures	93
6.8.2	Differences in Senescence Characteristics	80		7.4.5.2	CL Fitting Following Suture Removal	93
					Abbreviations	94
6.9	Identification of Mechanisms Responsible for Decreased Proliferative Capacity	80			References	94

Chapter 8
Allergic Disease of the Conjunctiva and Cornea

Andrea Leonardi

6.9.1	Are Critically Short Telomeres Responsible for Decreased Proliferative Capacity?	81
6.9.2	Is Sub-lethal Oxidative DNA Damage Responsible for Decreased Proliferative Capacity?	81
6.10	Future Directions	82
	References	83

8.1	Introduction and Classification	97
8.2	Clinical Forms	98
8.2.1	Seasonal and Perennial Allergic Conjunctivitis	98
8.2.2	Vernal Keratoconjunctivitis	98
8.2.3	Atopic Keratoconjunctivitis	100
8.2.4	Giant Papillary Conjunctivitis	101
8.2.5	Contact Blepharoconjunctivitis	101
8.2.6	Drug-Induced Conjunctivitis or Keratoconjunctivitis	101
8.2.7	Urban Eye Allergy Syndrome	102
8.3	Differential Diagnosis	103
8.4	Diagnostic Tests in Ocular Allergy	104
8.5	Ocular Immunity and the Allergic Reaction	104
8.5.1	Innate Immunity and Ocular Allergy	104
8.5.2	The Allergic Process	105
8.5.3	Allergic Inflammation	106
8.6	The Cornea in Allergic Diseases	107
8.6.1	Corneal Immunology	107
8.6.2	Allergic Inflammation and Corneal Damage	107
8.6.3	Tear Instability and Corneal Involvement	107
8.6.4	Corneal Clinical Manifestations	

Chapter 7
Current State of the Art of Fitting Gas-Permeable (GP) Contact Lenses

Silke Lohrengel and Dieter Muckenhirn

7.1	Corneal Topography and Automatic Fitting Programs	87
7.2	Fitting CLs	88
7.3	The Keratoconus	88
7.3.1	KC Peculiarities in Conjunction with CL	88
7.3.1.1	Corneal Sensitivity and Maximum Resilience	88
7.3.1.2	Corneal Contour: KC Stage: KC Type	89
7.3.2	Forms of Correction	89
7.3.2.1	Soft Lenses	89
7.3.2.2	GP Contact Lenses	89
7.3.2.3	Piggyback	89

	in Ocular Allergy	108	9.7.1	The Stimulus for Inflammation and Scarring in Trachoma	127
8.6.5	Confocal Microscopy and Allergic Keratoconjunctivitis	108	9.7.2	Histopathology	128
8.6.6	Keratoconus and Allergic Conjunctivitis	109	9.7.3	The Immune Response in Trachoma	128
8.6.7	Keratoglobus	109	9.7.4	Immunopathogenesis of Conjunctival Scarring	129
8.6.8	Allergic Keratoconjunctivitis and Corneal Infection	110	9.8	Trachoma Control	130
8.6.9	Allergy and Corneal Transplant	110	9.8.1	The SAFE Strategy	130
8.6.9.1	Immunology	110	9.8.2	Surgery for Trichiasis	130
8.6.9.2	Clinical Outcomes	111	9.8.3	Antibiotics	130
8.7	Treatment of Ocular Allergy	111	9.8.4	Face Washing	132
8.7.1	Nonpharmacological Management	112	9.8.5	Environmental Improvements	132
8.7.2	Treatment of Allergic Conjunctivitis	112	9.10	Conclusion	132
8.7.2.1	Topical Ocular Pharmacological Treatment	112		References	133

Chapter 10
Keratoprosthesis
Jason J. Jun, Donna E. Siracuse-Lee, Mary K. Daly, and Claes H. Dohlman

8.7.2.2	Topical Nonocular Pharmacological Treatment	113
8.7.2.3	Systemic Pharmacological Treatment	113
8.7.2.4	Specific Immunotherapy	114
8.7.3	Treatment of GPC	114
8.7.4	Treatment of Vernal Keratoconjunctivitis	114
8.7.4.1	Corticosteroids	114
8.7.4.2	Cyclosporine and Other Immunosuppressive Treatments	115
8.7.5	Treatment of AKC	115
8.7.5.1	Cyclosporine and Other Immunosuppressive Treatments	115
8.7.6	Surgical Treatment of Keratoconjunctivitis	116
	References	116

10.1	Introduction	137
10.2	Prognostic Hierarchy	138
10.3	Defining Patient Subtypes	138
10.3.1	Patient Subtype A: The Noninflamed Eye	138
10.3.2	Patient Subtype B: The Inflamed Eye	138
10.4	Experience with Kpro in Patient Subtype A	138
10.4.1	Boston Type 1 Kpro	138
10.4.1.1	Pediatric Application of Boston Type 1 Kpro	139
10.4.2	AlphaCor Kpro	140
10.5	Experience with Kpro in Patient Subtype B	140
10.5.1	Osteo-Odonto Keratoprosthesis (OOKP)	140
10.5.2	Boston Type 2 Kpro	141
10.6	Other Kpro Designs	141
10.6.1	Pintucci Kpro	141
10.6.2	Seoul-Type Kpro	141
10.6.3	Worst-Singh Kpro	141
10.6.4	Russian/Ukrainian Experience	142
10.7	New Directions in Kpro Research	142
10.7.1	Hydroxyapatite Biologic Haptics	142
10.7.2	Biologic Coatings	142
10.7.3	Biologic Scaffolds and Enhanced Hydrogels	142
10.8	Conclusion	142
	References	143

Chapter 9
Trachoma
Matthew J. Burton

9.1	Introduction	121
9.1.1	Overview	121
9.1.2	History	121
9.2	Clinical Features	122
9.2.1	Symptoms and Signs	122
9.2.2	Trachoma Grading Systems	123
9.2.3	Differential Diagnosis	123
9.3	Chlamydia Trachomatis	123
9.4	Laboratory Diagnosis	124
9.5	Clinical Signs and Infection	125
9.6	Epidemiology	125
9.6.1	Prevalence and Distribution	125
9.6.2	Age and Gender	126
9.6.3	Risk Factors for Active Trachoma and *C. Trachomatis* Infection	126
9.7	Pathophysiology of Trachoma	127

Chapter 11
Posterior Lamellar Keratoplasty in Perspective
Arnalich-Montiel F and Dart JKG

11.1	Introduction	145

11.2	Choosing Endothelial Keratoplasty Procedures..................	146	
11.2.1	Indications.............................	146	
11.2.2	Preoperative Considerations............	146	
11.2.2.1	Confirming the Extent of Endothelial Dysfunction	146	
11.2.2.2	Corneal Scarring	147	
11.2.2.3	Cataract and Intraocular Lens Status	147	
11.2.2.4	Lens/Iris Diaphragm Status	147	
11.2.2.5	Intraocular Pressure	148	
11.2.2.6	Retinal Function........................	148	
11.3	PLK Surgical Technique.................	148	
11.3.1	Donor Preparation	148	
11.3.2	Host Dissection for DSEK/DSAEK........	148	
11.3.3	Donor Insertion	149	
11.3.4	Techniques for Graft Centration.........	149	
11.3.5	Techniques for Promoting Donor Adhesion	150	
11.3.6	Post-operative Care	151	
11.3.7	Surgery for Complex Cases	151	
11.3.7.1	Failed Grafts	151	
11.3.7.2	Aniridics, Vitrectomised and Aphakic Eyes (Fig. 11.3e)	153	

11.3.7.3	Anterior Chamber Lens..................	153
11.4	Clinical Results and Complications.......	153
11.4.1	Visual Acuity	153
11.4.2	Astigmatism	153
11.4.3	Spherical Equivalent....................	153
11.4.4	Endothelial Cell Loss	154
11.4.5	Corneal Donor Dislocation (Fig. 11.4a–c)	155
11.4.6	Pupillary Block	156
11.4.7	Primary Graft Failure	156
11.4.8	Rejection	156
11.4.9	Other Complications	156
11.5	Conclusion.............................	157
	References.............................	157

Index *161*

Contributors

Matthew Burton
Department of Infectious and Tropical Diseases,
International Centre for Eye Health,
London School of Hygiene & Tropical Medicine,
Keppel Street,
London WC1E 7HT, UK

Douglas Coster
Department of Ophthalmology, NHMRC Centre for
Clinical Eye Research, Flinders Medical Centre,
Bedford Park, Adelaide, SA 5042, Australia

Mary Daly
Boston University Eye Associates Inc.,
Albany Street, Boston, MA 02118, USA
Veterans Affairs Boston Healthcare System,
Jamaica Plain, MA, USA
Department of Ophthalmology, Boston University
School of Medicine, Boston, MA, USA

Julie T. Daniels
Department of Ocular Biology and Therapeutics,
UCL Institute of Ophthalmology, 11-43 Bath Street,
London, EC1V 9EL, UK

John Dart,
Moorfields Eye Hospital,
162 City Road, London EC1V 2PD,
UK

Claas Dohlman
Massachusetts Eye and Ear Infirmary,
Harvard Medical School, MA, USA

Claire F. Jessup
Transplantation Immunology Laboratory,
University of Adelaide, SA 5005, Australia
Queen Elizabeth Hospital, 28 Woodville Road,
Woodville South SA 5011, Australia

Nancy C. Joyce
Schepens Eye Research Institute, 20 Staniford Street,
Boston, MA 02114, USA
Department of Ophthalmology, Harvard Medical School,
20 Staniford Street, Boston, MA 02114, USA

Jason J. Jun
Veterans Affairs Boston Healthcare System,
Jamaica Plain, MA, USA

Andrea Leonardi
Ophthalmology Unit, University of Padua, Via Giustiniani
2, I-35128 Padua, Italy

Silke Lohrengel
Hecht-Contactlinsen GmbH, Dorfstraße 2, 79280 Au,
Germany

Philipp Maier
University Eye Hospital Freiburg, Killianstraße 5,
79106 Freiburg, Germany

Dieter Muckenhirn
Hecht Contactlinsen GmbH, Dorfstraße 2-4,
79280 Au, Germany

Jerry Young Niederkorn
UT Southwestern Medical School, 5323 Harry Hines Blvd,
Dallas, TX 75390-9057, USA

Thomas Reinhard
Professor and Chairman of the University Eye Hospital,
Killianstraße 5, 79106 Freiburg, Germany

Alexander Reis
Augenwerk Optik, Landstraße 310,
FL-9495 Triesen/Vaduz, Principality of Liechtenstein

Alex J. Shortt
UCL Institute of Ophthalmology, 11-43 Bath Street,
London EC1V 9EL, UK

Donna E. Siracuse-Lee
Veterans Affairs Boston Healthcare System,
Jamaica Plain, MA, USA
Department of Ophthalmology, Boston University School
of Medicine, Boston, MA, USA

Stephen J. Tuft
Moorfields Eye Hospital, City Road,
London EC 1V 2PD, UK

Keryn A. Williams
Department of Ophthalmology, Flinders University,
Flinders Medical Centre, Bedford Park SA 5042, Australia

Chapter 1

Immune Privilege of Corneal Allografts

Jerry Y. Niederkorn

Core Messages

- Multiple anatomical, physiological, and immunoregulatory factors contribute to the immune privilege of corneal allografts. These factors conspire to prevent the induction and expression of immune responses to the histocompatibility antigens on the corneal allograft.
- Corneal allografts also elicit a dynamic immunoregulatory process that deviates the immune response from a destructive pathway to one of tolerance. Together, these conditions create an immune privileged environment and promote corneal allograft survival.
- Corneal allografts enjoy immune privilege that is unrivaled in the field of transplantation. However, this immune privilege is neither universal nor immutable. This has led some to dismiss immune privilege of corneal allografts out of hand. Moreover, the success of renal, cardiac, and liver transplants has improved over the past 3 decades and has reached levels similar to corneal allografts – an observation that has further fueled protests that corneal allografts are no different than other organ allografts, and that immune privilege is a misnomer. However, comparing survival rates among these categories of allografts is a bit like comparing an apple to an orange. For the comparisons to be valid, we must either compare the survival of corneal allografts in patients treated with the same intense systemic immunosuppressive agents that are used in renal, cardiac, or liver transplant patients, or compare all four categories of patients when the only treatment is topical corticosteroids (i.e., the standard prophylactic therapy in keratoplasty patients). The latter proposition, of course, is absurd, but does emphasize the importance of including all of the parameters when making comparisons relating to immune privilege.
- Prospective studies in animal models have unequivocally shown that in the absence of antirejection drugs, corneal allografts have dramatically higher acceptance and long-term survival rates than other categories of allografts such as skin transplants.

1.1 History of Corneal Transplantation and Immune Privilege

The notion that corneal tissues could be successfully transplanted was proposed three centuries ago by Erasmus Darwin, the grandfather of Charles Darwin. The first reported attempt at experimental corneal transplantation was performed in 1835 by Bigger, who transplanted a corneal allograft to a pet gazelle [1]. In 1838, Kissam attempted the first corneal transplant in a human subject and grafted a pig cornea onto a patient's eye using four interrupted sutures and without the use of anesthesia [2]! Almost half a century later corneal transplantation was once again attempted on humans when May transplanted rabbit corneal xenografts to humans and noted that the 24 attempts failed due to "imperfect technique and the inability to keep the eyes properly bandaged" [3]. It took almost seven decades before the first successful corneal transplant was grafted from a human donor to a human recipient [4, 5]. Since then, corneal transplantation has emerged as the most common form of solid tissue transplantation in the United States and the United Kingdom [6, 7].

The concept that the cornea and the anterior segment of the eye might be endowed with unusual immunological properties can be traced to Sir Peter Medawar, who noted the remarkable survival of orthotopic corneal allografts transplanted to the ocular surface and heterotopic skin allografts placed into the anterior chamber

Table 1.1 Immune rejection of corneal allografts and skin allografts in rats

Histocompatibility barrier	Incidence of rejection	
	Skin allograft (%)	Corneal allograft (%)
MHC + multiple minor histocompatibility antigens	100	38 to >90
MHC class I only	100	18–35
MHC class II only	100	0–10

(AC) of the rabbit eye. Medawar recognized the significance of the unusual properties of the corneal transplant and the anterior chamber over which it was transplanted, and coined the term "immune privilege" [8]. Clinical observations in human keratoplasty patients and results from experimental animal studies support the notion that corneal allografts enjoy immune privilege [5, 6, 9]. In routine human keratoplasty, no HLA matching is performed and topical corticosteroids are the only immunosuppressive agents administered. This is in sharp contrast to all other forms of solid tissue transplantation. Animal studies have provided perhaps the most compelling evidence for the immune privilege of orthotopic corneal allografts [5]. In rodent models of penetrating keratoplasty, the incidence of immune rejection of corneal allografts differing from the hosts at all known histocompatibility gene loci (i.e., MHC plus minor histocompatibility loci) can be as low as 38%, with the average being approximately 50%, even though immunosuppressive drugs are not used [5]. Corneal allograft survival is even more impressive when histocompatibility matching is applied. Corneal allografts mismatched with the host only at MHC class I loci enjoy long-term survival in 65 and 72% of the rat and mouse hosts, respectively [5]. Corneal allograft survival in rodents mismatched with the corneal allograft donor only at MHC class II loci display the most pronounced example of immune privilege, with graft rejection occurring in less than 10% of the hosts. In contrast, skin allografts in each of these categories are invariably rejected (Table 1.1). These remarkable findings have led to the misconception that the immune privilege of corneal transplants is universal and immutable.

1.2 How Successful Is Corneal Transplantation?

Although it is commonly stated that corneal allografts enjoy a first-year survival rate as high as 90%, the long-term survival rate is considerably lower and drops to 74% at 5 years and 62% at 10 years [7]. Moreover, graft survival is even worse in patients who are considered "high-risk" based on the presence of preexisting corneal neovascularization, ongoing ocular inflammation, or a history of previous corneal graft rejection. In these conditions, 10-year graft survival plummets to 35% [10]. In recent years, the success rate for renal, cardiac, and liver transplants has improved and has reached a level similar to corneal transplants, with approximately 75% of the grafts surviving at 5 years [7]. Unlike other categories of solid organ transplants, which have demonstrated improved survival over the past 10–15 years, the long-term survival of corneal transplants has not changed [7]. The improved survival of other organ transplants is largely a result of improved immunosuppressive drugs. In contrast, topical steroids continue to be the only immunosuppressive agents routinely used for preventing corneal allograft rejection and have been the mainstay among prophylactic immunosuppressive agents for decades. Unlike the rejection of cardiac, renal, and hepatic transplants, which pose a risk for survival and justify more aggressive immunosuppressive therapy, rejection of corneal allografts has far less serious consequences, which explains the ophthalmologist's reluctance to use systemic immunosuppressive drugs, which carry serious side effects and can significantly affect the patient's quality of life.

Summary for the Clinician:
Success of Corneal Allografts

- In the absence of risk factors, such as inflammation and neovascularization of the graft bed, corneal allografts enjoy immune privilege.
- Corneal allografts survive in the absence of HLA matching and without the use of systemic immunosuppressive drugs, which is further evidence of their immune privilege.
- Immune privilege of corneal allografts is not universal or immutable. Factors associated with corneal inflammation and neovascularization rob the cornea of its immune privilege and increase the risk for rejection.
- Topical application of corticosteroids is the mainstay prophylactic antirejection treatment. Risk to benefit ratio for keratoplasty patients precludes the use of more aggressive immunosuppressive protocols that have led to a steady improvement in the survival rates for kidney, liver, and heart transplants. In contrast, the success of corneal allografts has not improved over the past 3 decades.

1.3 Immune Rejection of Corneal Allografts

The beneficial effects of MHC matching in promoting the acceptance of other categories of allografts has been demonstrated, but remains controversial in corneal transplantation [7, 11]. One study has shown no benefit from MHC class I and class II matching on corneal allograft survival [6], while another study has reported a modest, albeit significant benefit of MHC class I matching, but an increased risk of rejection with MHC class II matching [12]. Studies in both humans and animals have clearly demonstrated that MHC class I antigens are expressed on all three layers of the cornea, while MHC class II antigens are conspicuously absent under nonpathological conditions. Minor histocompatibility antigens are also expressed in the cornea and can provoke corneal graft rejection [4, 5]. In fact, studies in both rats and mice suggest that minor histocompatibility antigens pose a greater barrier than MHC antigens for corneal allograft survival [13–15]. It has been estimated that 90% of the MHC antigens are expressed on the corneal epithelium, leading some to propose that removal of this layer might reduce the immunogenicity of corneal allografts and promote their survival. However, removal of donor epithelium prior to corneal transplantation did not enhance corneal allograft survival in 228 keratoplasty patients in one study [16]. Moreover, investigations in mice suggest that the corneal epithelium plays an active role in dampening inflammation, and that the removal of the corneal epithelium jeopardizes corneal allograft survival [9, 17].

Studies on the mechanisms of corneal graft rejection in patients have been largely inferential, as they have relied on in situ immunohistochemical phenotyping of cell surface markers on immune cells and the identification of cytokines in rejected corneal allografts. Animal studies, especially those in rodents, have provided the most useful insights into the mechanisms of immune rejection of corneal allografts. Maumenee was the first to unequivocally demonstrate that corneal allograft rejection was immune-mediated [18]. Using a rabbit model of penetrating keratoplasty, Maumenee demonstrated that rabbits that received skin grafts 2 weeks prior to the application of orthotopic corneal allografts from the same donor, rejected their corneal allografts at an accelerated tempo, thereby demonstrating immunological memory, and establishing the immunologic basis for corneal allograft rejection. In the late 1960s and mid 1970s, Khodadoust and Silverstein demonstrated that corneal allograft rejection was a cell-mediated process that could be adoptively transferred with lymphocytes that had been specifically sensitized to the corneal allograft donor's histocompatibility antigens [19, 20].

1.3.1 Role of CD4+ T Lymphocytes in Corneal Allograft Rejection

The development of the rat and, subsequently, the mouse model of penetrating keratoplasty paved the way for a series of studies exploring the immune mechanisms of corneal allograft rejection. Using these models, investigators have established that T cells, especially CD4+ T helper cells, were capable of mediating corneal allograft rejection [4]. Depletion of CD4+ T cells by in vivo antibody treatment or by gene deletion results in a steep reduction in the rejection of corneal allografts in rats and mice [4]. Likewise, there is a close correlation between corneal allograft survival and the down-regulation of CD4+ T cell immune responses [5]. CD4+ T cells can contribute to corneal allograft rejection in a number of ways. Delayed-type hypersensitivity (DTH) responses to alloantigens are mediated by CD4+ T cells and are closely correlated with corneal allograft rejection in mice. CD4+ T cells, especially the Th1 population, produce interferon-γ (IFN-γ) and tumor necrosis factor-α (TNF-α), which are known to induce apoptosis of corneal cells [4]. CD4+ T cells can also produce cell-contact-dependent apoptosis of corneal cells [21]. Although CD4+ T cells have been widely proclaimed as the sole mediators of corneal allograft rejection, it is noteworthy that depletion of CD4+ T cells by in vivo treatment with antibody or by deletion of the CD4 gene in mice does not abolish corneal allograft rejection; in fact, approximately 50% of the CD4+ T cell-deficient mice and rats go on to reject their corneal allografts [22–24]. In contrast, T cell-deficient mice do not reject corneal allografts, indicating that in addition to CD4+ T cells, one or more other T cell subsets can contribute to corneal allograft rejection.

1.3.2 Role of CD8+ T Lymphocytes in Corneal Allograft Rejection

CD8+ T cells are the other major subset of T lymphocytes that has been implicated in organ graft rejection. The notion that CD8+ cytotoxic T lymphocytes (CTL) mediate graft rejection has been embraced by numerous investigators. CD8+ CTL can kill allogeneic cells in vitro, including corneal cells. Moreover, CD8+ lymphocytes are among the mononuclear cells that are detected in rejected corneal allografts. However, rodent studies have shown that donor-specific CTL are not detected in hosts that have rejected corneal allografts. Moreover, corneal allograft rejection occurs unabatedly in CD8 knockout (KO) mice, perforin KO mice, or mice treated with anti-CD8 monoclonal antibody [4]. Unlike the condition with other allografts, corneal allograft rejection does not culminate in the development of donor-specific CTL. However, hosts with prevascularized corneal graft beds have a dramatically increased incidence and tempo of corneal allograft rejection. In these hosts, corneal allograft rejection elicits robust donor-specific CTL responses [25]. Moreover, CD8+ CTL collected from "high-risk" hosts that have rejected corneal allografts can induce corneal allograft rejection when adoptively transferred to severe combined immune deficient (SCID) mice, indicating that under certain conditions, CD8+ T cells can mediate corneal allograft rejection [26].

1.3.3 Role of Antibodies in Corneal Allograft Rejection

Although the weight of evidence suggests that corneal allograft rejection is T cell-mediated, there are reports suggesting a role for cytotoxic antibody. Antibodies specific for the donor's histocompatibility antigens can be detected in the serum of keratoplasty patients. An interesting correlation between ABO incompatibility and corneal allograft rejection in high-risk patients has been reported [6]. The incidence of rejection in patients with ABO-incompatible corneal allografts was twice that found in recipients who received ABO-compatible corneal grafts. ABO hemagglutinins are IgM antibodies, which are excellent complement-fixing immunoglobulins with potent cytolytic activity. ABO blood group antigens are expressed on human corneal epithelial and endothelial cells [27], and in vitro studies have shown that corneal endothelial cells are highly susceptible to cytolysis by complement-fixing antibodies [4, 28]. This is consistent with the notion that under certain conditions, antibody might contribute to corneal allograft rejection. Results from experiments in mice lend further support for this hypothesis. Donor-specific alloantibodies have been detected in the serum of mice at the time of corneal allograft rejection [28]. Passive transfer of alloantibodies to T cell-deficient mice, which normally do not reject corneal allografts, results in corneal allograft rejection [29, 30]. In contrast, corneal allograft rejection occurs in both B cell-deficient mice and complement-deficient mice, indicating that complement-fixing antibodies are not required for corneal allograft rejection, and that other immune effector mechanisms can also mediate graft failure in the absence of alloantibody [28, 31].

1.3.4 Role of Macrophages and NK Cells in Corneal Allograft Rejection

The immune system is composed of two distinctly different components: the adaptive and the innate immune systems. The adaptive immune system is characterized by exquisite antigen specificity and the participation of an intact T cell repertoire. Adaptive immune responses require several days to develop, but display long-term memory, which is manifested by swift responses to subsequent encounters with the original antigen. T lymphocytes, B lymphocytes, and antibodies are the primary elements of the adaptive immune system. The innate immune system is comprised of granulocytes, macrophages, natural killer (NK) cells, and the alternate pathway of the complement system. In contrast to the adaptive immune system, the innate immune system is characterized by its rapid activation by pathogens via recognition of toll-like receptors and pathogen-associated molecular patterns (PAMP) that are expressed on various microorganisms. Although the innate immune responses are swift, the responding cells lack antigen specificity and do not display memory.

Animal studies have provided compelling evidence that elements of the innate immune system indirectly contribute to corneal allograft rejection. DTH reactivity to donor histocompatibility antigens is closely correlated with corneal allograft rejection [4]. Macrophages are a major cell population in DTH lesions and are present in rejected corneal allografts. Studies in both the mouse and rat models of penetrating keratoplasty have shown that elimination of periocular macrophages by subconjunctival injection of liposomes containing the macrophagicidal drug clodronate prevents corneal allograft rejection [4]. However, further analysis has revealed that macrophages do not act as effector cells by damaging the donor corneal graft, but appear to be crucial antigen presenting cells (APC) that activate CD4+ T cells, which enter the graft and function as the end stage effector cells that deliver the lethal hit to the corneal allograft [4]. Neutrophils are also present in the inflammatory infiltrate of rejected corneal allografts, but there is little evidence to support an important role for them in corneal allograft rejection.

NK cells act as "first responders" to viral infections, and are believed to play an important role in the immune surveillance of neoplasms. Recent studies in the rat model of penetrating keratoplasty suggest that NK cells might also participate in corneal allograft rejection [32, 33]. Cells with surface markers that are characteristic of NK cells have been detected in the corneal stroma and the aqueous humor of hosts with rejected corneal allografts.

Moreover, NK cells have been shown to kill allogeneic corneal endothelial cells in vitro [34]. If NK cells participate in the destruction of corneal allografts, they most likely collaborate with CD4+ T cells or alloantibodies, which would provide the antigen specificity that is characteristic of corneal allograft rejection.

1.3.5 What are the Effectors of Corneal Allograft Rejection?

The weight of evidence indicates that multiple mechanisms and immune elements can be invoked to produce corneal allograft rejection. The use of various gene KO mouse strains and the selective depletion of immune cell populations have revealed an enormous redundancy in the immune effector mechanisms that can be enlisted to bring about corneal allograft rejection. B cell-deficient and complement-depleted hosts reject corneal allografts, indicating that complement-mediated cytolysis is not required for rejection. Likewise, the prompt rejection of corneal allografts transplanted to CD4 KO mice and CD8 KO mice demonstrates that neither of these two T lymphocyte populations is indispensable for the rejection of corneal allografts. Perforin KO mice lack the cytolytic protein that is utilized by CTL and NK cells, yet these mice are also fully capable of rejecting corneal allografts. Although depletion of ocular macrophages prevents corneal allograft rejection, macrophages alone cannot mediate rejection. These observations lead to the inescapable conclusion that multiple pathways exist for corneal allograft rejection, and that the immune privilege of corneal allografts involves multiple mechanisms and molecules that disable each of these effector pathways. Failure to disarm each of these immune effector mechanisms compromises immune privilege and leads to corneal allograft rejection.

1.4 Role of Atopic Diseases in Corneal Allograft Rejection

Anecdotal reports have suggested that atopic diseases, especially allergic conjunctivitis, increase the risk for corneal allograft rejection. Studies in the mouse model of penetrating keratoplasty have confirmed this suspicion and have shown that mice with either allergic conjunctivitis or allergic asthma have a dramatic increase in the incidence and tempo of corneal allograft rejection [35, 36]. Prospective studies in this model have demonstrated that the increased rejection was due to a systemic, not local, effect of the allergic diseases. That is, mice with allergic conjunctivitis in only one eye experienced a dramatically higher rejection in either the allergen-challenged eye or the contralateral eye that had not been exposed to allergens and did not display clinical or histological features of allergy. Moreover, mice with allergic asthma also experience a dramatic increase in the incidence of corneal allograft rejection, providing further evidence that the untoward effects of allergic diseases are systemic in nature and the increased rejection is not simply due to a "hot" inflamed graft bed. Interestingly, terminating the host's exposure to relevant allergens results in the restoration in immune privilege. That is, allergic mice that are isolated from the relevant allergen for 30 days display the same incidence of corneal allograft rejection as nonallergic mice. The underlying basis for the increased incidence and tempo of corneal graft rejection in allergic diseases remains a mystery. It is possible that atopic diseases such as allergic conjunctivitis or allergic asthma have an adjuvant effect and enhance the generation of CTL, DTH, or alloantibody responses. Another possibility is that allergic diseases disable one or more of the mechanisms that are crucial for the establishment of immune privilege (see below). In either case, atopy-associated exacerbation of corneal allograft rejection reminds us that seemingly benign immunological perturbations can rob the corneal allograft of its immune privilege.

Summary for the Clinician: Immune Mechanisms of Corneal Allograft Rejection

- Corneal allograft rejection is a T cell-dependent process.
- No single immune effector mechanism is solely responsible for corneal allograft rejection.
- Antibodies, CTL, and DTH can independently mediate corneal graft rejection
- Allergic diseases increase the risk of corneal allograft rejection.
- The immune system displays remarkable redundancy in the mechanisms that can mediate corneal allograft rejection.

1.5 Immune Privilege of Corneal Allografts Is a Tripartite Phenomenon

There are three distinct phases in the immune rejection of an allograft. The first step is initiated when donor-derived APC emigrate from the graft and enter a draining lymph node. The MHC antigens on the APC are capable of directly interacting with the T cell receptor (TCR) on the host T cells within the lymph node and eliciting robust immune responses. This is referred to as the "direct pathway" of alloactivation. The second, and perhaps more important, pathway for eliciting an immune response to corneal allografts is the "indirect pathway" in which the host's APC residing in the graft bed capture alloantigens shed from the corneal allograft. The host APC process the donor histocompatibility antigens and load alloantigenic peptide fragments onto MHC class II molecules, which engage the TCR on CD4+ T cells. The indirect pathway of alloantigen stimulation via presentation of minor histocompatibility antigens is believed by many to be more important than the direct pathway of alloantigenic stimulation [13, 15]. Both the direct and indirect pathways culminate in the activation and expansion of T lymphocyte populations that specifically recognize the histocompatibility antigens on the corneal allograft. In low-risk eyes, such as those in keratoconus patients, the corneal graft bed is avascular and is typically free of inflammation. Under these conditions, the corneal allografts and the graft beds into which they are grafted possess unique properties that delay, disrupt, or block the induction of the immune response – a process termed "afferent blockade."

The second phase of the immune response to foreign histocompatibility antigens occurs in the regional lymph nodes, which drain the corneal graft bed. In the mouse, these are the submandibular and cervical lymph nodes [37, 38]. Within the lymph nodes, either donor-derived (direct pathway) or host-derived APC (indirect pathway) present alloantigenic moieties to T cells, which undergo clonal expansion and activation. This is termed the "central processing" phase of the alloimmune response, and it culminates in the production of prodigious numbers of activated T cells that enter the bloodstream and migrate to the graft/host interface. B cells are also activated in the draining lymph node, and subsequently develop into plasma cells, which secrete antibodies that recognize the MHC histocompatibility antigens on the corneal allografts. As a general rule, minor histocompatibility antigens elicit little or no antibody response. Therefore, if alloantibodies play a role in graft rejection, they are most likely directed at the MHC or ABO antigens on the corneal allograft.

The third phase of the alloimmune response is the "efferent phase" in which the activated T cells and antibodies enter the bloodstream and are transported to the host/graft interface. After migrating to the host/graft interface, the immune effector elements can attack all three cell layers of the cornea, but it is the destruction of the corneal endothelium in particular that leads to the loss of corneal clarity and thus, graft failure.

The immune rejection of corneal allografts occurs by a three-step process that can be likened to a conventional sensory neuron/motor neuron reflex arc. This "immune reflex arc" includes an initial stimulus (antigen-laden APC), which activates a central processing region (regional lymph node). Within the central processing region, an effector response is generated (activated T cells and antibodies) and is transmitted back to the site of the original stimulus (corneal allograft). The immune privilege of corneal allografts relies on the disarming of each of these three components of the immune reflex arc.

1.5.1 Afferent Blockade of the Immune Response to Corneal Allografts

It is widely accepted that the avascular nature of the corneal graft bed contributes to corneal allograft survival. Studies in rodent models of penetrating keratoplasty have shown that maneuvers that induce hemangiogenesis and lymphangiogenesis of the corneal graft bed create a "high-risk" environment, which invariably leads to 100% graft rejection. It was originally believed that the presence of blood vessels in the corneal graft bed facilitated the entry of alloantigens into the bloodstream, thereby allowing them direct access to peripheral lymphoid tissues, such as the spleen and eventually the lymph nodes, where they elicited an immune response to the donor's histocompatibility antigens (= alloantigens). However, intravenous (IV) injection of alloantigens results in the down-regulation of cell-mediated immune responses to alloantigens and in fact, enhances rather than jeopardizes allograft survival [39, 40]. A more plausible explanation for the increased rejection of corneal grafts transplanted into vascularized graft beds lies in the induction of new lymph vessels. The same stimuli that induce formation of new blood vessels in the corneal graft bed coincidentally elicit lymphangiogenesis. In the generation of a conventional immune response, APC migrate to regional lymph nodes via afferent lymph vessels. Emerging evidence suggests that the stimuli that induce hemangiogenesis also induce the formation of lymph vessels in the corneal graft bed. In addition, these stimuli also recruit and activate host APC, which can enter the newly formed lymph vessels. These events enhance the afferent arm of the immune response and culminate in corneal graft rejection [41, 42].

One of the earliest explanations offered to explain the immune privilege of corneal allografts suggested that corneal cells did not express histocompatibility antigens and thus were invisible to the immune system. However, numerous studies in experimental animals and human subjects have unequivocally shown that all three cell layers of the cornea express MHC class I antigens, as well as multiple minor histocompatibility antigens [4]. It is estimated that the epithelium expresses over 90% of the MHC antigens on the corneal allografts. However, removal of the corneal epithelium does not enhance corneal graft survival in humans and appears to exacerbate corneal allograft rejection in mice [9, 16, 17]. Thus, corneal allografts express multiple histocompatibility antigens that can serve as targets for immune rejection. However, expression of these antigens alone is insufficient to provoke immune rejection, and other characteristics of the corneal allograft and graft bed are pivotal in the induction of the alloimmune response.

Epithelial tissues such as the skin contain a dense network of APC, namely Langerhans cells (LC), which act as sentinels sampling antigens such as pathogens that confront the epithelial surface. After capturing antigens, LC migrate via lymph vessels to regional lymph nodes where they process and present alloantigenic peptides to T cells. LC are also potent stimulators of alloimmune responses. As few as ten cutaneous allogeneic LC can prime mice for the generation of CTL against alloantigens (i.e., histocompatibility antigens)[43]. The central region of the corneal epithelium is normally devoid of mature LC that constitutively express MHC class II molecules. However, various stimuli that are associated with the development of "high-risk" conditions for corneal allograft survival (e.g., corneal neovascularization and inflammation) induce the swift appearance of MHC class II positive LC in the central corneal epithelium. These corneas contain MHC class II positive LC of donor origin and are highly immunogenic, and also experience an increased incidence and tempo of immune rejection (Table 1.2). Thus, the presence of donor-derived "passenger" MHC class II positive LC abolishes immune privilege by restoring the afferent arm of the immune reflex arc. This in turn promotes the generation of a robust alloimmune response that culminates in corneal allograft rejection. However, afferent blockade of the immune reflex arc can be reestablished by removing the MHC class II positive LC. Since LC are vulnerable to hyperbaric oxygen and ultraviolet B (UVB) irradiation, treating LC-containing corneal allografts in vitro with either hyperbaric oxygen or low dose UVB irradiation prior to orthotopic transplantation reduces their immunogenicity and restores their immune privilege.

Host LC reside in the limbus and are also an important consideration in the afferent arm of the immune response. Conditions that are closely associated with high-risk corneal grafts (e.g., inflammation and neovascularization) are also known to activate limbal LC and induce their centripetal migration into the corneal graft. Interleukin-1 (IL-1) is one of the stimuli that is upregulated in inflamed or vascularized eyes that beckons LC to enter the corneal allograft. Blocking IL-1 function by topical administration of IL-1 receptor antagonist inhibits LC migration into the corneal allograft and produces a dramatic reduction in the incidence of corneal allograft rejection [5].

As stated earlier, the induction or afferent arm of the immune response requires that antigen-laden APC migrate from the corneal allograft to the regional lymph node. Conceptually, the simplest method for preventing this inductive step is to either ligate the lymph vessels that drain the ocular surface or remove the regional lymph nodes that they serve. This has been proven in mouse experiments in which surgical removal of the ipsilateral cervical or submandibular lymph nodes prior to transplantation prevents the immune rejection of corneal allografts [37, 38].

Thus, blocking the afferent arm of the immune response by inhibiting the transmission of alloantigens from the corneal allograft to the regional lymph node pharmaceutically, surgically, or immunologically promotes immune privilege and ensures corneal allograft survival.

Table 1.2 Effect of MHC class II positive donor-specific Langerhans cells on corneal allograft rejection in rodents

Histocompatibility barrier	% Graft rejection	
	LC⁻ corneal allografts	LC⁺ corneal allografts
MHC + multiple minor histocompatibility antigens	50	>90
Minor histocompatibility antigens only	40	80
MHC class I only	18	20
MHC class II only	<10	<10

> **Summary for the Clinician: Afferent Blockade of the Immune Response**
>
> All three layers of the corneal allograft display MHC class I and minor histocompatibility antigens that can be targeted for immunologic attack.
>
> - Removing the corneal epithelium does not enhance corneal graft survival, and may in fact increase the risk for rejection.
> - In normal corneas, the central corneal epithelium lacks mature MHC class II positive APC.
> - Corneas from inflamed or vascularized eyes contain large numbers of activated APC that elicit intense immune responses that culminate in graft rejection. In vitro treatment with UVB or oxygen can rid these corneas of "passenger APC" and enhance corneal allograft survival.
> - The absence of lymphatic vessels in the corneal graft bed prevents the induction of immune responses to the corneal allograft
> - Factors that are associated with increased risk of corneal graft rejection invariably enhance the afferent arm of the immune response.
> - Simple removal of the draining lymph node blocks the afferent arm of the immune response, promotes immune privilege, and ensures corneal allograft survival.

1.5.2 Immune Deviation in the Central Processing Component of the Immune Reflex Arc

The orthotopic corneal allograft lies over the AC of the eye and is in direct contact with the aqueous humor. It has been recognized for over 100 years that the AC of the eye possesses immune privilege. Various categories of tumor and tissue allografts experience prolonged and sometimes, permanent survival when transplanted into the AC, yet are promptly rejected if transplanted to other body sites [44, 45]. Since the orthotopic corneal allograft is in direct juxtaposition to the AC, it benefits from its immune privilege. Numerous factors contribute to the immune privilege of the AC. The aqueous humor contains a myriad of immunosuppressive and antiinflammatory molecules. The cells lining the inside of the eye are decorated with cell membrane-bound molecules such as FasL (CD95L), tumor necrosis factor-related apoptosis-inducing ligand (TRAIL), and programmed death ligand-1 (PD-L1), which inhibit T cell proliferation, down-regulate the production of proinflammatory cytokines, and induce apoptosis of T cells that enter the AC.

Allogeneic cells that are either injected into the AC or that reside in tissue allografts that are transplanted into the AC elicit a unique form of immune regulation that deviates the systemic immune response from a destructive pathway to one of tolerance. That is, allogeneic cells and allografts placed subcutaneously or intraperitoneally elicit the production of complement-fixing antibodies, CTL, and DTH responses against the alien histocompatibility antigens. In contrast, allogeneic cells and allografts placed into the AC of the eye, do not elicit the development of DTH, and in fact induce T regulatory cells that actively suppress DTH responses to the alloantigens that were introduced into the AC. Moreover, AC injection of antigen results in the preferential production of noncomplement-fixing antibodies and the absence of complement-fixing antibodies. This immunoregulatory phenomenon has been termed anterior chamber-associated immune deviation (ACAID) and is believed to be crucial for the maintenance of immune privilege in the eye. ACAID culminates in the generation of T regulatory cells that down-regulate both Th1- and Th2-based immune-mediated inflammation and DTH responses to alloantigens. The antigen-specific suppression of DTH has important implications for corneal allograft survival, as the appearance of DTH responses to the alloantigens on corneal allografts is closely correlated with corneal allograft rejection [4]. Likewise, hosts with long-term clear corneal allografts do not display DTH responses to the alloantigens expressed on the corneal allografts, and in fact develop T regulatory cells that actively suppress DTH responses to these alloantigens. Significant numbers of corneal cells are sloughed into the AC during orthotopic corneal transplantation, and since the corneal allograft is in direct contact with the AC, it is reasonable to propose that events surrounding orthotopic corneal transplantation are conducive for the induction of ACAID. Moreover, studies in both the rat and mouse models of penetrating keratoplasty have shown that AC injection of donor-specific cells prior to corneal transplantation enhances corneal allograft survival. In addition, the selective silencing of complement-fixing antibody production reduces the risk for antibody-mediated rejection of corneal allografts.

The induction of ACAID is a complex process that involves the participation of three organs and one organ system: (a) eye, (b) thymus, (c) spleen, and (d) sympathetic nervous system. The generation of ACAID is initiated when ocular macrophages capture antigens that enter the AC. The F4/80+ ocular macrophages emigrate from the eye to the thymus and spleen. Within the thymus, they induce the generation of NK1.1+ T cells (NKT cells), which then emerge from the thymus and enter the bloodstream where they migrate to the spleen. Other F4/80+ ocular macrophages are believed to migrate directly from the eye to the spleen. In the spleen, the F4/80+ ocular macrophages engage in a complex series of cellular interactions with B lymphocytes, γδ T lymphocytes, NKT cells, CD4+ T lymphocytes, CD8+ lymphocytes, and the third component of complement (C3). These interactions culminate in the generation of CD8+ T regulatory cells that suppress both Th1 and Th2 immune-mediated inflammation, as well as DTH to the antigens that entered the AC. Importantly, the suppression of immune-mediated inflammation and DTH is antigen-specific. If ACAID is crucial for corneal allograft survival, then it stands to reason that disruption of the cell populations that are needed for the induction of ACAID should jeopardize corneal allograft survival. Studies in rodent models of penetrating keratoplasty have confirmed this suspicion and shown that corneal allograft rejection is dramatically increased in the hosts treated by: (a) splenectomy; (b) depletion of γδ T cells; (c) depletion of IL-10; or (d) depletion of B cells [46].

Data from rodent models of penetrating keratoplasty strongly support the notion that the immune privilege of corneal allografts relies on the generation of ACAID or an ACAID-like immunoregulatory process that suppresses T cell-mediated immune responses (especially DTH) to the donor's histocompatibility antigens [46].

Summary for the Clinician: Immune Deviation and Corneal Allograft Survival

- Orthotopic corneal allografts induce a deviation in the immune response that inhibits T cell-mediated immunity to the corneal alloantigens, and favors graft survival.
- This immune deviation is termed ACAID, and can be induced by AC injection of donor cells or by orthotopic transplantation of corneal allografts.
- ACAID produces antigen-specific suppression of T cell-mediated immunity and a deviation of the antibody response from complement-fixing antibodies to noncomplement-fixing antibodies. Complement-fixing antibodies can kill corneal cells. Therefore, the selective silencing of complement-fixing antibodies eliminates this form of graft rejection and provides the corneal allograft an additional level of immune privilege.
- An intact spleen is necessary for the induction of ACAID and the survival of corneal allografts in rodents. Do patients with a history of a previous splenectomy have an increased risk for corneal allograft rejection?

1.5.3 Efferent Blockade of the Immune Response to Corneal Allografts

One of the original explanations for the immune privilege of corneal allografts proposed that the absence of blood and lymph vessels in the corneal graft bed isolated the corneal graft from immune effector elements (T lymphocytes and antibodies) that were present in the blood. Although this sequestration hypothesis has been unequivocally disproven, the notion that the corneal allograft is shielded from immune effector elements does have merit. Corneal endothelial and epithelial cells express an interesting array of cell membrane molecules that disarm activated T lymphocytes and disable the complement system. FasL (CD95L) is expressed on both corneal endothelial and epithelial cells and induces apoptosis of neutrophils and activated T cells, which express its receptor (Fas, CD95). The importance of FasL-induced apoptosis in corneal allograft survival was demonstrated in two independent studies, which showed that corneal allografts prepared from mutant mice that failed to express functional FasL invariably underwent immune rejection [47, 48]. The cornea also expresses another apoptosis-inducing cell membrane molecule called programmed death domain ligand-1 (PD-L1). When PD-L1 engages its receptor (PD-1) on T lymphocytes, it induces T lymphocyte apoptosis, inhibits T lymphocyte proliferation, and prevents the production of the proinflammatory cytokine interferon-γ (IFN-γ). Corneal allografts prepared from gene KO mice that fail to express PD-L1 have twice the incidence of rejection as corneal grafts that express functional PD-L1 [49, 50]. Moreover, in vivo administration of anti- PD-L1 antibody into normal mice results in a sharp increase in the incidence of corneal allograft rejection [49, 50].

Although there is some evidence that cytotoxic antibodies can produce corneal allograft rejection in mice, their role in the rejection of corneal allografts in humans remains unresolved and controversial. The capacity of antibodies to produce complement-mediated cytolysis of corneal allografts is severely limited by the expression of complement regulatory proteins (CRP) that are expressed on the cell membranes of corneal epithelial cells and are present in the aqueous humor. Corneal epithelial cells express CRP and are impervious to in vitro cytolysis by complement-fixing antibodies [28]. In contrast, corneal endothelial cells do not express CRP and are vulnerable to cytolysis by complement-fixing alloantibodies in vitro. However, the aqueous humor contains soluble CRP, which disable the complement system and protect corneal endothelial cells from complement-mediated injury. Thus, antibody-mediated corneal allograft rejection is severely limited by CRP that are present in the aqueous humor and expressed on the corneal epithelium.

The aqueous humor also contains a myriad of soluble factors that suppress immune-mediated inflammation (Table 1.3). NK cells have been implicated in corneal allograft rejection in the rat. However, the aqueous humor contains at least two soluble factors that affect the function of NK cells and may restrict the capacity of NK cells to contribute to corneal allograft rejection. Macrophage migration inhibitory factor (MIF) and TGF-β are present in the AH at concentrations that inhibit NK cell cytolytic activity in vitro and in vivo. MIF produces an immediate inhibition of the cytolytic machinery of NK cells, while TGF-β produces inhibition of NK cell-mediated cytolysis that is equally strong, but is delayed until 18 h after exposure to NK cells.

> **Summary for the Clinician: Efferent Blockade of Corneal Allograft Rejection**
>
> - The corneal allograft and aqueous humor expresses molecules that block the expression of immune effector elements at the graft/host interface.
> - Cells on the corneal allograft express cell membrane-bound molecules, FasL and PD-L1, which disable and delete T lymphocytes that enter the corneal transplant.
> - CRP are also expressed on the cell membranes of corneal cells and are present in the aqueous humor, and act as buffers to reduce the risk for complement-mediated graft rejection.

Table 1.3 Immunosuppressive and immunoregulatory molecules in the aqueous humor

Molecule	Effect on immune system
TGF-β	Suppresses activation of T cells; promotes immune deviation; down-regulates MHC class I expression on corneal cells; suppresses NK cells
VIP	Inhibits T cell activation and proliferation; inhibits DTH
CGRP	Inhibits production of proinflammatory factors by macrophages
MIF	Inhibits NK cells
FasL	Suppresses neutrophil recruitment and activation
CRP	Disables complement cascade
IDO	Depletes tryptophan and "starves" T lymphocytes
α-MSH	Inhibits DTH and production of proinflammatory factors by macrophages
SOM	Suppresses IFN-γ production by activated T cells; induces production of α-MSH

TGF-β transforming growth factor beta; *VIP* vasoactive intestinal peptide; *CGRP* calcitonin gene-related peptide; *MIF* macrophage migration inhibitory factor; *FasL* Fas ligand; *CRP* complement regulatory proteins; *IDO* indoleamine dioxygenase (this is a cytoplasmic enzyme that is not present in the aqueous humor, but depletes tryptophan within the eye); *α-MSH* alpha-melanocyte stimulating hormone; *SOM* somatostatin

References

1. Bigger SL (1837) An inquiry into the possibility of transplanting the cornea with the view of relieving blindness (hitherto deemed incurable) caused by several diseases of that structure. Dublin J Med Sci 11:408–447
2. Kissam R (1844) Ceratoplastice in man. N Y J Med 2: 281–289
3. May CH (1887) Transplantation of a rabbit's eye into the human orbit. Arch Ophthalmol 16:47–53
4. Niederkorn JY (2007) Immune mechanisms of corneal allograft rejection. Curr Eye Res 32:1005–1016
5. Niederkorn JY (2003) The immune privilege of corneal grafts. J Leukoc Biol 74:167–171
6. Group CCTSR (1992) The collaborative corneal transplantation studies (CCTS). Effectiveness of histocompatibility matching in high-risk corneal transplantation. Arch Ophthalmol 110:1392–1403
7. Waldock A, Cook SD (2000) Corneal transplantation: how successful are we? Br J Ophthalmol 84:813–815
8. Medawar PB (1948) Immunity to homologous grafted skin. III. The fate of skin homografts transplanted to the brain, to subcutaneous tissue, and to the anterior chamber of the eye. Br J Exp Pathol 29:58–69
9. Streilein JW (2003) New thoughts on the immunology of corneal transplantation. Eye 17:943–948
10. Williams KA, Muehlberg SM, Lewis RF et al (1997) Long-term outcome in corneal allotransplantation. The Australian corneal graft registry. Transplant Proc 29:983
11. George AJ, Larkin DF (2004) Corneal transplantation: the forgotten graft. Am J Transplant 4:678–685
12. Vail A, Gore SM, Bradley BA et al (1994) Influence of donor and histocompatibility factors on corneal graft outcome. Transplantation 58:1210–1216

13. Boisgerault F, Liu Y, Anosova N et al (2001) Role of cd4(+) and cd8(+) t cells in allorecognition: lessons from corneal transplantation. J Immunol 167:1891–1899
14. Nicholls SM, Bradley BA, Easty DL (1995) Non-MHC antigens and their relative resistance to immunosuppression after corneal transplantation. Eye 9(Pt 2):208–214
15. Sonoda Y, Streilein JW (1992) Orthotopic corneal transplantation in mice–evidence that the immunogenetic rules of rejection do not apply. Transplantation 54:694–704
16. Stulting RD, Waring GO III, Bridges WZ et al (1988) Effect of donor epithelium on corneal transplant survival. Ophthalmology 95:803–812
17. Hori J, Streilein JW (2001) Role of recipient epithelium in promoting survival of orthotopic corneal allografts in mice. Invest Ophthalmol Vis Sci 42:720–726
18. Maumenee A (1951) The influence of donor-recipient sensitization on corneal grafts. Am J Ophthalmol 34:142–152
19. Khodadoust AA, Silverstein AM (1976) Induction of corneal graft rejection by passive cell transfer. Invest Ophthalmol 15:89–95
20. Khodadoust AA, Silverstein AM (1969) Transplantation and rejection of individual cell layers of the cornea. Invest Ophthalmol 8:180–195
21. Hegde S, Beauregard C, Mayhew E et al (2005) CD4(+) T-cell-mediated mechanisms of corneal allograft rejection: role of Fas-induced apoptosis. Transplantation 79:23–31
22. Ayliffe W, Alam Y, Bell EB et al (1992) Prolongation of rat corneal graft survival by treatment with anti-CD4 monoclonal antibody. Br J Ophthalmol 76:602–606
23. He YG, Ross J, Niederkorn JY (1991) Promotion of murine orthotopic corneal allograft survival by systemic administration of anti-CD4 monoclonal antibody. Invest Ophthalmol Vis Sci 32:2723–2728
24. Niederkorn JY, Stevens C, Mellon J et al (2006) CD4+ T-Cell-independent rejection of corneal allografts. Transplantation 81:1171–1178
25. Ksander BR, Sano Y, Streilein JW (1996) Role of donor-specific cytotoxic T cells in rejection of corneal allografts in normal and high-risk eyes. Transpl Immunol 4:49–52
26. Niederkorn JY, Stevens C, Mellon J et al (2006) Differential roles of CD8+ and CD8− T lymphocytes in corneal allograft rejection in 'high-risk' hosts. Am J Transplant 6:705–713
27. Salisbury JD, Gebhardt BM (1981) Blood group antigens on human corneal cells demonstrated by immunoperoxidase staining. Am J Ophthalmol 91:46–50
28. Hegde S, Mellon JK, Hargrave SL et al (2002) Effect of alloantibodies on corneal allograft survival. Invest Ophthalmol Vis Sci 43:1012–1018
29. Hegde S, Niederkorn JY (2000) The role of cytotoxic T lymphocytes in corneal allograft rejection. Invest Ophthalmol Vis Sci 41:3341–3347
30. Holan V, Vitova A, Krulova M et al (2005) Susceptibility of corneal allografts and xenografts to antibody-mediated rejection. Immunol Lett 100:211–213
31. Goslings WR, Yamada J, Dana MR et al (1999) Corneal transplantation in antibody-deficient hosts. Invest Ophthalmol Vis Sci 40:250–253
32. Claerhout I, Kestelyn P, Debacker V et al (2004) Role of natural killer cells in the rejection process of corneal allografts in rats. Transplantation 77:676–682
33. Mayer K, Reinhard T, Reis A et al (2003) Differential contribution of natural killer cells to corneal graft rejection in 3-week-old versus mature rats. Transplantation 76:578–582
34. Apte RS, Niederkorn JY (1996) Isolation and characterization of a unique natural killer cell inhibitory factor present in the anterior chamber of the eye. J Immunol 156:2667–2673
35. Beauregard C, Stevens C, Mayhew E et al (2005) Cutting edge: atopy promotes Th2 responses to alloantigens and increases the incidence and tempo of corneal allograft rejection. J Immunol 174:6577–6581
36. Flynn TH, Ohbayashi M, Ikeda Y et al (2007) Effect of allergic conjunctival inflammation on the allogeneic response to donor cornea. Invest Ophthalmol Vis Sci 48:4044–4049
37. Plskova J, Duncan L, Holan V et al (2002) The immune response to corneal allograft requires a site-specific draining lymph node. Transplantation 73:210–215
38. Yamagami S, Dana MR (2001) The critical role of lymph nodes in corneal alloimmunization and graft rejection. Invest Ophthalmol Vis Sci 42:1293–1298
39. Ayliffe W, McLeod D, Hutchinson IV (1992) The effect of blood transfusions on rat corneal graft survival. Invest Ophthalmol Vis Sci 33:1974–1978
40. Ishii N, Aoki I, Ishii T et al (1988) Suppressor T cells in mice made unresponsive to skin allografts. J Invest Dermatol 91:333–335
41. Chen L, Hamrah P, Cursiefen C et al (2004) Vascular endothelial growth factor receptor-3 mediates induction of corneal alloimmunity. Nat Med 10:813–815
42. Cursiefen C, Cao J, Chen L et al (2004) Inhibition of hemangiogenesis and lymphangiogenesis after normal-risk corneal transplantation by neutralizing VEGF promotes graft survival. Invest Ophthalmol Vis Sci 45:2666–2673
43. McKinney EC, Streilein JW (1989) On the extraordinary capacity of allogeneic epidermal Langerhans cells to prime cytotoxic T cells in vivo. J Immunol 143:1560–1564
44. Niederkorn JY (2006) See no evil, hear no evil, do no evil: the lessons of immune privilege. Nat Immunol 7:354–359
45. Streilein JW (2003) Ocular immune privilege: therapeutic opportunities from an experiment of nature. Nat Rev Immunol 3:879–889

46. Niederkorn JY (2006) Anterior chamber-associated immune deviation and its impact on corneal allograft survival. Curr Opin Organ Transplant 11:360–365
47. Stuart PM, Griffith TS, Usui N et al (1997) CD95 ligand (FasL)-induced apoptosis is necessary for corneal allograft survival. J Clin Invest 99:396–402
48. Yamagami S, Kawashima H, Tsuru T et al (1997) Role of Fas-Fas ligand interactions in the immunorejection of allogeneic mouse corneal transplants. Transplantation 64:1107–1111
49. Hori J, Wang M, Miyashita M et al (2006) B7–H1-induced apoptosis as a mechanism of immune privilege of corneal allografts. J Immunol 177:5928–5935
50. Shen L, Jin Y, Freeman GJ et al (2007) The function of donor versus recipient programmed death-ligand 1 in corneal allograft survival. J Immunol 179:3672–3679

Chapter 2

Mechanisms of Corneal Allograft Rejection and the Development of New Therapies

Douglas J. Coster, Claire F. Jessup, Keryn A. Williams

Core Messages

- Effective suppression of corneal inflammation provides some insurance against subsequent graft rejection. Postoperative inflammation must be diagnosed promptly and treated energetically.
- Avoid high-risk corneal transplants if at all possible. A failed graft may create more problems than the original disease.
- There is an increasing evidence of a small benefit of tissue matching in corneal transplantation.
- HLA matching is recommended if logistics allow.
- Patients with severe visual disability and who understand the risks involved may benefit from systemic immunosuppression.
- When systemic immunosuppression is employed, management of the patient should be shared with a transplant physician experienced in the field.

2.1 Status of Corneal Transplantation

Corneal transplantation is a paradox. For some patients – those with keratoconus and some dystrophies – the procedure is remarkably successful. For others – those with poor vision, following inflammatory diseases of the cornea – the procedure is remarkably unsuccessful. The tragedy is that inflammatory diseases of the cornea are the second largest cause of blindness world-wide [1]. For those with this problem who receive a corneal graft, failure is common and allograft rejection is the usual cause of failure. For millions of others, the poor prognosis precludes surgery – they are never offered a transplant.

Patients who have had inflammatory eye disease and who receive a corneal transplant are considered to be at "high risk" – attention must be paid to lowering their risk of rejection. This is not readily achieved, and improvements in graft survival have not been seen in corneal transplantation in recent years. On the other hand, the outcome of transplantation of vascularised solid organs has improved steadily over the last 40 years. This improvement has been due to the development of more effective ways of preventing and treating allograft rejection. For the most part, the strategies that have been so important in organ transplantation are not applicable to corneal transplantation. New approaches are needed to reduce the impact of corneal allograft rejection – strategies that take into account the unique biology of the cornea and the clinical context in which corneal transplantation is practiced.

2.2 Success Rate of Corneal Transplantation

The survival of corneal grafts is 86% at 1 year and 73% at 5 years (Fig. 2.1a) [2]. This compares unfavorably with the results of vascularised solid organ grafts such as kidney allografts (Fig. 2.1b) [3, 4]. A number of factors have contributed to the improvement in outcomes of solid organ transplantation. Tissue matching has become more accurate with the development of molecular techniques, and systemic immunosuppression is increasingly effective. An increasing proportion of patients receive transplants from living-related donors, and this too contributes to the improved survival rates. None of these approaches is readily applicable to corneal transplantation. Tissue matching is not as effective for corneal transplantation because of the relative importance of minor

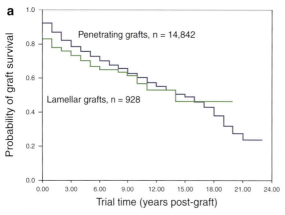

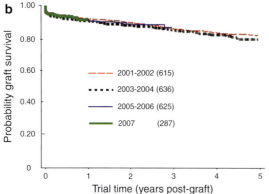

Fig. 2.1 Kaplan–Meier graft survival plots. (**a**) Survival of penetrating and lamellar corneal grafts over 24 years, from 1985 to 2009; *n* represents the number of eyes initially at risk. Data from the Australian Corneal Graft Registry, with permission. (**b**) Survival of first renal allografts from deceased unrelated donors, stratified by year of transplantation from 2001 to 2007 ("modern era" grafts). Data from the 31st report of the Australia and New Zealand dialysis and transplant registry 2008 [4], with permission. Disclaimer: these data reported have been supplied by the Australia and New Zealand Dialysis and transplant registry, but the interpretation and reporting of these data in no way should be seen as an official policy or interpretation by the Australia and New Zealand dialysis and transplant registry

histocompatibility antigens. Corneal transplantation is performed for visual disability, and because blindness is not a potentially fatal condition (unlike heart or liver failure), the risks of systemic immunosuppression can seldom be justified. For this reason, regional (ocular) immunosuppression rather than systemic immunosuppression is required. The advantage derived from using living related donors for renal transplantation is not available for corneal transplantation. It is not possible to use living-related donors in corneal transplantation because this cannot be done without damaging the sight of the donor.

2.3 Maintenance and Erosion of Corneal Privilege

The cornea has long been recognized as an immunologically privileged site. Perhaps this privilege has evolved as a consequence of its conflicting, dual roles. It is both an optical element of the eye, for which it must remain transparent and of an appropriate shape, and it is exposed to the environment, and thus has a protective function. Challenges to the cornea resulting in a brisk inflammatory response with scarring sequelae might alter corneal structure, which depends on an undisturbed ultrastructure for good optical function. Immunological privilege may act to minimize the impact of inflammation. Corneal privilege is eroded in diseased corneas in which inflammation has occurred, and grafts placed in such recipient corneas are rejected promptly. In between the "virgin" cornea and the situation described above, there is a spectrum: corneal privilege is relative. It varies in extent across species. For example, the normal rabbit cornea is similar to the normal human cornea, with a weak tendency to spontaneous rejection of allografts. On the other hand, the normal sheep spontaneously rejects allografts after 3 weeks, probably because it is naturally somewhat vascularised.

Various factors contribute to corneal privilege in humans. The normal cornea has no blood vessels or lymphatics. Furthermore, the vessels in the eye have tight junctions, which form the basis of the blood–eye barrier [5]. As a consequence of the avascularity and the blood–eye barrier, the cornea is somewhat sequestered from systemic immune responses. It is also relatively acellular, particularly with respect to cells capable of processing and presenting antigen, crucial to the initiation of an allograft response. The normal cornea has some Langerhans cells in the epithelium, and a small population of interstitial dendritic cells and macrophages in the peripheral stroma [6, 7]. Some species, notably mice, have a larger population of antigen presenting cells (APCs) in the stroma. Mice also have a tendency to spontaneous rejection of allografts. There is limited expression of major histocompatibility complex (MHC) determinants on the surface of corneal cells. Class I antigens are present on epithelial cells, stromal keratocytes, and endothelium. Class II expression is limited primarily to bone-marrow derived cells [8]. Corneas along with other privileged sites such as testes do, however, constitutively express Fas ligand, which provides a mechanism for eliminating immunocompetent cells that find their way into the cornea. In addition, the anterior chamber fluid is relatively rich in immunomodulatory cytokines [9].

Acute inflammation results in breakdown of the blood–eye barrier, providing access for cells and large molecules [10]. With chronic inflammation, new blood vessels and lymphatics are formed, forever connecting the cornea to the vascular and lymphatic circulations [3] Inflammation also increases histocompatibility antigen expression [11]. Through wound healing and postoperative inflammatory events such as inflammation around a loose stitch, or intercurrent conjunctivitis or uveitis, the cornea acquires a population of bone marrow-derived cells capable of processing and presenting antigen. This population persists for years after the initial inflammation has subsided, and the number of these cells in a recipient cornea correlates well with allograft rejection and graft failure – the larger the number of cells in the recipient bed, the greater the risk of graft failure [12]. These cells are capable of processing foreign donor antigen, thereby initiating an allograft response.

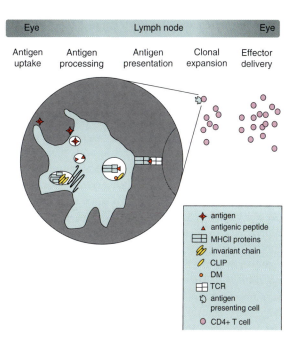

Fig. 2.2 The antigen uptake, processing and presentation pathway leading to clonal expansion of T cells. In the context of sensitization to cornea-derived antigen, the precise location of processing and presentation remain unclear

2.4 The Corneal Allograft Response

A detailed knowledge of the corneal allograft response is required if alternative approaches to suppressing the corneal allograft response are to be developed and the outcome of corneal transplants improved. Important elements are the erosion of privilege, a necessary precedent to the establishment of an allograft response, the preponderance of indirect over direct presentation of antigen, and the importance of the corneal endothelium, which has little capacity for repair, as the primary target of the effector arm of the immune response. There are several steps of the activation cascade during corneal allograft rejection that may be amenable to therapy including (1) antigen uptake, (2) antigen processing, (3) antigen presentation, (4) T cell expansion and (5) effector cell influx into the eye (Fig. 2.2). The first two are likely to occur, at least to some extent, locally in the ocular environs, and may be particularly in useful targets for topically applied therapeutics or gene therapy.

2.5 Antigen Uptake in the Eye

For antigens to be "seen" by T cells, they must be taken up and presented by APCs. Graft-derived antigen can be phagocytosed by many cells within the eye, including macrophages and dendritic cells. Proteins shed from the graft or remnants of dead donor cells may be engulfed in this way. In addition, dendritic cells are able to sample small amounts of live cell membranes (termed "nibbling"). While there is evidence that soluble protein antigens in the anterior chamber may disseminate as widely as the spleen [13] and mesenchymal lymph node [14], the relevance of this to responses against transplanted corneal tissue is yet to be determined.

There are numerous populations of potential APC within the eye that may capture alloantigen. Macrophages and dendritic cells are resident not only in the iris, but also throughout the trabecular meshwork, choroid, and episclera [10]. Langerhans cells have long been recognized as important ocular dendritic cells that reside in the peripheral cornea and migrate into the graft upon transplantation. More recently, a heterogeneous population of bone marrow-derived cells including immature dendritic cells and macrophages has been described in the central cornea. These cells upregulate MHC Class II following transplantation, but do not traffic to the regional lymph nodes [15]. Instead, resident host APC that take up graft-derived antigen and traffic to the nodes within hours of transplant are probably most important for sensitisation [15]. Intravital microscopy techniques have provided direct evidence that resident ocular APC take up antigen effectively, but many of these cells are observed to remain in situ. Thus, sensitisation that occurs in the lymph node may be facilitated by the escape of a small number of potent antigen-bearing dendritic cells. Alternatively, ocular APC may "communicate" via newly described nanotubes [16], passing antigen to more mobile dendritic cells that can then migrate to lymph nodes.

Despite the identification of various populations of ocular cells that can engulf antigen, the population that is the most important for mediating corneal allograft rejection remains unknown. While dendritic cells are very effective at initiating immune responses, the population of resident macrophages may be important as a local antigen "bank," recruiting and interacting with effector cells, as well as enhancing the development of corneal vessels and lymphatics for effector cell delivery.

Therapeutically, ocular antigen uptake can be most effectively achieved by depleting the cornea of APC. In rodent models, depletion of resident macrophages by subconjunctival injection of clodronate-containing liposomes early in the post-transplant period delays onset of rejection [17]. However, cells such as macrophages are very important for ocular antiviral responses, and their large-scale removal would likely incur a severe infection risk. Also, since only a small number of antigen-laden dendritic cells would be required to migrate to the regional lymph node to cause sensitisation, therapeutic benefit via this approach may be difficult to achieve.

2.6 Antigen Processing

For an exogenous antigen to be presented on the surface of an APC, it must first be processed within the cell. The preponderance of the indirect pathway of antigen presentation during corneal allograft rejection means that proteins involved in MHC Class II processing may be ideal therapeutic targets. APCs, such as B cells, macrophages, and dendritic cells contain all the machinery to process and present antigen on MHC Class II molecules on their surface. Phagocytosed graft-derived antigen is degraded by proteases in intracellular endosomes within the first hour after uptake. In the endoplasmic reticulum, the peptide cleft of the MHC Class II dimer is occupied by an invariant chain protein, which later degrades to form a minimal CLIP protein. The late endosome then fuses with a MHC Class II-containing vesicle, and a degraded antigen fragment is loaded into the peptide-binding cleft in place of the CLIP protein. This substitution requires another molecule, DM. The stable MHC II–antigen complex is then transported to the cell surface, where it can interact with a host CD4 T cell bearing the cognate T cell receptor (TCR).

A number of opportunities exist for therapeutic manipulation of antigen processing. While APC maturation and antigen processing are likely to occur during transit to the lymph node, local therapies applied to the eye prior to or during surgery may have an effect on ocular resident APC. Cathepsin S is an enzyme that causes the degradation of the invariant chain for subsequent removal of CLIP from the peptide-binding cleft of MHC Class II. Inhibitors of cathepsin, such as the cysteine protease inhibitor family of cystatins, halt the processing of antigen. In the context of corneal transplantation, a delay in sensitisation, due to inefficient antigen processing, may be sufficient to prevent acute rejection events and improve corneal graft survival.

2.7 Antigen Presentation

Antigen presentation is the process in which the processed alloantigen/MHC complex is presented in association with MHC molecules to the TCR on a T cell. It is the first allospecific step in the allograft response. This occurs along with many other interactions between the APC and T cell, which influence the impact of antigen presentation, including co-receptor and co-stimulatory interactions that may enhance or impede the impact of presentation (Fig. 2.3). It remains unclear how the interaction of the TCR with its cognate peptide/MHC results in the appropriate response for the T cell. Even though the cell surface molecule interactions are well defined, a number of models exist for TCR triggering, and the real situation is probably a combination of these. Whatever the mechanism of receptor triggering, it is likely that the final outcome of T cell-APC interactions is impacted by (1) the temporal expression and density of co-stimulatory molecules, (2) the phosphorylation state of immunoreceptor intracellular tails, (3) the spatial organization of phosphatases (e.g., CD45) and kinases (e.g., Lck), and (4) the cytokine milieu at the time of presentation [18].

Despite the complexity of the process, the interaction between APCs and host immunocytes offers the prospect of allospecific therapeutic intervention, but this has not yet been achieved in clinical transplantation. Antibodies to key elements of antigen presentation, for example, anti-CD4 and anti-CD3 antibodies and CTLA4-Ig fusion protein, have been used clinically with some success, but these agents work in a nonspecific rather than an alllospecific way to suppress immune responses [19–21]. Because they are administered systemically and result in systemic immunosuppression, this approach has not been widely employed in corneal transplantation. Biologics of the molecular size of whole antibody molecules are too large to cross into the cornea, and therefore cannot be delivered topically.

Because antigen presentation following corneal transplantation occurs distally in the regional lymph nodes, most locally applied ocular therapies targeting this process are unlikely to have a significant effect. However, one promising approach to prevention of presentation of cornea-derived alloantigen is to interrupt cell-chemokine

2.11 Prevention of Allograft Rejection

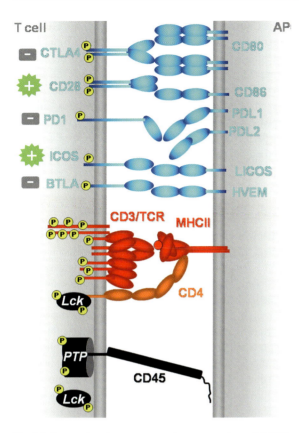

Fig. 2.3 Interactions between an antigen presenting cell (APC) and a CD4+ T cell. The overall outcome of the MHC-bound peptide/T cell receptor (TCR) interaction (*red*) is impacted by coreceptors (*orange*), co-stimulatory molecules (*cyan blue*), the phosphorylation state and density of immunoreceptor tyrosine motifs in intracellular tails (*yellow circles*), and the organization of protein tyrosine phosphatases (e.g., CD45) and kinases (e.g., Lck). Activatory (+) or inhibitory (−) signals delivered by co-stimulatory molecules are shown

interactions involved in trafficking the antigen-loaded APC out of the eye and into the lymph node. Experimentally, blockade of the CCR7–CCL21 pathway decreases the number of ocular-derived APC in the node [22]. Other approaches, such as the local expression of interleukin 10 (IL-10), probably work by inhibiting the maturation and/or trafficking of ocular APC. IL10 promotes the development of monocytes with high phagocytic ability but poor antigen presentation capabilities [23].

2.8 T Cell Activation, Proliferation, and Clonal Expansion

T cell activation, proliferation, and clonal expansion are consequences of antigen presentation. Clonal expansion occurs in draining lymph nodes and other related lymphoid tissues, and is driven by interleukin 2 (IL2). The most potent effect of calcineurin blockers such as cyclosporin A and FK 506 is on IL2-controlled clonal expansion in lymph nodes and other lymphoid tissue, beyond the reach of eye-drop therapy. Hence, systemic administration of calcineurin blockers is required to prolong corneal graft survival. Neither cyclosporin A nor FK506 has been shown to extend graft survival when delivered topically.

2.9 Effector Arm of the Allograft Response

The effector arm of the immune response brings destructive cells and proteins into the donor cornea. Damage is mediated primarily through cellular mechanisms. Antibody plays little if any part in corneal graft rejection. CD4+ cells play a central role in the recruitment of a wide range of cells with destructive capability. These include macrophages, polymorphonuclear granulocytes, and NK cells via a range of cytokines, including tumor necrosis factor-alpha (TNFα), and interferon gamma. CD8+ T lymphocytes, although present in rejecting grafts, are not necessary for the rejection process, and CD8-deficient animals reject corneal grafts in the normal way.

The effector arm is directed at all cellular components of the cornea, but the endothelium is the crucial target. This important cellular monolayer has no capacity for repair, and remains of donor origin as long as the graft survives. In contrast, donor corneal epithelium and stromal keratocytes are eventually replaced with cells of recipient origin.

2.10 Current Management of Corneal Transplants

The clinical management of patients with corneal transplants is somewhat arbitrary – like much of clinical medicine. This is because of a paucity of high-level evidence, and a wide range of clinical entities and circumstances. Despite this, there is general agreement on many aspects of management. Topical corticosteroids, the mainstay of contemporary treatment of corneal allograft rejection, discourage the movement of the effector cells into the graft. This nonspecific treatment is very effective, and is unlikely to be supplanted by more specific antibody-based therapies because so many different cells play a role in graft destruction.

2.11 Prevention of Allograft Rejection

Not all cases requiring a corneal allograft are at high risk of rejection. Patients in whom there has been no previous corneal inflammation – those with keratoconus and some corneal dystrophies – have a low risk of rejection. No special measures need to be taken for these patients, and topical glucocorticosteroids remain the mainstay of prophylaxis for rejection. On the other hand, patients who have had previous corneal inflammation, particularly if the host bed is vascularised, or have had previous grafts in the same eye are at high risk of rejection and graft failure. Clinicians need to evaluate the risk of allograft rejection prior to surgery so that the risks are minimized – particularly if the patient is monocular. Patients with a high risk of rejecting their grafts may be candidates for therapeutic interventions that cannot be justified for low-risk cases.

2.12 Stratification of Risk

There are good grounds for avoiding high-risk corneal transplantation in cases where the contralateral eye is normal. In such cases, there may be little to gain. Visual disability is limited by the quality of vision in the better eye, not how poor it is in the worse eye. Unless the vision achieved in the grafted eye exceeds the vision in the contralateral eye, which is difficult to achieve when the contralateral eye is normal, there is little functional benefit to be had. Furthermore, should the graft fail, the inconvenience and disruption from the failed graft may exceed the problems which brought the patient to surgery. In addition to this problem, when it is decided to offer someone a corneal allograft, the degree of risk needs to be assessed. Survival tables exist to assist with this assignment [2].

2.13 Protecting Immune Privilege

Erosion of corneal immune privilege is a consequence of inflammation, and so the control of inflammation is a key element of any antirejection strategy. Two aspects of corneal immune privilege can be managed clinically, at least to some degree: the accumulation of bone marrow-derived APCs in the graft and the maintenance of avascularity. Effective management of keratitis early in the disease process may limit the recruitment of inflammatory cells and prevent vascularization, a consequence of chronic inflammation. Use of topical corticosteroid is the only therapy likely to be effective in this regard.

2.14 Minimizing Antigenic Differences Between Donor and Recipient

Debate continues about the role of tissue matching in corneal transplantation. HLA matching has little support in the United States but has majority support in Europe. It is generally conceded that the effect of current tissue matching strategies is not as effective for corneal transplants as for renal transplantation, because of the importance of minor histocompatibility antigens in the former. Nevertheless, enough studies demonstrate a modest improvement with Class I and II matching to warrant this approach if it is available – or at least to keep an open mind on the subject [11, 12, 24].

2.15 Systemic Immunosuppression

Systemic immunosuppression is not widely employed in corneal transplantation, even for patients who are at high risk of rejecting their graft. The well-recognized risks associated with systemic immunosuppression can seldom be justified. The exceptions are patients who are blind for the want of a functioning corneal transplant, who are able to understand the risks of long-term systemic immunosuppression, and who are so affected by their blindness that they are prepared to accept the likely morbidities.

Another factor dissuading the use of systemic immunosuppression is the limited evidence supporting its use. Some investigators report a beneficial effect [25, 26], others do not [27–29]. For those who qualify for systemic immunosuppression, the choice of regimen is somewhat arbitrary, and there is no evidence that any one regimen is any better than any other. Under these circumstances, it is reasonable to extrapolate from what has proven to be effective in other clinical situations. Currently, the most widely employed regimens in organ transplantation employ use of a calcineurin blocker, either cyclosporin A or FK506, and an antiproliferative agent such azathioprine or mycophenolate. It can only be assumed that the same dose and length of administration needs to be adhered to in patients with corneal grafts. Over the years, we have found it preferable to manage patients with corneal transplants needing immunosuppression with the help of transplant physicians who treat patients with organ transplants, and to manage them similarly.

2.16 Surgical Techniques and Postoperative Management

Surgical approaches that reduce inflammation as far as possible should be employed. Inflammation is often the immediate precedent of a rejection episode. The nylon sutures used to secure the graft can be the cause of postsurgical inflammation. At the time of surgery, some consideration needs to be given to the suture pattern to be employed.

If there is, or has been, focal inflammatory disease, it may be preferable to use interrupted rather than a continuous suture. Areas of the host cornea that have been inflamed tend to have a low threshold for subsequent inflammation. The presence of a suture may be enough to induce an inflammatory response, which may lead to vascularization. When this occurs, it can be managed by removing a single stitch, something, which cannot be done if a continuous suture has been employed. For the same reason, it is important to remove loose sutures. Sutures tend to loosen as a consequence of inflammation. An "inflammatory canal" around a suture shortens the intracorneal path of the suture and results in loosening of the suture, which further irritates the epithelium resulting in more inflammation. The consequences are revealed in graft survival statistics. Corneal grafts from which the sutures are removed very early – within 6 months – often fail [2]. This is because early suture removal in these cases is usually forced by suture loosening occurring as a consequence of inflammation.

Management of wound healing and inflammation in the postoperative period has much to do with ultimate outcomes. A feature of corneal transplantation is the centre effect – the marked differences in graft survival between centers that cannot be explained by differences in case mix. It is likely that an important factor is the way intercurrent inflammation is managed. Patients with better access to experienced clinicians are likely to be treated more promptly and effectively.

Any intercurrent inflammation occurring in the postoperative phase demands early diagnosis and treatment. Uveitis, blepharitis, conjunctivitis, or similar conditions should be managed effectively and promptly. This amounts to identifying and negating any stimulus to inflammation, for example, removing a loose stitch or treating bacterial conjunctivitis with antibiotics. It may also be necessary to suppress the inflammatory process with topical corticosteroids.

2.17 Management of Acute Rejection Episodes

Rejection episodes occur frequently in patients with corneal transplants. They may be so minor that patients do not report them, and they settle spontaneously, or if they are apparent clinically, they may respond to corticosteroids with the graft regaining normal function. At worst, they result in irreparable damage to the graft endothelium and graft failure. Intense treatment with topical steroids is employed by the majority of surgeons. However, current treatments are inadequate; too many grafts fail. New approaches specifically developed for the cornea that are appropriate for the clinical context are required.

2.18 New Therapies with Novel Mechanisms

For the reasons set out above, it is desirable to find a way of providing loco-regional immunosuppression for corneal transplantation. Two approaches could be antibody-based therapy delivered as eye-drops, and, alternatively, utilizing gene therapy.

2.19 Antibody-based Immunosuppressive Agents in Transplantation

Antibody-based treatments are used extensively in organ transplantation. Virtually all the steps in the allograft response are amenable to manipulation with antibodies. T cells and their products are central elements in the allograft response. As described previously, antigen presentation involves two associated molecular events, the interaction of the TCR and adjacent CD3 and CD4 molecules with the foreign antigen (signal 1), and the reaction of CD80 and CD86 on APCs with the corresponding receptors CD28 and CTLA4 on T cells (signal 2). Anti-CD3, anti-CD4, and anti-CD52 antibodies are frequently used in organ transplantation. CD52 is a receptor on T cells, B cells, monocytes, and natural killer cells. Its function is unknown. Activated T cells produce IL2, which functions as an autostimulant, driving T cell activation and clonal expansion through its interaction with the IL2 receptor (IL2R). Antibodies directed at the receptor prolong graft survival, and are used in clinical organ transplantation. The efferent arm of the allograft response involves a range of cellular and noncellular destructive processes. TNFα seems to have a central role in these processes. It is being used to treat uveitis, and may find a role in the treatment of allograft rejection.

2.20 Engineered Antibodies for Eye Disease

Although used extensively in organ transplantation, antibody-based therapies have not so far found a place in clinical corneal transplantation [30]. Currently, the antibodies used in clinical organ transplantation are systemically administered and produce systemic immunosuppression. Further, whole antibodies are too large to be absorbed across the cornea, so local administration as eye drops is not likely to be effective – even if the target of the antibody were in the eye.

Until recently, therapeutic polyclonal or monoclonal antibodies were produced by immunizing animals or culturing murine hybridoma cell lines, respectively. Developments in molecular biology mean that customized chimeric human or fully human antibodies can now be produced from synthetic DNA libraries. Antibody engineering allows for the creation of small antibody fragments much smaller than the whole antibody, so small that they can pass across the cornea easily and enter the eye in therapeutic doses [31, 32]. A mouse anti-rat CD4 single chain variable region (scFv) fragment and a mouse anti-rat CTLA4 construct have both been shown to prolong cornel graft survival in experimental animals, but only when administered systemically, despite there being high levels of the antibody fragment in the aqueous and vitreous compartments of the eye [33–35]. This highlights a limitation of the concept of topically administered regional immunosuppression. The target molecule must have a role early in the allograft response – prior to antigen presentation – as it would appear to occur primarily outside the eye and the reach of topical therapy. An antibody fragment against TNFα is currently undergoing clinical trials. This shows promise, in that it is likely to suppress some elements of the complex effector phase of graft rejection.

2.21 Gene Therapy of the Donor Cornea

Another possible way to thwart the corneal allograft response is by gene therapy. The cornea is an attractive prospect for gene therapy. Prior to corneal transplantation, the donor cornea is stored for days or even weeks ex vivo, during which time transduction with a vector can be achieved without any urgency. In addition, the anterior segment of the eye is somewhat sequestered from the general circulation and immune system, which lessens the risk of systemic complications arising from the transgene or the vector. The endothelium is an ideal cellular monolayer for gene therapy vectors. It is easily accessible and can be examined clinically without difficulty. Two important considerations in gene therapy are the vector and the transgene.

2.22 Vectors for Gene Therapy of the Cornea

An extensive range of viral and nonviral vectors has been used in experimental corneal transplantation studies, but there is no consensus as to the usage of the optimal vector. However, viral vectors are being increasingly preferred by researchers in the field [36]. The most widely used include recombinant adenoviral, lentiviral, and adeno-associated viral vectors. Our preference is for an HIV-1-based lentiviral vector, which integrates into genomic DNA and can rapidly produce stable transgene expression within the eye [37–40]. Safety concerns around the possibility of recipients developing AIDS can be dismissed: the viruses used for gene therapy have been stripped of the genes responsible for replication of the virus. There is a theoretical risk of insertional mutagenesis, but there are no reports to date of oncogene activation or any other serious adverse events with any lentiviral vector.

2.23 Transgenes for Prolonging Corneal Graft Survival

At this stage, gene therapy approaches for corneal transplantation have been restricted to laboratory studies using animal models. No clinical studies have been undertaken. Most of the work has been done in inbred rodents, and some in larger outbred animals such as sheep. Species differences have considerable influences on outcomes. A variety of transgenes has been shown to prolong corneal allograft survival significantly (Table 2.1) [41–52]. For the most part, gene therapy in rats and mice has produced rather modest prolongation of corneal graft survival, but the results are sufficiently encouraging to suggest that ex vivo transduction of corneas prior to transplantation is worthy of exploration in pre-clinical models. In this regard, studies in sheep are particularly encouraging because the extension of graft survival with ovine IL-10 or p40-IL12 transgenes was considerable [41, 42]. Presumably, the products of these genes operate in the earliest (most proximal) phase of the allograft response, which occurs in the eye. Genes that produce proteins acting later in the allograft response cannot be expected to have a significant effect on graft survival when the genes are delivered to the eye because the processes they are directed at occur outside the eye.

2.24 Future Prospects

The need to improve the outcome of corneal transplantation is obvious to all those involved in the field. As the mechanisms of corneal transplantation have been better defined, so too have the opportunities for therapeutic intervention. Regional immunosuppression targeting those phases of the corneal allograft response that occur most proximally (antigen uptake and APC maturation and migration) or most distally (graft destruction) may be the key. This may be achieved through topical administration of therapeutic agents or by gene therapy. Both options offer prospects for an overdue improvement in corneal transplantation outcomes.

Table 2.1 Transgenes demonstrated to prolong corneal allograft survival significantly in animal models

Transgene	Vector	Model	Outcome	Reference
Cellular interleukin-10 (IL10)	Adenovirus	Sheep	Median survival extended from 20 days (controls) to 55 days (treated)	41
Cytotoxic lymphocyte antigen 4-Ig fusion protein (CTLA4-Ig)	Adenovirus	Rat	Ex vivo transduction of cornea extended median graft survival from 9 to 10 days; systemic injection extended survival from 9 to 18 days	43
Interleukin-4 (IL4) and CTLA4	MIDGE	Mouse	Treatment of recipient cornea extended survival from 27 ± 19 to 64 ± 28 days	44
IL4 with CTLA4	MIDGE	Mouse	Survival extended from 27 ± 6 to 62 ± 26 days	45
Endostatin-kringle 5 fusion protein (EK5)	HIV-based lentivirus	Rabbit	Controls failed at 14–18 days; none of EK5-treated grafts failed by 39 days	46
p40 subunit of interleukin 12 (p40-IL12)	Adenovirus	Sheep	Median survival extended from 20 days (controls) to 45 days (treated)	42
CTLA4-Ig and viral IL10 (vIL10)	Adenovirus	Rat	Ex vivo transduction of cornea extended mean survival from 13 to 16 days (Ad-CTLA4-Ig) or to 15 days (Ad-CTLA4-Ig and Ad-vIL10); intraperitoneal injection Ad-CTLA4-Ig extended survival to 23 days (low dose) or 40 days (high dose)	47
Indoleamine 2,3-dioxygenase (IDO)	EIAV-based lentivirus	Mouse	Median survival extended from 11 to 21 days	48
Viral IL10	Adenovirus	Rat	Ex vivo transduction of cornea did not extend survival; intraperitoneal injection extended mean survival from 11 to 15 days	49
Nerve growth factor (NGF), CTLA4-Ig	Adenovirus	Rat	Ex vivo transduction of cornea with Ad-NGF extended mean survival from 13 to 17 days; intraperitoneal injection of Ad-NGF did not prolong survival; ex vivo transduction of cornea with Ad-NGF plus intraperitoneal Ad-CTLA4-Ig extended survival to 70 days in 6 of 7 animals	50

(continued)

Table 2.1 (continued)

Transgene	Vector	Model	Outcome	Reference
Bcl-xL	HIV-based lentivirus	Mouse	90% survival rate at 8 weeks in LV-Bcl-xL-treated corneas, compared with 40% in unmodified controls and 30% in LV-controls	51
Viral macrophage inflammatory protein II (vMIP II)	Liposomes plus transferrin	Mouse	Median graft survival prolonged to 21 days compared with untransfected or control-transfected donor corneas	52

Ad adenovirus; *MIDGE* minimalistic immunologically defined gene expression plasmid vector; *HIV* human immunodeficiency virus; *LV* lentivirus; *EIAV* equine infectious anemia virus

Acknowledgments The authors acknowledge the support of the National Health & Medical Research Council of Australia and the Ophthalmic Research Institute of Australia.

References

1. World Health Organization (WHO) Report (1998) The world health report 1998: life in the 21st century. Geneva, WHO, p 47
2. Williams KA, Lowe MT, Bartlett CM et al (2007) The Australian corneal graft registry 2007 report. Flinders University Press, Adelaide
3. Wolfe RA (2004) Long-term renal allograft survival: a cup half-full and half-empty. Am J Transplant 4:1215–1216
4. Campbell S, McDonald S, Excell L et al (2008) 31st report from the Australia and New Zealand dialysis and transplant registry. In: McDonald S, Excell L, Livingston B (eds) Transplantation. ANZDATA Registry, Adelaide, p pp 7
5. Bill A (1986) The blood aqueous barrier. Trans Ophthalmol Soc UK 105:149–155
6. Catry L, Van den Oord J, Foets B et al (1991) Morphologic and immunophenotypic heterogeneity of corneal dendritic cells. Graefes Arch Clin Ex Ophthalmol 229:182–185
7. Jager MJ (1992) Corneal Langerhans cells and ocular immunology. Reg Immunol 4:186–195
8. Whitsett CF, Stulting RD (1984) The distribution of HLA antigens on human corneal tissue. Invest Ophthalmol Vis Sci 25:519–524
9. Streilein JW (2003) Ocular immune privilege: the eye takes a dim but practical view of immunity and inflammation. J Leukoc Biol 74:179–185
10. Camelo S, Shanley AC, Voon AS et al (2004) An intravital and confocal microscopic study of the distribution of intracameral antigen in the aqueous outflow pathways and limbus of the rat eye. Exp Eye Res 79:455–464
11. Pepose JS, Gardner KM, Nestor MS et al (1985) Detection of HLA class I and II antigens in rejected human corneal allografts. Ophthalmology 92:1480–1484
12. Williams KA, White MA, Ash JK et al (1989) Leukocytes in the graft bed associated with corneal graft failure. Analysis by immunohistology and actuarial graft survival. Ophthalmology 96:38–44
13. Streilein JW, Niederkorn JY (1981) Induction of anterior chamber-associated immune deviation requires an intact, functional spleen. J Exp Med 153:1058–1067
14. Camelo S, Shanley A, Voon AS et al (2004) The distribution of antigen in lymphoid tissues following its injection into the anterior chamber of the rat eye. J Immunol 172:5388–5395
15. Kuffova L, Netukova M, Duncan L et al (2008) Cross presentation of antigen on MHC class II via the draining lymph node after corneal transplantation in mice. J Immunol 180:1353–1361
16. Chinnery HR, Pearlman E, McMenamin PG (2008) Cutting edge: membrane nanotubes in vivo: a feature of MHC class II+ cells in the mouse cornea. J Immunol 180:5779–5783
17. Slegers TP, Broersma L, van Roojen N et al (2004) Macrophages play a role in the early phase of corneal allograft rejection in rats. Transplantation 77:1641–1646
18. Choudhuri K, van der Merwe P (2007) Molecular mechanisms involved in T cell receptor triggering. Semin Immunol 19:255–261
19. Casadei DH, del C Rial M, Opelz G et al (2001) A randomized and prospective study comparing treatment with high-dose intravenous immunoglobulin with monoclonal antibodies for rescue of kidney grafts with steroid-resistant rejection. Transplantation 71(1):53–58
20. Cooperative Clinical Trials in Transplantation Research Group (1997) Murine OKT4A immunosuppression in

cadaver donor renal allograft recipients: a cooperative clinical trials in transplantation pilot study. Transplantation 63(9):1243–1251
21. Salomon B, Bluestone JA (2001) Complexities of CD28/B7: CTLA-4 costimulatory pathways in autoimmunity and transplantation. Annu Rev Immunol 19:225–252
22. Jin Y, Shen L, Chong EM et al (2007) The chemokine receptor CCR7 mediates corneal antigen-presenting cell trafficking. Mol Vis 13:626–634
23. Mosser DM, Zhang X (2008) Interleukin-10: new perspectives on an old cytokine. Immunol Rev 226:205–218
24. Cursiefen C, Chen L, Borges LP et al (2004) VEGF-A stimulates lymphangiogenesis and hemangiogenesis in inflammatory neovascularization via macrophage recruitment. J Clin Invest 113:1040–1050
25. Hill JC (1994) Systemic cyclosporine in high-risk keratoplasty: short versus long-term therapy. Ophthalmology 101:128–133
26. Sundmacher R, Reinhard T, Heering P (1992) Six years' experience with systemic cyclosporin. A prophylaxis in high-risk perforating keratoplasty patients. A retrospective study. Ger J Ophthalmol 1:432–436
27. Poon AC, Forbes JE, Dart JK et al (2001) Systemic cyclosporin A in high-risk penetrating keratoplasties: a case-control study. Br J Ophthalmol 85:1464–1469
28. Inoue KC, Amano S et al (2001) Long-term outcome of systemic cyclosporine treatment following penetrating keratoplasty. Jpn J Ophthalmol 45:378–382
29. Rumelt S, Bersudsky V, Blum-Hareuveni T et al (2002) Systemic cyclosporin A in high failure risk, repeated corneal transplantation. Br J Ophthalmol 86:988–992
30. Kirk AD (2006) Induction immunosuppression. Transplantation 82:593–602
31. Chatenoud L (2006) Monoclonal antibody-based strategies in autoimmunity and transplantation. Methods Mol Med 109:297–328
32. Filpula D (2007) Antibody engineering and modification technologies. Biomol Eng 24:201–215
33. Thiel MA, Coster DJ, Standfield SD et al (2002) Penetration of engineered antibody fragments into the eye. Clin Exp Immunol 128:67–74
34. Williams KA, Brereton HM, Farrall A et al (2005) Topically applied antibody fragments penetrate into the back of the rabbit eye. Eye 19:910–913
35. Ottiger M, Thiel MA, Feige U et al (2009) Efficient intraocular penetration of topical anti-TNF-alpha single-chain antibody (ESBA105) to anterior and posterior segment without penetration enhancer. Invest Ophthalmol Vis Sci 50:779–786
36. Parker DG, Brereton HM, Coster DJ et al (2009) The potential of viral-vector mediated gene transfer to prolong corneal allograft survival. Curr Gene Ther 9(1):33–44
37. Poeschla EM (2003) Non-primate lentiviral vectors. Curr Opin Mol Ther 5:529–540
38. Saenz DT, Poeschla EM (2004) FIV: from lentivirus to lentivector. J Gene Med 6(Suppl 1):S95–S104
39. Parker DGA, Kaufmann C, Brereton HM et al (2007) Lentivirus-mediated gene transfer to the rat, ovine and human cornea. Gene Ther 14:760–767
40. Anson DS, Fuller M (2003) Rational development of a HIV-1 gene therapy vector. J Gene Med 5:829–838
41. Klebe S, Sykes PJ, Coster DJ et al (2001) Prolongation of sheep corneal allograft survival by ex vivo transfer of the gene encoding interleukin-10. Transplantation 71:1214–1220
42. Klebe S, Coster DJ, Sykes PJ et al (2005) Prolongation of sheep corneal allograft survival by transfer of the gene encoding ovine IL-12–p40 but not IL-4 to donor corneal endothelium. J Immunol 175:2219–2226
43. Comer RM, King WJ, Ardjomand N et al (2002) Effect of administration of CTLA4-Ig as protein or cDNA on corneal allograft survival. Invest Ophthalmol Vis Sci 43:1095–1103
44. Muller A, Zhang EP, Schroff M et al (2002) Influence of ballistic gene transfer on antigen-presenting cells in murine corneas. Graefes Arch Clin Exp Ophthalmol 240:851–859
45. Zhang EP, Franke J, Schroff M et al (2003) Ballistic CTLA4 and IL-4 gene transfer into the lower lid prolongs orthotopic corneal graft survival in mice. Graefes Arch Clin Exp Ophthalmol 241:921–926
46. Murthy RC, McFarland TJ, Yoken J et al (2003) Corneal transduction to inhibit angiogenesis and graft failure. Invest Ophthalmol Vis Sci 44:1837–1842
47. Gong N, Pleyer U, Yang J et al (2006) Influence of local and systemic CTLA4Ig gene transfer on corneal allograft survival. J Gene Med 8:459–467
48. Beutelspacher SC, Pillai R, Watson MP et al (2006) Function of indoleamine 2, 3-dioxygenase in corneal allograft rejection and prolongation of allograft survival by over-expression. Eur J Immunol 36:690–700
49. Gong N, Pleyer U, Volk HD et al (2007) Effects of local and systemic viral interleukin-10 gene transfer on corneal allograft survival. Gene Ther 14:484–490
50. Gong N, Pleyer U, Vogt K et al (2007) Local overexpression of nerve growth factor in rat corneal transplants improves allograft survival. Invest Ophthalmol Vis Sci 48:1043–1052
51. Barcia RN, Dana MR, Kazlauskas A (2007) Corneal graft rejection is accompanied by apoptosis of the endothelium and is prevented by gene therapy with Bcl-xL. Am J Transplant 7:2082–2089
52. Pillai RG, Beutelspacher SC, Larkin DF et al (2008) Expression of the chemokine antagonist vMIP II using a non-viral vector can prolong corneal allograft survival. Transplantation 85:1640–1647

Chapter 3

New Developments in Topical and Systemic Immunomodulation Following Penetrating Keratoplasty

Alexander Reis, Thomas Reinhard

Core Messages

- Immunologic rejection is the main cause of corneal graft failure.
- Acute rejection is mainly mediated by T cells, and can be prevented with steroids, IL-2 inhibitors (cyclosporine, tacrolimus), mycophenolate mofetil, and TOR-inhibitors (everolimus, rapamycin).
- Based on their risk of immunologic rejection, corneal transplants are rated as either normal-risk or high-risk transplants.
- In a normal-risk situation, the postoperative application of topical steroids accompanied by a short course of systemic steroids is sufficient to prevent acute graft rejection in most cases.
- In high-risk keratoplasty, systemic immunosuppression with mycophenolate mofetil or cyclosporine has to be used to maintain clear graft survival.
- Topical immunosuppression with either cyclosporine A or tacrolimus might present an attractive therapeutic approach to reduce drug-specific systemic side effects.
- More specific approaches using monoclonal antibodies, which target only selected aspects of the host's immune response, have failed to safely and sufficiently prolong graft survival in experimental settings, and have therefore not gained clinical relevance.

3.1 Introduction

Immunologic graft rejection is the single most important reason for graft failure following corneal transplantation.

In a normal-risk-situation (e.g., keratokonus, Fuchs endothelial dystrophy), the risk for corneal graft failure due to rejection is less than 10% within the first 5 years after transplantation. This makes penetrating keratoplasty the most successful transplantation when compared with transplantation of solid organs. Nevertheless, we do lose almost 10% of the transplants within the first 5 years. Several strategies might enhance graft survival in this setting.

The most promising approach is matching for the donor–host immune-relevant antigens: if the graft does not generate any immune response, there is no need to interfere with the host immune system.

Another approach might be a topical one: by using immunomodulatory drugs, antibodies or gene therapy, graft survival might be enhanced without systemic side effects.

A completely different scenario is corneal transplantation in a high-risk situation: without the use of systemic immunosuppression, corneal graft failure has to be expected in as many as 50% or more patients within the first 5 postoperative years.

Despite the privilege that the transplanted organ can directly (and not via the vascular system) be reached with topical steroids in extremely high concentrations, thereby interfering with the host's immune system right at the "battlefield" of graft rejection, this strategy is only sufficient to prevent graft rejection in a normal-risk situation.

Especially in a high-risk situation with a vascularized host cornea, the clonal expansion of alloreactive T cells happens in lymphoid organs (i.e., lymph nodes and spleen): after the recognition of the foreign tissues by T cells, these specific T cells start to proliferate and generate an immunological army against the graft. It is therefore crucial not only to work with topical immunomodulatory strategies, but to employ immunosuppressive substances systemically in a high-risk situation.

To understand the possible targets of immunosuppression and immunomodulation we have to take a look at the underlying immunology.

3.2 Immunology

Immunological responses against the transplanted cornea remain the major cause of allograft injury and loss. The innate and adaptive immune systems are variously involved in rejection. Several factors determine the strength and nature of the immune response: (1) the nature of the grafted cornea (i.e., whether it is a clear corneal button or a limbo-corneal transplant); and (2) the nature of the recipient's graft bed (i.e., whether it is clear, vascularized, or has a limbal stem cell insufficiency). Additionally, inflammatory responses (and graft rejection is a form of an inflammatory response) are physiologically suppressed in the anterior chamber: on the one hand, antigens injected intraocularly elicit deviant systemic immune responses that are devoid of immunogenic inflammation (a phenomenon called anterior chamber-associated immune deviation, ACAID). On the other hand, the ocular microenvironment (aqueous humor, secreted by cells that surround this chamber) suppresses intraocular expression of immunogenic inflammation [1].

These special anatomical features are responsible for the excellent results in normal-risk corneal transplantation when compared to solid organ transplantation or high-risk corneal transplantation.

The nature of the host's immune response can be determined by its histopathology and time course as acute or chronic rejection.

3.2.1 Acute Rejection

Acute rejection, which may occur weeks to years after transplantation, involves both humoral and cell-mediated immune reactions. T cells play a central role in acute rejection by responding to alloantigens, predominantly MHC molecules, presented on endothelial, epithelial, or stromal cells. Both CD4+ and CD8+ T cells contribute to acute rejection. CD4+ T cells mediate acute rejection by secreting cytokines and inducing delayed-type of hypersensitivity-like reactions in the graft. Recognition and lyses of foreign cells by cytotoxic CD8+ T cells is an important mechanism of acute rejection. T cells may be activated by two distinct mechanisms: the direct and the indirect pathway.

Based on the target, immune reactions against the transplanted cornea may be divided into endothelial, stromal of epithelial rejection. The most frequent and most severe form of an immune response is against the endothelium. The reason is that the immunogenic epithelial cells are replaced within approximately 1 year by the host's epithelium, and the stroma mostly consists of intracellular substance and only a small number of cells.

3.2.2 Major Histocompatibility Complex (MHC)

3.2.2.1 Direct Pathway of Allorecognition

Direct recognition of foreign MHC antigens by T cells might be a cause of acute rejection: donor antigen-presenting cells (which are transplanted with the graft) present donor MHC class I and class II molecules to recipient T cells, resulting in the generation and clonal proliferation of helper and cytotoxic T cells.

3.2.2.2 Indirect Pathway of Allorecognition

This is the primary cause of graft rejection. It occurs when the MHC molecules of the donor tissues are taken up and processed by the host's antigen-presenting cells, which present the foreign peptides to T cells.

Since MHC molecules are highly polymorphic in nature, they are mainly responsible for allograft rejection. But transplantation between individuals with identical MHC molecules may also fail in the late phase because at this time the so-called minor-histocompatibility antigens come into play.

3.2.3 Chronic Rejection

This term is not widely used in corneal transplantation and it is not clearly defined. The pathogenesis of chronic rejection is not clear. Chronic rejection is up to now only characterized by accelerated endothelial cell loss; however, this question is still not answered sufficiently [2, 3]. Chronic rejection cannot be prevented sufficiently with current immunosuppressive drugs (which mainly work through their interference with T cells), so the present strategy is to limit the number of acute rejection episodes. Many risk factors may possibly increase the incidence of chronic rejection, e.g., the number and severity of acute rejection episodes and recurrence of herpetic ocular disease.

3.3 Normal-risk vs. High-risk Transplantation

Based on their risk of graft rejection, corneal transplants can be divided into normal-risk or high-risk transplants.

3.3.1 Normal-risk Transplantation

In a normal-risk situation (e.g., first transplant in keratokonus or Fuchs` endothelial dystrophy) a 5-month course of topical steroids (e.g., prednisolone acetate 1%) 5 times a day, reduced by one drop every month) accompanied by systemic steroids (prednisolon 1 mg/kg tapered within 3 weeks) is sufficient to maintain a 5-year clear graft survival of more than 90%. Up to 20% of normal-risk corneal transplants experience an acute rejection episode, which can be converted in about 50% of cases with topical and systemic steroids.

3.3.2 High-risk Transplantation

Postoperative systemic immunosuppression is widely accepted as the treatment of choice in immunologic high-risk groups. The definition of high-risk corneal transplantation includes the following:

- History of previous graft rejections
- Deep vascularization of the recipient cornea in more than three quadrants
- Limbal stem cell deficiency, which requires a corneolimbal graft
- Severe atopic dermatitis

In addition to topical and systemic application of steroids as mentioned earlier, systemic immunosuppression should be used for at least 6 months following transplantation.

3.3.3 Rationale for Systemic Immunosuppression

The first goal of a timely limited systemic immunomodulation is the prevention of acute rejection episodes. The second goal is the interference with the initial graft-host interaction in a way that graft-protective cells and cytokines are promoted, hence enabling a clear graft survival without any further medication. We have already shown clinically that we can reach the first goal in most patients when using cyclosporine or mycophenolate mofetil (MMF) systemically.

3.3.4 Why Is Immunomodulation with Topical Steroids Not Sufficient to Prevent Immunologic Graft Rejection in High-Risk Patients?

The cornea is a privileged place for transplantation, both for its anatomical features (see above) and the possibility to bring a medication directly to the transplanted organ, thereby reducing systemic side effects. In a high-risk situation, the immunological privilege is diminished and there is over 50% risk of graft loss within 1 year without the use of systemic immunosuppression.

Why Are Topical Steroids Not Enough?

The activation of the recipient's immune system against the transplanted cornea (i.e., the priming of naïve T cells) occurs in lymphoid tissues. This hypothesis is supported by experiments in which T cell activation, and therefore graft rejection, did not occur when secondary lymphoid organs were absent [4]. These experimental data indicate that leucocytes participate in host T cell priming by migrating from the graft to the host's lymph node and/or spleen, where they activate alloreactive host T cells in the direct and indirect pathway. Such primed T cells circulate and target MHC molecules expressed by cells of the graft.

As topical steroids do not reach the secondary lymphoid organs, and even systemic steroids do not interfere sufficiently with the clonal expansion of activated T cells, it is essential to administer systemic immunosuppressives in order to achieve clear graft survival.

3.3.5 Rationale for Topical Immunomodulation

The cornea is a privileged tissue to transplant: its accessibility makes it particularly suitable for topical therapeutic strategies. Two strategies might be employed:

a. Immunomodulatory strategies which interfere either with allograft recognition (afferent part of the immune response) or
b. Strategies which interfere with allograft rejection (efferent part of the immune system).

These strategies have until today been realized in experimental settings in three different ways by using either drugs, monoclonal antibodies, or gene therapy, and are described in the following chapters.

> **Summary for the Clinician**
>
> - If corneal transplantation is performed in a high-risk situation without the use of systemic immunosuppression, corneal graft failure can be expected in as many as 50% cases within the first postoperative year.
> - Definition of High-risk Corneal Transplantation:
>   - History of previous graft rejections
>   - Deep vascularization of the recipient cornea in more than three quadrants
>   - Limbal stem cell deficiency, which requires a corneo-limbal graft
>   - Severe atopic dermatitis
> - In a high-risk situation, it is crucial not only to work with topical or systemic steroids but to employ immunosuppressive substances systemically.
> - T cells play a central role in rejection by responding to alloantigens, predominantly MHC molecules, presented on endothelial, epithelial, or stromal cells.
> - The activation of the recipient's immune system against the transplanted cornea i.e., the priming of naïve T cells occurs in lymphoid tissues.
> - As topical steroids do not reach the secondary lymphoid organs, and even systemic steroids do not interfere sufficiently with the clonal expansion of activated T cells, it is essential to administer systemic immunosuppressives in order to achieve clear graft survival.
> - The first goal of a timely limited systemic immunomodulation is the prevention of acute rejection episodes.
> - The second goal is the interference with the initial graft-host interaction in a way that graft-protective cells and cytokines are promoted, hence enabling a clear graft survival without any further medication.

3.4 Immunosuppressive Agents

3.4.1 History

Along with the increase in the number of solid organ transplants our therapeutic armamentarium and knowledge of immunosuppressive drugs in corneal transplantation has been improved.

In the 1950s, the selection of immunosuppressive drugs was limited to corticosteroids and azathioprine. In the 1960s, polyclonal antilymphocyte (ALG) and antithymocyte (ATG) globulins supplemented the repertoire. In the late 1970s, cyclosporine A (CSA) lead to a real breakthrough in clinical solid organ transplantation. Motivated by the encouraging results in graft survival, the research in this immunological field led us now to a wide range of potent immunosuppressive agents with highly specific sites of action.

According to their mode of action, these new drugs can be divided up into agents that selectively inhibit cytokine gene transcription/expression (cyclosporine, tacrolimus), antiproliferative agents (MMF), and agents that interfere with intracellular signal transduction (rapamycin, everolimus). Immunosuppressives might also be classified as biologics, which are defined as naturally occurring or genetically engineered mammalian proteins (thymoglobulin, basiliximab, and daclizumab) or xenobiotics (drugs produced from micro-organisms, e.g., cyclosporine, tacrolimus).

Despite the tremendous breath of the discipline of immunosuppressive molecules only a small number of drugs have gained access to experimental or clinical corneal transplantation. We have decided to focus only on these agents.

Corticosteroids
CSA
Tacrolimus (FK506)
MMF
RAD (Everolimus)
Rapamycin (Sirolimus)
FTY720
FK778
Pimecrolimus
Biological agents

3.4.2 Corticosteroids

Corticosteroids prevent interleukin (IL)-1 and IL-6 production by macrophages and inhibit all stages of T cell activation. Adverse effects of systemic steroids include Cushing disease, bone disease (e.g., osteoporosis, avascular necrosis), cataracts, glucose intolerance, infections, hyperlipidemia, and growth retardation. Adverse effects of topically applied steroids include cataract, glaucoma, and in the case of epithelial defects – steroid ulcers.

3.4.3 Cyclosporine A

The fermentation product from the fungi Tolypocladium inflatum gams was first isolated in 1970 by Thiele and Kis. Its immunosuppressive properties were discovered in 1972 by Borel.

CSA binds to the intracellular immunophilin cyclophilin (immunophilins are proteins, which bind to immunosuppressive drugs). The CSA-cyclophilin complex blocks calcineurin-calmodulin-induced phosphorylation of NFAT (nuclear factor of activated T cells) transcription factor for IL-2 and other early T-cell-specific genes, and hence is highly T-cell-specific.

Clinical efficacy and safety data have mostly been acquired in solid organ transplantation, and it is still the golden standard in all forms of solid organ transplantation (except liver transplantation), mainly in combination with steroids, azathioprine, or MMF.

3.4.3.1 CSA in Corneal Transplantation

The first documented experiences in corneal transplantation date back to the mid 1980s with exceptional efforts undertaken by Hill and colleagues [5, 6] in South Africa. These initial positive clinical experiences with systemic CSA to prevent corneal allograft rejection in high-risk keratoplasty have been confirmed by Sundmacher and Reinhard [7–9].

Despite the significant improvement of outcome in high-risk keratoplasty, the use of CSA is limited due to its considerable toxicity and the need for costly drug monitoring. The toxicity is mostly caused by the CSA-cyclophilin-calcineurin-calmodulin complex, which interferes with tubular and endothelial cell functions: nephro- and hepatotoxicity, alterations in glucose metabolism, hypertension, and gingival hyperplasia. To avoid the systemic toxicity, attempts have been undertaken to apply CSA in topical formulations [10–14]. The encouraging results of these mostly experimental studies in preventing corneal graft rejection did not hold true clinically till date. However, we have shown that topical CSA is efficient in the treatment of distinct immunological disorders of the cornea (e.g., M. Thygeson, persistent nummuli following adenovirus infections) [15, 16].

A new approach to apply CSA topically is the LX201 (LUCIDA) subconjunctival implant. A multicenter trial has started in 2007 and will end in 2009 to evaluate its efficacy in preventing corneal graft rejection in a high-risk setting. LX201 is a sustained release silicone implant containing 30% CSA by weight. The LX201 implant releases the cyclosporine at steady doses over the course of a year.

3.4.4 Tacrolimus (fk506)

Tacrolimus has been proven clinically superior to CSA following solid organ transplantation [17, 18]. Tacrolimus, like CSA, is a macrolide antibiotic (structurally related to erythromycin and rapamycin) derived from a fungus, *Streptomyces tsukubaensis* [19]. Its immunosuppressive properties were discovered by Ochai in 1985. In vitro studies have shown that, even in concentrations 40–200 times lower than CSA, Tacrolimus possesses extremely powerful immunosuppressive effectiveness [20, 21]. Although the final step in modulating the immune system is the same for CSA and Tacrolimus, i.e., interfering with the intracytoplasmatic calcineurin system, and hence the interleukin IL-2 production, both drugs manage this in a different manner. Tacrolimus binds to the intracellular FKBP-12 (FK binding protein)-12. The Tacrolimus-FKBP-12 complex blocks calcineurin-calmodulin-induced phosphorylation of the cytoplasmic component of NFAT transcription factor for IL-2 and other "early" genes. Like CSA, tacrolimus is a highly specific inhibitor of lymphocyte activation. Its toxicities are similar to CSA (probably due to its calcineurin mediated interference with tubular and endothelial cells) i.e., nephro-, neurotoxicity, arterial hypertension, diabetogenicity.

3.4.4.1 Tacrolimus in Corneal Transplantation

Up to now, there are only limited clinical data available about the efficacy of tacrolimus in corneal transplantation [22, 23]. This might partially be explained by its relatively narrow safety margins. While CSA might be given in a body weight-adjusted dose (a sub-optimal therapeutic approach), Tacrolimus has to be closely monitored because there is a greater risk of over-immunosuppression. This is also the reason for the initial, rather unjustified, bad reputation of this drug: initially, blood levels of 20–30 ng/ml have been targeted (with corresponding adverse events), whereas today blood levels of 5–10 ng/ml are considered as the optimal range.

The potency of this drug to inhibit experimental corneal allograft rejection has been proven [24–26]. As the corneal penetration of FK506 is better than that of CSA, there is much hope in finding an efficient topical administration to prevent systemic side effects. Experimentally, the efficacy of topical Tacrolimus has yet been proven [27–31] and clinical studies of topical Tacrolimus in atopic conjunctivitis are under way.

We have tested FK506 eyedrops in a clinical trial with normal-risk patients. Although we found this therapeutic approach to be efficient, the galenic formulation we used resulted in local side effects (itching and burning) [32, 33].

3.4.5 Mycophenolate Mofetil (MMF)

MMF is the bioavailability-enhanced morpholinoethyl-ester of mycophenolic acid (MPA), which was originally isolated from Penicillium spp. MMF is rapidly converted to MPA, its active compound. Its safety and effectiveness in combination with CSA following kidney transplantation has been proven in several clinical studies [34–37]. Unlike CSA or Tacrolimus, MMF does not interfere with IL-2 pathways. MPA reversibly inhibits the de novo formation of guanosine nucleotides [38] by inhibiting the enzyme inosine monophosphate dehydrogenase (with high affinity to the isoform II, which is expressed in activated lymphocytes). As T and B cells are predominantly dependent on the de novo synthesis of guanosine nucleotides, the purine biosynthesis of these cells is selectively inhibited [39]. As MMF is not an antimetabolite and does not lead to genetic miscoding, it is not carcinogenic (in contrast to antimetabolites like azathioprine).

MMF in Corneal Transplantation

We have been able to prove the potency of this drug, and its synergistic effect to CSA and FK506 in delaying corneal allograft rejection in the rat keratoplasty model [40]. Following these initial positive experiences, we conducted a prospective clinical trial with MMF and CSA in high-risk keratoplasty patients. The data of this study show a similar efficacy of MMF and CSA in preventing allograft rejection [41]. But due to the large therapeutic margin and favorable safety profile of MMF, costly drug monitoring is not indicated [42, 43]. Additionally, we used this substance in immunological disorders of the eye, again with favorable results [44].

There are no published data about the topical application of MMF in corneal transplantation.

3.4.6 Rapamycin (Sirolimus)

Sirolimus is an immunosuppressive agent previously known as rapamycin. It has been under development for more than 20 years before it gained FDA approval in 1999. Sirolimus is a macrocyclic lactone produced by Streptomyces hygroscopicus found in the soil of Easter Island. Structurally, sirolimus resembles tacrolimus, and binds to the same intracellular binding protein or immunophilin known as FKBP-12. However, sirolimus has a novel mechanism of action. While tacrolimus and cyclosporine block lymphokine (e.g., IL2) gene transcription, sirolimus acts later to block IL2-dependent T lymphocyte proliferation and the stimulation caused by cross-linkage of CD28, possibly by blocking activation of a kinase, referred to as mammalian target of rapamycin or *"mTOR"*, a serine–threonine kinase that is important for cell cycle progression. Therefore, sirolimus is believed to act in synergy with cyclosporine (or tacrolimus) to suppress the immune system.

Rapamycin has been shown to be highly efficient in preventing experimental solid organ [45, 46] and clinical renal transplantation [47, 48]. It is noteworthy to mention that rapamycin is not nephrotoxic, which makes this drug especially interesting for renal transplant recipients.

Rapamycin in Corneal Transplantation

A couple of experimental studies have shown the efficacy of sirolimus in inhibiting murine corneal allograft rejection [49–52]. We have conducted a small clinical study with sirolimus in high-risk corneal transplantation. We have started Rapamune® at the day of transplantation in a dose of 2 mg/day. The dose was adjusted to reach plasma levels of 4–10 ng/ml on the following days, trying to keep plasma levels close to 4 ng/ml. We have seen that the efficacy of Rapamune® in preventing corneal allograft rejection is comparable to cyclosporine and MMF. But it is noteworthy to mention that we have seen a high incidence of side effects in this small group of patients.

There are no published data about the topical administration of rapamycin in corneal transplantation.

3.4.7 RAD (Everolimus)

Everolimus is an oral Rapamycin derivative. It is chemically derived from rapamycin, which has been obtained by fermentation of an actinomycetes strain. It has been found that everolimus (40-0-[2-hydroxyethyl])-RPM is stable in oral formulations, and that its efficacy after oral dosing is at least equivalent to that of rapamycin [53, 54]. The mode of action is equivalent to rapamycin i.e., binding to FKBP, inhibiting TOR1 and 2, and hence inhibiting cell cycle progression of activated t cells.

Everolimus and sirolimus are also called *proliferation signal inhibitors* (PSI), because they prevent proliferation of T cells.

Everolimus may have a special role in solid organ transplantation as it has been shown to reduce chronic allograft vasculopathy in such transplants [55].

Everolimus in Corneal Transplantation

Everolimus has been tested in the rat model of corneal transplantation, both as a single therapy and in combination with CSA and MMF. It appears that the potency of everolimus to prevent corneal allograft rejection is comparable to CSA. Additionally, a synergistic effect of everolimus has been found in a double-drug regimen with CSA as well as with MMF [56–58].

Everolimus might also be used in a topical formulation to prevent corneal allograft rejection [59].

There are up to now no clinical data on the efficacy and safety of everolimus in clinical corneal transplantation.

3.4.8 FTY 720

The chemical 2-amino-2[2-(4-octylphenyl)ethyl]-1,3, propane diol is one of a class of small-molecule immunosuppressive agents. This compound was chemically synthesized in an effort to minimize the toxic in vivo properties of a structurally related and highly potent immunosuppressive agent, myriocin. FTY 720's mechanism of action, although not fully characterized, appears to be unique among immunosuppressants. In vivo, FTY 720 induces a significant reduction in the number of circulating lymphocytes. It is thought to act by altering lymphocyte trafficking/homing patterns through modulation of cell surface adhesion receptors. Although much research has yet to be done to unravel the nature of the mechanism of action of FTY 720, its efficacy has been sufficiently proven in numerous animal models, especially when administered in combination with cyclosporine. It has been shown that FTY 720 is efficacious in a variety of transplant and autoimmune models without inducing a generalized immunosuppressed state, and is effective in human kidney transplantation.

FTY 720 in Corneal Transplantation

We have been able to show the efficacy of FTY 720 in inhibiting murine corneal allograft rejection [60]. There are up to now no data of FTY 720 in clinical corneal transplantation.

3.4.9 FK788

The immunosuppressive drug FK778, a malononitrilamide, is a derivative of the active metabolite of leflunomide A77 1726. Its main mechanism of action is the inhibition of the dehydroorotate dehydrogenase. The resulting reduced capacity of the de novo pyrimidine synthesis leads to inhibition of T and B cell proliferation.

FTY 778/FK778 in Corneal Transplantation

Systemic immunosuppression with FK778 prolongs graft survival in the rat keratoplasty model. FK778's efficacy is comparable with that of MMF in preventing immunologic graft rejection [61].

There are no published data about the topical administration of FK778 in corneal transplantation.

3.5 Pimecrolimus

The ascomycin macrolactam derivative pimecrolimus (SDZ ASM 981) is a cell-selective inhibitor of inflammatory cytokines specifically developed for the treatment of inflammatory skin diseases, such as atopic dermatitis. Pimecrolimus is an immunophilin ligand, which binds specifically to the cytosolic receptor, immunophilin macrophilin-12. This pimecrolimus-macrophilin complex effectively inhibits the protein phosphatase calcineurin by preventing calcineurin from dephosphorylating the nuclear factor of activated T cells. This results in the blockage of signal transduction pathways in T cells and the inhibition of the synthesis of inflammatory cytokines [62].

3.5.1 Pimecrolimus in Corneal Transplantation

We have tested pimecrolimus in a murine model of corneal transplantation. Pimecrolimus did not prolong corneal allograft survival when applied topically [63].

3.5.2 Biologic Agents

Reports about the clinical use of biological agents in corneal transplantation are very rare. To complete this overview, their mode of action is outlined shortly. To prevent corneal allograft rejection in experimental settings, various strategies have been used:

- Anti-T-cell receptor and T cell depletion therapy [64, 65]
- Manipulation of costimulatory membrane-receptors by down-regulation of stimulatory molecules and/or upregulation of inhibitory molecules [66, 67]
- Overproduction of tumor necrosis factor-related, apoptosis-induced ligand [68]
- Interference with proinflammatory cytokines or chemoattractants (tumor necrosis factor alpha, IL-1, IL-12, CXCL9/Mig, and CXCL10/IP10) [69]
- Increasing graft-protective cytokines (nerve growth factor, IL-4, IL-10) [70]
- Macrophage depletion [71]

3.5.2.1 Basiliximab and Daclizumab

Basiliximab is the only biologic agent that has been tested in a clinical setting of corneal transplantation.

Basiliximab and daclizumab are humanized monoclonal antibodies that target the IL-2 receptor. Clinically, both agents are very similar, and both are used for induction therapy in solid organ transplantation.

These agents have a very low prevalence of adverse effects, although hypersensitivity reactions have been reported with basiliximab, albeit rarely.

Perioperative basiliximab has been tested in combination with CSA postoperatively, in a small clinical study with favorable results [72]. In 2008, a prospectively randomized clinical trial of basiliximab as monotherapy compared to cyclosporine was completed. These data suggest that basiliximab has a lower efficacy in preventing immune reactions after risk keratoplasty than CSA. However, the side effect profile of basiliximab is more favorable than that of CSA [73].

> **Summary for the Clinician**
>
> - Until today, the efficacy to prevent corneal graft rejection has only been proven for cyclosporine, MMF, and rapamycin in prospective clinical trials.
> - The efficacy and safety of tacrolimus in high-risk corneal transplantation has been described in a retrospective manner.
> - It is important to weigh the pros and cons of any immunosuppressive regimen, especially in high-risk corneal transplantation, as it is not a life-saving procedure.
> - With respect to the profile of side effects, we prefer MMF and cyclosporine over rapamycin, tacrolimus, and basiliximab.
> - Tacrolimus is the only immunosuppressive agent, which has been shown to efficiently prevent corneal allograft survival when applied topically in a clinical setting.

3.6 Guidelines for Practitioners

3.6.1 Systemic Immunosuppression with Drugs with Proven Efficacy in Corneal Transplantation

3.6.1.1 Preoperative Evaluation

As systemic immunosuppression might promote tumor growth or reactivation of a chronic infection, patients have to be checked by their internists to rule out neoplasms and infections (blood chemistry, abdominal ultrasound, chest X-ray) before immunosuppression is started. Additionally, due to possible drug-specific side effects of immunosuppressive agents, renal and hepatic functions have to be controlled. The patients should undergo these examinations at the time of entering the waiting list for transplantation. If any contraindications against systemic immunosuppression are found, these conditions have to be cleared before transplantation. If the conditions cannot be cleared, the indication for high-risk corneal transplantation has to be reconsidered. In this situation, the use of an optimally matched graft might be an interesting alternative to systemic immunosuppression. In the case of drug-specific contraindications, alternative drugs should be used (e.g., in the case of renal impairment, MMF should be used instead of CSA).

3.6.1.2 How to Use Cyclosporine in High-risk Corneal Transplantation

Additionally to perioperative topical and systemic steroids, CSA is started at the day of operation in a dosage of 100 mg twice daily. Within the first postoperative week, full blood levels of CSA have to be checked daily, and the dose adjusted to reach serum levels of 120–150 ng/ml. We adjust the dose by using increasing or decreasing steps of 25 mg. If serum levels appear to be stable, we reduce drug monitoring to once a week in the first few months, and afterwards once a month. Additionally, we check for liver and kidney functions. Depending on the risk situation, we continue the therapy for at least 6 or 12 months, and taper therapy by reducing CSA in 25 mg steps daily.

CSA is especially helpful in high-risk patients who suffer additionally from atopic dermatitis. CSA should only be used with great caution in patients with renal impairment, diabetes, and arterial hypertension.

3.6.1.3 How to Use MMF in High-risk Corneal Transplantation

The application of MMF following high-risk corneal transplantation is easier than the use of CSA. Additionally to perioperative topical and systemic steroids, MMF is started at the day of operation in a dosage of 1 g twice daily. Drug monitoring is not mandatory as it has broad safety margins. We perform blood chemistry once a month as MMF might be myelosuppressive and might lead to a rise in liver-enzymes. If side effects occur, we reduce MMF to 0.5 g twice daily. In the case of drug-specific side effects or graft rejection, drug monitoring is indicated to rule out inadequate dosing.

MMF is especially valuable in herpetic ocular disease when combined with Acyclovir due to its synergistic antiherpetic effect [74].

In cases of

- Arterial hypertension
- Diabetes
- Chronic renal disease
- Low compliance

MMF is preferred to CSA or tacrolimus because of its safety margins and the profile of possible side effects.

After at least 6 or 12 months following transplantation, MMF is tapered and discontinued within 1 week. In case of drug-specific side effects, we monitor blood levels.

3.6.2 Topical Immunosuppression

After steroids, FK506 is the only drug with proven clinical efficacy in preventing corneal allograft rejection when administered topically. However, topical FK506 is still not commercially available for ophthalmic use.

CSA has until now not proven its efficacy when applied topically. A multicenter trial with a subconjunctival implant (LUCIDA) will end in 2009.

3.7 Conclusion

CSA, which has long been the golden standard in organ and high-risk corneal transplantation, is now accompanied by MMF.

The first decade of the new millenium has been disappointing for transplant therapeutics: no new immunosuppressive agents have been approved for clinical use. Several high-profile drugs and biologics failed the rigors of clinical trials or had disappointing preclinical results (FTY720, FK778, anti-CDI54, anti-IL15, anti-CD28). Several challenges face the industry and clinical investigators in bringing novel drugs to the clinic, including the difficulty in targeting new endpoints for toxicities or chronic allograft disease since acute rejection has been reduced to below 15% in solid organ and high-risk corneal transplantation [75].

As this is the case for systemic immunosuppression, it is also true for topical immunosuppression. Until now, the only immunosuppressive agent, which has been approved for clinical use in ophthalmology is CSA 0.05% eye drops. But this formulation has no beneficial effect on corneal allograft survival.

Some ophthalmologists still neglect the importance of systemic immunosuppression to enhance graft survival in a high-risk setting by arguing that "it is not justified to risk potentially life-threatening complications that go with shutting down the immune system for a prolonged period."

This is a very important aspect. What is justified? Is it more justified to oppose a patient with renal deficiency and well-established therapy (dialysis) to a kidney transplant with a life-long immunosuppressive therapy than a patient with blindness to a timely limited immunosuppression?

Since we started routinely using systemic immunosuppression in our high-risk patients nearly 20 years ago, no patient ever died during the timely limited course of immunosuppression following corneal transplantation.

Today's systemic immunosuppression does not shut down the immune system, as it did 50 years ago. Even in solid organ transplantation with high-dose triple-drug immunosuppression, the risk of death from drug-related side effects is low.

We think it is very important that the transplant surgeon explains the pros and cons of any therapeutic regimen to the patient. He also has to outline the faith of a high-risk graft with or without systemic immunosuppression. It is the patient who has to judge whether he wants to have a high-risk transplant done with or without systemic immunosuppression. And it is for the surgeon to decide whether it is justified for the society to perform a high-risk transplantation without proper treatment, and thereby losing a precious corneal graft donated from a deceased member of the society.

It is extremely important to understand the necessity of systemic immunosuppression in high-risk keratoplasty with the armamentarium we have at hand today.

Nevertheless, innovations in topical immunomodulation might be a very useful strategy for supporting systemic therapy in high-risk keratoplasty, and it might lead to even better graft survival in normal-risk keratoplasty.

References

1. Streilein JW, Okamoto S, Sano Y, Taylor AW (2000) Neural control of ocular immune privilege. Ann NY Acad Sci 917:297–306
2. Birnbaum F, Reinhard T, Bohringer D, Sundmacher R (2005) Endothelial cell loss after autologous rotational keratoplasty. Graefes Arch Clin Exp Ophthalmol 243(1): 57–59
3. Reinhard T, Bohringer D, Enzmann J, Kogler G, Wernet P, Bohringer S, Sundmacher R (2004) HLA class I/II matching and chronic endothelial cell loss in penetrating normal risk keratoplasty. Acta Ophtahmol Scand 82(1):13–18
4. Lakkis FG, Arakelov A, Koniecny BT, Inoue Y (2000) Immunologic "ignorance" of vascularized organ transplants in the absence of secondary lymphoid tissue. Nat Med 6:686–688
5. Hill JC, Maske R (1988) An animal model for corneal graft rejection in high-risk keratoplasty. Transplantation 46(1):26–30
6. Hill JC (1995) Systemic cyclosporine in high-risk keratoplasty: long-term results. Eye 9(Pt 4):422–428
7. Reinhard T, Moller M, Sundmacher R (1999) Penetrating keratoplasty in patients with atopic dermatitis with and without systemic cylocsporin A. Cornea 18(6):645–651

8. Reinhard T, Sundmacher R (1992) Perforating keratoplasty in endogenous eczema. An indication for systemic cyclosporin A – a retrospective study of 18. Klin Monatsbl Augenheilkd 201(3):159–163
9. Reinhard T, Sundmacher R, Godehardt E, Heering P (1997) [Preventive systemic cyclosporin A after keratoplasty at increased risk for immune reactions as the only elevated risk factor] Systemische Cyclosporin-A-Prophylaxe nach Keratoplastiken mit erhohtem Risiko fur Immunreaktionen als einzigem erhohten Risikofaktor. Ophthalmologe 94(7):496–500
10. Hoffmann F, Wiederholt M (1986) Topical cyclosporin A in the treatment of corneal graft reaction [editorial]. Cornea 5(3):129
11. Perry HD, Donnenfeld ED, Acheampong A, Kanellopoulos AJ, Sforza PD, D'Aversa G, Wallerstein A, Stern M (1998) Topical cyclosporine A in the management of postkeratoplasty glaucoma and corticosteroid-induced ocular hypertension (CIOH) and the penetration of topical 0.5% cyclosporine A into the cornea and anterior chamber. CLAO J 24(3):159–165
12. Chen YF, Gebhardt BM, Reidy JJ, Kaufman HE (1990) Cyclosporine-containing collagen shields suppress corneal allograft rejection. Am J Ophthalmol 109(2):132–137
13. Gokce EH, Sandri G, Bonferoni MC, Rossi S, Ferrari F, Güneri T, Caramella C (2008) Cyclosporine A loaded SLNs:evaluation of cellular uptake and cornealcytotoxicity. Int J Pharm 364(1):76–86
14. Bourges JL, Lallemand F, Agla E, Besseghir K, Dumont JM, BenEzra D, Gurny R, Behar-Cohen F (2006) Evaluation of a topical cyclosporine A prodrug an corneal graft rejection in rats. Mol Vis 12:1461–1466
15. Reinhard T, Sundmacher R (1996) Local cyclosporin A therapy in thygeson superficial punctate keratitis–a pilot study. Klin Monatsbl Augenheilkd 209(4):224–227
16. Reinhard T, Sundmacher R (1999) Topical cyclosporin A in thygeson`s superficial punctate keratitis. Graefes Arch Clin Exp Ophthalmol 237(2):109–112
17. Bussutil RW, Holt CD (1997) Tacrolimus (FK506) is superior to cyclosporine in liver transplantation. Transplant Proc 29:534–538
18. Woodle ES, Thistlethwaite JR, Gordon JH (1996) A multicenter trial of FK506 (tacrolimus) therapy in refractory acute renal allograft rejection. A report of FK506 Kidney Transplant Rescue Study Group. Transplantation 62: 594–599
19. Kino T, Hatayama H, Hashimoto M et al (1987) FK-506, a novel immunosuppressant isolated from Streptomyces: 1: fermentation, isolation, and physio-chemical and biological characteristics. J Antibiot 40:1249–1255
20. Sawada S, Suzuki G, Kawase Y, Takaku F (1987) Novel immunosuppressive agent, FK-506: in vitro effects on the cloned T cell activation. J Immunol 40:1249–1255
21. Yoshimura N, Matsui S, Hamashima T, Oka T (1989) Effects of a new immunosuppressive agent, FK-506, on human lymphocyteresponsiveness in vitro: 1: inhibition of expression of alloantigen-activated suppressor cells, as well as induction of alloreactivity. Transplantation 47:351–356
22. Sloper CM, Powell RJ, Dua HS (2001) Tacrolimus (FK506) in the management of high-risk corneal and limbal grafts. Ophthalmology 10:1838–1844
23. Joseph A, Raj D, Shanmuganathan V, Powell RJ, Dua HS (2007) Tacrolimus immunosuppression in high-risk corneal grafts. Br J Ophthalmol 91(1):51–55
24. Reis A, Reinhard T, Sundmacher R, Godehard E, Braunstein C (1998) FK506 and mycophenolatemofetil: two novel immunosuppressants in murine corneal transplantation. Transplant Proc 30(8):4344–4347
25. Benelli U, Lepri A, Del-Tacca M, Nardi M (1996) FK-506 delays corneal graft rejection in a model of corneal xenotransplantation. J Ocul Pharmacol Ther 12(4):425–431
26. Reis A, Reinhard T, Sundmacher R, Godehard E, Braunstein C (1998) A comparative investigation of the effect of FK506 (Prograf*) and cyclosporin A (sandimmun*, CSA) in murine corneal transplantation. Graefes Arch Clin Exp Ophthalmol 236:785–789
27. Hikita N, Lopez JS, Chan C, Mochizuki M, Nussenblatt RB, de Smet MD (1997) Use of topical FK506 in a corneal graft rejection model in lewis rats. Invest Ophthalmol Vis Sci 38:901–909
28. Minamoto A, Sakata H, Okada K, Fujihara M (1995) Suppression of corneal graft rejection by subconjunctival injection of FK-506 in a rat model of penetrating keratoplasty. Jpn J Ophthalmol 39(1):12–19
29. Mills RA, Jones DB, Winkler CR, Wallace GW, Wilhelmus KR (1995) Topical FK-506 prevents experimental corneal allograft rejection. Cornea 14(2):157–160
30. Dickey JB, Cassidy EM, Bouchard CS (1993) Periocular FK-506 delays allograft rejection in rat penetrating keratoplasty. Cornea 12(3):204–207
31. Fei WL, Chen JQ, Yuan J, Quan DP, Zhou SY (2008) Preliminary study of the effect of FK506 nanospheric-suspension eye droops on rejection of penetrating keratoplasty. J Ocul Pharmacol Ther 24(2):235–244
32. Reinhard T, Mayweg S, Reis A, Sundmacher R (2005) Topical FK506 as immunoprophylaxis after allogeneic penetrating normal-risk keratoplasty: a randomized clinical pilot study. Transpl Int 18(2):193–197
33. Reis A, Mayweg S, Birnbaum F, Reinhard T (2008) Long-term results of FK 506 eye drops following corneal transplantation. Klin Monatsbl Augenheilkd 225(1):57–61
34. The Tricontinental Mycophenolate Mofetil Renal Transplantation Study Group (1996) A blinded, randomized clinical trial of mycophnolate mofetil for the prevention of acute rejection in cadaveric renal transplantation. Transplantation 61(7):1029–1037

35. Deierhoi M, Sollinger H, Diethelm A et al (1993) One-year follow-up results of a phase 1 trial of mycophenolate mofetil (RS-61443) in cadaveric renal transplantation. Transplant Proc 25:693f
36. European Mycophenolate Mofetil Cooperative Study Group (1995) Placebo controlled study of mycophenolate mofetil combined with cyclosporin and corticosteroids for the prevention of acute rejection. Lancet 345(8961): 1321–1325
37. Simmons WD, Rayhill SC, Sollinger HW (1997) Preliminary risk-benefit assessment of mycophonlate mofetil in transplant rejection. Drug Saf 17(2):75–92
38. Allison A, Hovi R, Watts A, Webster A (1977) The role of de novo purine synthesis in lymphocyte transformation. Ciba Found Symp 48:207
39. Morris R, Hoyt E, Murphy P (1990) Mycophenolic acid morpholinoethylester (RS-61443) is a new immunosuppressant that prevents and halts heart allograft rejection by selevtive inhibition of T- and B-cell purine synthesis. Transplant Proc 22:1659
40. Reis A, Reinhard T, Sundmacher R, Braunstein C, Godehardt E (1998) Effect of mycophenolate mofetil, cyclosporin A, and both in combination in a murine corneal graft rejection model. Br J Ophthalmol 82:700–703
41. Reis A, Reinhard T, Voiculescu A, Kutkuhn B, Godehardt E, Spelsberg H, Althaus C, Sundmacher R (1999) Mycophenolatemofetil versus cyclosporin A in high-risk keratoplasty patients: a prospectively randomized clinical trial. Br J Ophthalmol 83:1268–1271
42. Birnbaum F, Reis A, Böhringer D, Sokolowska Y, Mayer K, Voiculescu A, Oellerich M, Sundmacher R, Reinhard T (2006) An open prospective pilot study on the use of rapamycin after penetrating high-risk keratoplasty. Transplantation 81(5):767–772
43. Reinhard T, Mayweg S, Sokolovska Y, Seitz B, Mittelviefhaus H, Engelmann K, Voiculescu A, Godehardt E, Sundmacher R (2005) Systemic mycophenolate mofetil avoids immune reactions in penetrating high-risk keratoplasty: preliminary results of an ongoing prospectively randomized multicentre study. Transpl Int 18(6):703–708
44. Reis A, Reinhard T, Sundmacher R, Althaus C, Voiculescu A, Kutkuhn B (1998) Mycophenolatemofetil in ocular immunological disorders. A survey of the literature with 3 case reports, Mycophenolatmofetil (CellCept) bei okularen immunologischen Störungen. Literaturübersicht mit 3 Kasuistiken. Klin Monatsbl Augenheilkd 5:257–261
45. Morris RE, Huang X, Gregory CR, Billingham ME, Rowan R, Shorthouse R (1995) Berry-studies in experimental models of chronic rejection: use of rapamycin (sirolimus) and isoxazole derivatives (leflunomide and its analogue) for the suppression of graft vascular disease and obliterative bronchiolitis. Transplant Proc 27(3):2068–2069
46. Vu MD, Qi S, Xu D, Wu J, Peng J, Daloze P, Sehgal S, Leduc B, Chen H (1998) Synergistic effects of mycophenolate mofetil and sirolimus in prevention of acute heart, pancreas, and kidney allograft rejection and in reversal of ongoing heart allograft rejection in the rat. Transplantation 66(12): 1575–1580
47. Brattstrom C, Tyden G, Sawe J, Herlenius G, Claesson K, Groth CG (1996) A randomized, double-blind, placebo-controlled study to determine safety, tolerance, and preliminary pharmacokinetics of ascending single doses of orally administered sirolimus (rapamycin) in stable renal transplant recipients. Transplant Proc 28(2):985–986
48. Murgia MG, Jordan S, Kahan BD (1996) The side effect profile of sirolimus: a phase I study in quiescent cyclosporine-prednisone-treated renal transplant patients. Kidney Int 49(1):209–216
49. Olsen TW, Benegas NM, Joplin AC, Evangelista T, Mindrup EA, Holland EJ (1994) Rapamycin inhibits corneal allograft rejection and neovascularization. Arch Ophthalmol 112(11):1471–1475
50. Thompson P, Xu D, Brunette I, Chen H (1998) Combined effect of rapamycin and cyclosporine in the prevention of rat corneal allograft rejection. Transplant Proc 30(4): 1033–1035
51. Yuan XB, Yuan YB, Jiang W, Liu J, Tian EJ, Shun HM, Huang DH, Yuan XY, Li H, Sheng J (2008) Preparation of rapamycin-loaded chitosan/PLA nanoparticles for immunosuppression in corneal transplantation. Int J Pharm 349(1–2):241–248
52. Shi W, Gao H, Xie L, Wang S (2006) Sustained intraocular rapamycin delivery effectively prevents high-risk corneal allograft rejection and neovascularization in rabbits. Invest Ophthalmol Vis Sci 47(8):3339–3344
53. Crowe A, Lemaire M (1998) In vitro and in situ absorption of SDZ-RAD using a human intestinal cell line (Caco-2) and a single pass perfusion model in rats: comparison with rapamycin. Pharm Res 15(11):1666–1672
54. Schuurman HJ, Schuler W, Ringers J, Jonker M (1998) The macrolide SDZ RAD is efficacious in a nonhuman primate model of allotransplantation. Transplant Proc 30(5): 2198–2199
55. Eisen HJ, Tuzcu EM, Dorent R et al (2003) Everolimus for the prevention of allograft rejection and vasculopathy in cardiac-transplant recipients. N Eng J Med 349:847–858
56. Reis A, Megahed M, Reinhard T, Godehardt E, Spelsberg H, Braunstein C, Sundmacher R (2000) Coadministration of the new macrolide immunosuppressant RAD and mycophenolate mofetil in experimental corneal transplantation. Transplantation 70(9):1397–1401
57. Reis A, Megahed M, Reinhard T, Braunstein C, Godehardt E, Sundmacher R (2001) RAD, a new immunosuppressive macrolide in murine corneal transplantation. Graefes Arch Clin Exp Ophthalmol 239(9):689–692

58. Reis A, Megahed M, Reinhard T, Godehardt E, Braunstein C, Sundmacher R (2002) Synergism of RAD and cyclosporin A in prevention of acute rat corneal allograft rejection. Cornea 21(1):81–84
59. Baspinar Y, Bertelman E, Pleyer U, Buech G, Siebenbrodt I, Borchert HH (2008) Corneal permeation studies of everolimus microemulsion. J Ocul Pharmacol Ther 24(4): 399–402
60. Mayer K, Birnbaum F, Reinhard T, Reis A, Braunstein S, Claas F, Sundmacher R (2004) FTY720 prolongs clear corneal allograft survival with a differential effect on different lymphocyte populations. Br J Ophthalmol 88(7):915–919
61. Birnbaum F, Schwartzkopff J, Scholz C, Reis A, Reinhard T (2007) The new malononitrilamide immunosuppressant FK778 prolongs corneal allograft survival in the rat keratoplasty model. Eye 21(12):1516–1523
62. Gupta AK, Chow M (2003) Pimecroliums: a review. J Eur Acad Dermatol Venereol 17:493–503
63. Birnbaum F, Schwartzkopff J, Scholz C, Reinhard T (2007) Topical pimecrolimus does not prolong clear graft survival in a rat keratoplasty model. Graefes Arch Clin Exp Ophthalmol 245(11):1717–1721
64. Pleyer U, Milani JK, Dukes A, Chou J, Lutz S, Rückert D, Thiel HJ, Mondino BJ (1995) Effect of topically applied anti-CD4 monoclonal antibodies on orthotopic corneal allografts in a rat model. Invest Ophthalmol Vis Sci 36(1):52–61
65. Fu H, Larkin DF, George AJ (2008) Immune modulation in corneal transplantation. Transplant Rev 22(2):105–115
66. Comer RM, King WJ, Ardjomand N, Theoharis S, George AJT, Larkin DFP (2002) Effect of administration of CTLA4-Ig as Protein or cDNA on corneal allograft survival. Invest Ophthalmol Vis Sci 43(4):1095–1103
67. Watson MP, George AJ, Larkin DF (2006) Differential effects of costimulatory pathway modulation on corneal allograft survival. Invest Ophthalmol Vis Sci 47(8): 3417–3422
68. Xie L, Shi W, Guo P (2003) Roles of tumor necrosis factor-related apoptosis-inducing ligand in corneal transplantation. Transplantation 76(11):1556–1559
69. Amescua G, Collings F, Sidani A, Bonfield TL, Rodriguez JP, Galor A, Medina C, Yang X, Perez VL (2008) Effect of CXCL-1/KC production in high risk vascularized corneal allografts on T cell recruitment and graft rejection. Transplantation 85(4):615–625
70. Gong N, Pleyer U, Vogt K, Anegon I, Flügel A, Volk HD, Ritter T (2007) Local overexpression of nerve growth factor in rat corneal transplants improves allograft survival. Invest Ophthalmol Vis Sci 48(3):1043–1052
71. Slegers TP, van der Veen G, Hermans LJ, Broersma L, van Rooijen N, Völker-Dieben HJ, van Rij G, van der Gaag R (2003) Adhesion molecule expression in local-macrophage-depleted rats bearing orthotopic corneal allografts. Graefes Arch Clin Exp Ophthalmol 241(5):432–438
72. Schmitz K, Hitzer S, Behrens-Baumann W (2002) Immune suppression by combination therapy with basiliximab and cyclosporin in high risk keratoplasty. A pilot study. Ophthalmologe 99(1):38–45
73. Birnbaum F, Jehle T, Schwartzkopff J, Sokolovska Y, Böhringer D, Reis A, Reinhard T (2008) Basiliximab following penetrating risk-keratoplasty–a prospective randomized pilot study. Klin Monatsbl Augenheilkd 225(1):62–65
74. Mayer K, Reinhard T, Reis A, Voiculescu A, Sundmacher R (2003) Synergistic antiherpetic effect of acyclovir and mycophenolate mofetil following keratoplasty in patients with herpetic eye disease: first results of a randomised pilot study. Graefes Arch Clin Exp Ophthalmol 241(12): 1051–1054
75. Vincenti F, Kirk AD (2008) What's next in the pipeline. Am J Transplant 8(10):1972–1981

Chapter 4

Cytokine Analysis of the Aqueous Humor in the Context of Penetrating Keratoplasty

Philip Maier, Thomas Reinhard

Core Messages

- The immune privilege of the eye manifests with an anti-inflammatory and immunosuppressive microenvironment, with an extended survival of allogeneic allografts, and with the induction of tolerance to eye-derived antigens. In this context, TGF-β2 is the most important factor for the maintenance of the anterior chamber-associated immune deviation (ACAID).
- The determination of cytokines in the aqueous humor raises many pitfalls regarding puncture of the anterior chamber and handling of the samples prior to analysis.
- Corneal graft rejection leads not only to a change of the local cytokine profile in the anterior chamber but also to a systemic cytokine response.
- Until now, there have been very rare investigations on cytokine profiles in human aqueous humor showing heterogeneous results. Therefore, further studies are necessary to find out whether cytokine profiles in the aqueous humor might allow us in the future to predict the risk of endothelial immune reactions following penetrating keratoplasty (PK).
- From animal models, we know that Interleukin 1b is able to prevent the ACAID. Its role in human corneal transplantation remains unclear. Its natural antagonist, Interleukin 1 receptor antagonist, is able to antagonize the effects of IL-1a and IL-1b. Therefore, the balance between these two factors may be important for the development of immune reactions.
- The potent pro-inflammatory effects of Interleukin 2 known from in vitro experiments may be lower in vivo as Interleukin 2 levels do not seem to be increased in human aqueous humor during endothelial immune reactions following PK.
- Levels of pro-inflammatory Interleukin 6 seem to be increased in human aqueous humor during endothelial immune reactions following PK.

- IL-10 is able to limit and terminate inflammatory responses. However, it seems to be increased in human aqueous humor following PK in cases of accepted grafts, as well as in cases showing signs of graft rejection. This could be a result of an "activation of the ocular immune privilege" to avoid corneal tissue damage following PK.
- IFN-γ antagonizes many effects of TGF-β2. Furthermore, IFN-γ seems to be increased whereas TGF-β2 seems to be decreased in human aqueous humor during graft rejection. This further emphasizes their importance in the development and maintenance of endothelial immune reactions following PK.
- TNF-α seems to be increased in human aqueous humor during graft rejection following PK, reinforcing its function in initiating and maintaining immune responses.
- sFasL is up-regulated in some patients following PK, particularly in the scenario of corneal graft rejection. It seems to play a role in transplant immunology; the exact function, however, remains unclear.
- It is only from in vitro experiments and animal models of organ transplantation that we know that IL-4 as well as IL-5 may have graft protective effects. However, their importance in human corneal transplantation needs further investigation.
- IL-12 favors the differentiation of Th1 cells; however, its function regarding transplant immunology is not fully understood.
- Thrombospondin, somatostatin, a-MSH or CGRP are further important regulators regarding the immune privilege of the anterior ocular segment, but more investigations are needed regarding their importance in the context of corneal transplantation.

The remainder of the chapter will focus on the function of pro- and anti-inflammatory factors in the context of corneal transplantation. At first, we give a short overview on the immune privilege of the anterior ocular segment and discuss various pitfalls regarding the determination of cytokine levels in the aqueous humor. Following that, we describe general effects of various important cytokines known from in vitro experiments, and we discuss results from animal models of corneal transplantation. Finally, we present results regarding the relevance of cytokines in human corneas and human aqueous humor regarding penetrating keratoplasty (PK). One major goal of the determination of cytokines levels in the aqueous humor of patients prior to PK may be that a distinct cytokine pattern in the aqueous humor might allow us to predict the risk for immune reactions following PK.

4.1 Immune Privilege of the Anterior Ocular Segment

In the eye, a precise microanatomy and clear media are mandatory to maintain sufficient visual acuity; therefore, the ocular immune privilege allows for protection of the eye by avoiding tissue damage due to immunogenic inflammation. There are three different manifestations of the immune privilege with an anti-inflammatory and immunosuppressive microenvironment, with an extended survival of allogeneic allografts, and with the induction of tolerance to eye-derived antigens.

The whole concept is presented and discussed in chapter 1 by Jerry Niederkorn.

4.1.1 Anterior Chamber-Associated Immune Deviation (ACAID)

The anterior chamber-associated immune deviation (ACAID), which is one important part of the ocular immune privilege, is characterized by a typical, systemic immune response to antigens in the anterior chamber where the delayed-type hypersensitivity (Th1 response) is suppressed [1]. In normal aqueous humor, a specific pattern of cytokines, growth factors, and neuropeptides is found that contributes to the maintenance of the ocular immune privilege [2–5]. Transforming growth factor beta 2 (TGF-β2) has been identified as the most important factor in the aqueous humor for the maintenance of ACAID [2, 4], whereas interleukin 1(IL-1), interferon gamma (INF-γ), and tumor necrosis factor alpha (TNF-α) are able to destroy the ocular immune privilege and prevent ACAID induction when injected into the anterior chamber [6].

4.1.2 The Th1/Th2 Paradigm

The differentiation between the Th1 phenotype, which is strongly associated with cell-mediated immunity, and the Th2 phenotype, which is associated with humoral immunity, is called the Th1/Th2 paradigm. Th1/Th2 cell function is mainly regulated by individual cytokines where Th1 cytokines can inhibit Th2 responses and vice versa. Th1 responses represent cell-mediated immunity including activation of B cells, macrophages, NK-cells, cell-mediated cytotoxicity, and delayed-type hypersensitivity, leading to severe tissue damage. Th2 responses represent humoral immunity including B-cell activation, mast-cell activation, eosinophil cytotoxicity, IgE production, and IgG production, leading to less tissue damage (Fig. 4.1). Acute allograft rejection is supposed to be a Th1 cell-dependent process.

> **Summary for the Clinician**
> - The immune privilege of the eye manifests with an anti-inflammatory and immunosuppressive microenvironment, with an extended survival of allogeneic allografts, and with the induction of tolerance to eye-derived antigens.
> - Acute allograft rejection is supposed to be a Th1 cell-dependent process.
> - TGF-β2 is one of the most important factors for the maintenance of the ocular immune privilege.

4.2 Pitfalls in the Determination of Cytokine Levels from Aqueous Humor

Regarding the relevance of specific cytokines in the context of corneal transplantation, most conclusions are drawn from in vitro experiments or animal models where cytokine levels are determined in corneal tissue. However, it is rarely possible to conclude from such results on the human situation in aqueous humor. The determination of cytokine levels in the human aqueous humor, however, has even more pitfalls than cytokine determination in serum [7]. At first, only very small sample volumes of human aqueous humor can be drawn out of the anterior

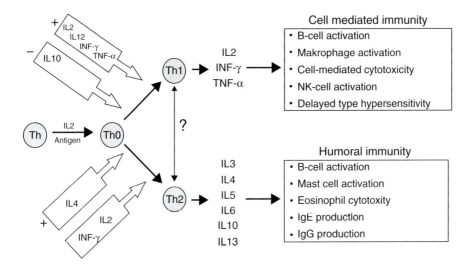

Fig. 4.1 The Th1/Th2 paradigm resulting in different cytokine production by T cells. Antigen stimulation may lead to the production of a wide range of cytokines in naive T cells. A variety of mechanisms and signals (including cytokines) start a more restricted T cell differentiation resulting in a cytokine production pattern by distinct cells, the Th1 and Th2 cells. This differentiation finally modifies the effector mechanisms of Th1 and Th2 cells further influencing the expression of each other through regulatory cytokines that they produce

chamber at the beginning of intraocular surgery. The problem of small sample volumes is one reason why it is very difficult to isolate inflammatory cells in the aqueous humor. In an attempt to find these cells in human aqueous humor, we found an increased amount of immune cells with increasing severity of endothelial immune reactions. Mainly macrophages and monocytes followed by lymphocytes were identified. However, we could not find any immune cells in the aqueous humor of patients with cataract, with a corneal graft without signs for immune reaction, and in patients with a corneal graft following complete resolution of an endothelial immune reaction [8]. Therefore, we concluded that cellular analysis of human aqueous humor might not be helpful in finding prognostic parameters regarding the occurrence of immune reactions following PK. Furthermore, during the puncture of the anterior chamber, contacts of the syringe with the iris or bleedings from limbal vessels may falsify the cytokine analysis and must, therefore, be avoided. Otherwise, the sample has to be discarded. Moreover, the kind of instruments and materials used for anterior chamber puncture or for storage of the samples is important, e.g., specific cytokine levels may be increased or decreased by the usage of either glass or plastic cups or syringes. The storage method may also influence cytokine levels. For example, partial activation of TGF-β2 takes place in vitro when samples are frozen and thawed. We found that TGF-β2 levels determined in fresh samples of aqueous humor are lower compared to the ones in samples that have been frozen and thawed [9]. Therefore, active TGF-β2 levels should always be determined from fresh samples to receive correct values. As the sample volumes are very small, it is possible to determine only one single cytokine in the aqueous humor by conventional ELISA techniques, limiting the possible predictive power of each sample. However, newly developed technologies, namely microparticle-based flow cytometric analysis [10], allow the simultaneous determination of various cytokines from only a few microliters of human aqueous humor. In this context, new 3D biochips based on microstructured surface-attached polymer networks may enhance the sensitivity compared to multiparametric immunoassays by a noncompetitive ELISA on-chip technology.

Summary for the Clinician

- Many different parameters such as the technique of puncture of the anterior chamber and the materials used for this procedure, as well as handling of the samples prior to the analysis, have to be considered for the determination of cytokines in human aqueous humor.

4.3 Relevance of Individual Cytokines in Corneal Transplantation

4.3.1 Interleukin 1b

4.3.1.1 General Functions from In Vitro Experiments

Interleukin 1b (IL-1b) is a pro-inflammatory cytokine that can activate dendritic cells (DCs) and macrophages [11]. In the cornea, IL-1 initiates the inflammatory cascade and the immunological response [12], and eventually induces corneal tissue damage. Although IL-1 is a key player in the inflammatory response in the cornea, it seems also to contribute to tissue repair processes [13].

4.3.1.2 Effects in Animal Models of Corneal Transplantation

Following IL-1b treatment, cells reveal an enhanced capacity to present antigens to T cells that secrete other pro-inflammatory cytokines such as INF-γ or TNF-α. The injection of IL-1b into the anterior chamber has been shown to prevent the ACAID in an animal model. This demonstrates the capacity of IL-1b to stimulate the activity of antigen-presenting cells (APC) and to activate T cells [6].**

4.3.1.3 Interleukin 1b Levels in Human Aqueous Humor

The results of investigations on Interleukin 1b levels in human aqueous humor are heterogeneous. One study showed an increase of IL-1b levels in human aqueous humor during endothelial immune reactions following PKP compared to control patients [14]. However, in a multiplex analysis of human aqueous humor, we found comparable IL-1b levels in patients prior to PK, in patients with an accepted graft, and in patients during an endothelial immune reaction (see Sect. 4.4)

> **Summary for the Clinician**
> - IL-1b has the capacity to stimulate the activity of APC and T cells, initiating an immunological response in the cornea. Its role in corneal transplantation is not fully understood.

4.3.2 Interleukin 2

4.3.2.1 General Functions from In Vitro Experiments

Interleukin 2 (IL-2) is a potent pro-inflammatory cytokine that is secreted following antigen-binding to T cells. It stimulates growth, differentiation, and survival of antigen-specific T cells [15]. Moreover, corneal endothelial cells were shown to inhibit T-cell proliferation by blocking IL-2 production in vitro [16].

4.3.2.2 Effects in Animal Models of Corneal Transplantation

In organ transplantation, IL-2 is thought to be a barrier towards tolerance, and thus one factor leading to immune reactions [17]. However, it has been shown that IL-2 is not necessary for allograft rejection, as IL-2 knockout mice revealed only modestly reduced survival times of islet cells [18].

4.3.2.3 Interleukin 2 Levels in Human Aqueous Humor

As IL-2 is believed to induce immune reactions [17], one would anticipate higher IL-2 levels during an endothelial immune reaction, and an anti IL-2 treatment to be effective. However, we did not find higher, but rather somewhat lower levels of the pro-inflammatory, Th1-related cytokine IL-2 in the aqueous humor of patients with endothelial immune reaction compared to controls. Furthermore, we found that antagonizing IL-2 by basiliximab in a pilot study was less effective in preventing endothelial immune reactions than the treatment with cyclosporin A [19]. Thus, the potential immune reaction-inducing effect of IL-2 may be strong in vitro, but somewhat less profound in vivo, following PK. However, IL-2 levels may also have been influenced by the time point of gaining aqueous humor for analysis in our studies, as increased IL-2 levels might be responsible for the induction and the beginning of immune reactions, but not for their maintenance when they are clinically visible.

> **Summary for the Clinician**
> - IL-2 is one of the most potent pro-inflammatory cytokines. Its immune response inducing effects found in vitro might be lower in vivo.

4.3.3 Interleukin 6

4.3.3.1 General Functions from In Vitro Experiments

Interleukin 6 (IL-6) is a multifunctional cytokine with pro- and anti-inflammatory activities [20]. It is produced by T cells, macrophages, fibroblasts, and endothelial cells [21].

4.3.3.2 Effects in Animal Models of Corneal Transplantatoin

King et al. found increased mRNA expression of IL-6 in corneas during allograft rejection in rats [22].

4.3.3.3 Interleukin 6 Levels in Human Aqueous Humor

Interleukin 6 (IL-6) levels have been reported to rise during corneal endothelial immune reactions [23, 24]. However, we did not find elevated levels of pro-inflammatory IL-6 in the aqueous humor during an endothelial immune reaction. This is in contrast to the findings by Funding et al. [23], who demonstrated, that increased levels of IL-6 during an endothelial immune reaction are a result of IL-6 production by the intraocular environment as a reaction to the rejection process, and not a result of plasma influx. The reason for this incongruency is most likely the lack of statistical power from multiple comparisons in our experiments (see Sect. 4.4). Although Funding et al. [14] did not correct their statistical analysis for multiple comparisons, their results would not be altered by so doing, due to the very low p-values. It seems unlikely that the use of different multiplex array kits by us and Funding et al. [14] is responsible for the different results, as the underlying testing technique was the same. However, we noted overall higher IL-6 levels in our control patients than Funding et al. did in their patients, which might partially explain the different statistical results.

Summary for the Clinician

- IL-6 levels have been reported to rise during corneal endothelial immune reaction.

4.3.4 Interleukin 10

4.3.4.1 General Functions from In Vitro Experiments

Interleukin 10 (IL-10) is a multifunctional cytokine with diverse effects on most hemopoietic cell types. The principal function of IL-10 appears to be the limitation and ultimate termination of inflammatory responses. It also plays a key role in the differentiation and function of T-regulatory cells, which may figure prominently in the control of immune responses and tolerance in vivo [25]. In addition to these anti-inflammatory effects, IL-10 can up-regulate CD-163 expression [26] in monocytes and macrophages that represent a significant portion of the immune cell population in rejected grafts [8, 27].

4.3.4.2 Effects in Animal Models of Corneal Transplantation

Although IL-10 is considered one of the most promising immunosuppressive cytokine candidates, exogenous IL-10 administration did not prolong corneal graft survival in a rat model of allotransplantation [28]. Animals that were injected subconjunctivally with IL-10 even showed a trend towards earlier rejection when compared to controls [28]. As it is known that cytokines can show paradoxical effects [29], further investigation is required in order to determine a role for IL-10 in corneal graft acceptance. It has been shown that the gene transfer of IL-10 can lead to prolonged graft survival in different animal transplantation models including corneal transplantation [30, 31]. Gong et al. [32] demonstrated that only systemic, but not topical application of IL-10 gene vectors, prolonged corneal graft survival in a rat keratoplasty model. They concluded that IL-10 modulates cytokine expression in the draining lymph nodes, leading to graft-protecting effects. However, the mechanism of IL-10 gene transfer, promoting increased corneal graft survival, is not yet fully understood. In contrary to the graft protecting effects, IL-10 is able to promote cytotoxic cell activity in vitro [33], and prolonged administration of IL-10 apparently has a detrimental effect on graft survival in mice [34].

4.3.4.3 Interleukin 10 Levels in Human Aqueous Humor

We found increased levels of IL-10 in the aqueous humor of patients with and without signs of immune reactions following PK. This seems to stand in contrast to the functions of IL-10, in that it has primarily immunosuppressive effects by inhibiting the production of pro-inflammatory cytokines such as IL-1, IL-2, or TNF-α. Increased IL-10 levels during an endothelial immune reaction might be a consequence of IL-10 production by the local environment in the anterior chamber, so as to restrict the inflammatory process by maintaining "some" immunological privilege in the presence of an acute inflammation.

> **Summary for the Clinician**
>
> - IL-10 is able to limit and terminate the inflammatory responses. However, its effects regarding corneal allograft rejection are still not fully understood.

4.3.5 Interferon Gamma (IFN-γ)

4.3.5.1 General Functions from In Vitro Experiments

IFN-γ is secreted by activated T cells and natural killer cells. It activates APC and promotes Th1 differentiation. By antagonizing many TGF-β2 effects, it can destroy the eye's immune privilege [6], and might therefore be responsible for the induction of immune reactions following PK.

4.3.5.2 Effects in Animal Models of Corneal Transplantation

Nicholls et al. found no INF-γ producing cells on corneal endothelium during immune reactions in animal experiments [35]. King et al. found an increased expression of INF-γ mRNA in rejected corneal allografts in a rat model of PK [22]

4.3.5.3 INF-γ Levels in Human Aqueous Humor

We found increased levels of INF-γ in the aqueous humor of patients with clinical signs of endothelial immune reactions following PK. As INF-γ is a strong pro-inflammatory cytokine, strengthening the Th-1 immune response, increased levels during the acute phase of an endothelial immune reaction do not seem surprising. This reinforces our findings that TGF-β2, the counterpart of INF-γ, is statistically significantly decreased during immune reactions following PK [36]. However, the source of increased INF-γ levels in the aqueous during endothelial immune reactions remains unclear.

> **Summary for the Clinician**
>
> - IFN-γ activates APC, promotes Th1 differentiation, and antagonizes many effects of TGF-β2. It seems to be increased in human aqueous humor during endothelial immune reactions following PK.

4.3.6 Tumor Necrosis Factor Alpha (TNF-α)

4.3.6.1 General Functions from In Vitro Experiments

Regarding inflammatory processes leading to graft rejection, TNF-α is supposed to be important for the initiation, maintenance, and resolution? of inflammation. Upon stimulation by infectious agents, IL-1, INF-γ, or endotoxins TNF-α may be produced by macrophages, T and B cells, as well as by keratinocytes. The effects of TNF-α are analogous to T-cell-derived cytokines in the Th1 subset, and may lead to the activation of T cells, macrophages and neutrophils, MHC expression, as well as IL-1 and IL-6 production.

4.3.6.2 Effects in Animal Models of Corneal Transplantation

Up-regulation of TNF-α has been demonstrated in several allograft rejection models. Rayner et al. demonstrated that bioactive TNF can be found in aqueous humor following rabbit corneal allotransplantation. However, TNF levels did not correlate directly with endothelial rejection onset, but showed pulsatile peak levels that preceded and followed the observed onset of endothelial rejection. Blockade of TNF activity was able to prolong corneal allograft survival in some animals [37, 38]. In a mouse model of corneal transplantation, Zhu et al. showed that TNF-α expression generally decreases during the first postoperative week, and remains significantly elevated in allogeneic but not in syngeneic grafts, implicating TNF-α as a mediator of the alloimmune response in corneal transplantation.

4.3.6.3 TNF-α Levels in Human Aqueous Humor

Funding et al. showed increased TNF-α levels in human aqueous humor during endothelial immune reactions following PKP, compared to control patients in a multiplex analysis of human aqueous [14]. However, we found comparable TNF-α levels in the aqueous humor of patients prior to PK, of patients with an accepted graft, and of patients during an endothelial immune reaction. This difference might be because of a lack of statistical power due to multiple comparisons in our study. This is discussed in Sect. 4.4.

> **Summary for the Clinician**
>
> ■ TNF-α triggers the release of pro-inflammatory cytokines such as IL1, IL-6, IL-8, and INF-γ. Therefore, it might be responsible for the induction and maintenance of immune reactions.

4.3.7 Transforming Growth Factor Beta (TGF-β)

4.3.7.1 General Functions from In Vitro Experiment

Transforming growth factor-β2 (TGF-β2) is an approximately 25 kDa polypeptide encoded by a unique gene located on chromosome 1q41 [39]. This dimeric peptide is ubiquitously distributed in human tissues and synthesized by many different human cells. In the eye, it has been detected in tear fluid, in the vitreous, and in aqueous humor [2, 40, 41]. It is secreted as an inactive precursor (latent TGF-β2 complex, L-TGF-β2) by cell types such as corneal endothelial cells, cells of the trabecular meshwork, and the ciliary body [16, 42–48]. This precursor (200 kDa) is complexed with latency-associated peptide (LAP) and bound to latent TGF-β binding protein (LTBP). L-TGF-β2 is not able to bind to its receptor until LAP and LTBP are removed extracellularly via proteolytic cleavage. The exact mechanisms by which latent TGF-β2 is physiologically activated are not completely understood. One model of activation has been proposed in which latent TGF-β is released from the extracellular matrix (ECM) by proteases localized to cell surfaces, and activated, for example, by thrombospondin-1 [49] or specific integrins [50]. Following activation, TGF-β2 exerts its biological functions via binding to a membrane-bound heteromeric receptor (see Fig. 4.2) [42]. In addition to TGF-β2, two further isoforms of TGF-β have been identified in mammals, TGF-β1, and TGF-β3, which play an only minor role in immunomodulation of the anterior ocular segment

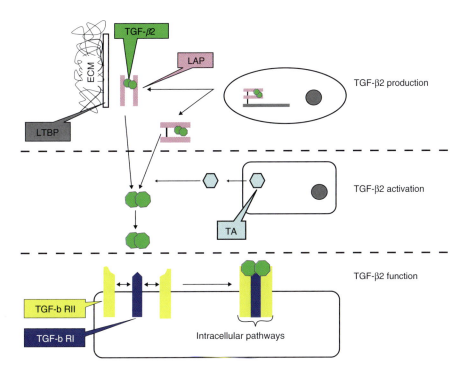

Fig. 4.2 TGF-β2 activation. TGF-β2 is produced as an inactive precursor consisting of a heterodimer with latency-associated protein (LAP). This latent TGF-β2 heterodimer can additionally build a complex with latent TGF-β2-binding protein (LTBP) resulting in a deposition to the extracellular matrix (ECM). TGF-β2 is activated by a TGF-β2 activator (TA) that induces LAP degradation or changes latent TGF-β2's conformation. Following activation TGF-β2 binds to a complex consisting of TGF-β receptor II (TGF-βRII) and TGF-β receptor I (TGF-β2RI) leading to the initiation of intracellular signaling pathways depending on the kinase activity of the receptors

[51]. TGF-β2 is known to play an important role in wound healing and the production of the ECM. It inhibits cell proliferation, and exerts various immunosuppressive effects.

4.3.7.2 Effects in Animal Models of Corneal Transplantation

In the anterior chamber, TGF-β2 is relevant for the maintenance of an immunosuppressive climate, as it alters the activities of APC, and suppresses T-cell proliferation, IFN-γ production, and the inflammatory activity of macrophages [2, 3, 52]. Antisera to TGF-β2 have been demonstrated to reverse the inhibitory activity of aqueous humor [2]. King et al. [22] found, in a rat model of keratoplasty, total TGF-β2 levels to be increased in eyes that had immune reactions. In their study, however, only TGF-β2 levels of the graft, but not of the aqueous humor, were determined. Moreover, animal experiments in endotoxin-induced uveitis revealed a regulation of active but not of total TGF-β2 levels in the aqueous humor [53, 54].

4.3.7.3 TGF-β2 Levels in Human Aqueous Humor

We found that total TGF-β2 could be detected in cataract patients, in patients following PK, with or without signs of endothelial immune reactions, irrespective of the underlying condition. However, there was no difference in total TGF-β2 levels between the different groups [55]. In patients, with newly diagnosed endothelial immune reactions following PK, lower TGF-β2 levels might have been expected if graft rejection was caused by a failure of the immunological privilege. In case of a longstanding immune reaction, on the other hand, an up-regulation of total TGF-β2 would have been conceivable, to restrain immunological graft destruction. The high steady-state levels of total TGF-β2 in the aqueous humor are compatible with its proposed role in the maintenance of the immunological privilege [56]. However, the anterior chamber appears to be unable to regulate total TGF-β2 levels to react to immunological challenges, as it was found in an animal model of endotoxin-induced uveitis [53, 54]. Therefore, we determined active TGF-β2 in fresh samples of aqueous humor to avoid activation of TGF-β2 by freezing and thawing [9]. We found that active TGF-β2 levels were decreased in the aqueous humor of patients following PK, newly diagnosed as having endothelial immune reactions [57]. As an endothelial immune reaction is usually accompanied by mild anterior uveitis, reduced levels of active TGF-β2 might be explained by dilution due to influx into the anterior chamber as part of the breakdown of the blood-aqueous barrier. If this was the case, total protein levels and total TGF-β2 levels were supposed to be decreased as well. However, we could show that total TGF-β2 levels [55] as well as total protein levels (unpublished data) are comparable in the aqueous humor of patients with and without immune reactions. In corneal transplantation, immune reactions mostly occur within the first 24 months following PK [58, 59]. Afterwards, endothelial immune reactions are rarely observed. Therefore, during this time, an immunosuppressive environment in the anterior chamber, maintained by high levels of active TGF-β2, seems to be exceptionally important. One could speculate that levels of active TGF-β2 decrease with time following PK, as the host might develop some kind of graft-induced tolerance to the donor tissue. If this assumption was correct, higher levels of active TGF-β2 prior to PK would lead to better clear graft survival. This is furthermore supported by the fact that we found highest levels of active TGF-β2 in keratoconus patients, who have the best prognosis following PK [36]. These findings might be interpreted as a hint towards a primarily altered immunological privilege in eyes that develop immune reactions following PK. The question thus arises whether only eyes with decreased TGF-β2 levels develop endothelial immune reactions following PK. If that was the case, active TGF-β2 might serve as a predictive parameter if determined prior to PK. Then, decreased TGF-β2 levels should force the surgeon to use HLA matched grafts, or to administer effective (topical and/or systemic) immunomodulative measures in the long run.

Summary for the Clinician

- TGF-β2 is the most important factor for the immunosuppressive climate in the anterior chamber, where it alters the activities of APC, and suppresses T-cell proliferation, IFN-γ production, and the inflammatory activity of macrophages. It exerts its effects only in its activated form. Active, but not total TGF-β2 levels are decreased in human aqueous humor during endothelial immune reactions following PK.

4.3.8 Fas, Fas Ligand and Soluble Fas Ligand

4.3.8.1 General Functions from In Vitro Experiments

Fas and its ligand (FasL) are transmembrane proteins that are responsible for peripheral lymphocyte homeostasis during immune responses [60]. Interaction between

Fas+ cells and FasL+ cells leads to apoptosis of Fas+ cells [60, 61]. Abundant amounts of FasL are found in the retina, the uvea, and the cornea of mice and humans [61]. Fas is expressed on the surface of several types of immunocompetent and nonimmunocompetent cells, while FasL is the natural ligand for Fas. Fas+ T cells can, for instance, undergo apoptosis when they bind to a cell expressing FasL. A soluble form of Fas ligand (sFasL) is released by the shedding of membrane-bound FasL. Soluble FasL has been demonstrated to be released by activated lymphocytes [61, 62], and it is most probably incapable of inducing apoptosis [63]. On the contrary, it may even interfere with induction of apoptosis by membrane-bound FasL [63]. In the cornea, FasL is constitutively expressed in the epithelium and endothelium. Apoptotic cell death of T lymphocytes entering the anterior chamber (and reacting with corneal endothelial FasL) is thought to result in the release of IL-10, which may play a role in the ACAID phenomenon [64]. It also confers protection to the cornea against inflammatory cells entering through the conjunctiva, limbal vessels, or via the anterior chamber. Whether T cells invading the corneal stroma also undergo apoptosis is not clear, since this layer of corneal cells has not been shown to express FasL. Taken together, corneal FasL is thought to play a role in immune privilege induction and in corneal allograft acceptance [65].

controls. The discrepancy between the study by Sugita et al. and ours may have been caused by the circumstances of anterior chamber puncture, or by the assay used for sFasL determination. In patients, with endothelial immune reactions, sFasL concentrations were higher than in those without immune reactions. It thus seems that the concentration of sFasL is up-regulated in some patients following PK, particularly in the scenario of corneal graft rejection. As sFasL blocks Fas without inducing apoptosis, Fas mediated apoptosis of T cells is inhibited. Therefore, overexpression of sFasL in patients with immune reactions following PK might not suppress but even reinforce inflammatory processes. While it is tempting to believe that sFasL may play a role in the immunological privilege and its failure, just what this role might be remains a matter of speculation.

> **Summary for the Clinician**
>
> ■ FasL is thought to play a role in immune privilege induction and in corneal allograft acceptance. sFasL concentrations in human aqueous humor were higher during endothelial immune reactions. However, its function in this context is not fully understood.

4.3.8.2 Effects in Animal Models of Corneal Transplantation

In the cornea, FasL, expressed on endothelial and epithelial cells, was demonstrated to be capable of killing Fas+ lymphoid cells. In a mouse keratoplasty model, FasL+ orthografts were accepted at a rate of 45%, whereas FasL- grafts were all rejected [65].

4.3.8.3 sFasL Levels in Human Aqueous Humor

The corneal endothelium has been suggested to be capable of releasing sFasL [66]. We determined soluble Fas ligand in the aqueous humor of patients undergoing sole cataract extraction (control group), of patients following PK, who did not have immune reactions, and of patients following PK, who were newly diagnosed as having endothelial immune reactions. None of the patients with cataract, 35% of patients without immune reaction, and 67% of patients with endothelial immune reaction had detectable sFasL concentrations. In contrast to our findings, Sugita et al. [66] reported detectable concentrations of sFasL in 11 out of 20 healthy

4.3.9 Further Cytokines and Immunomodulative Factors

The functions and effects of the following immunmodulative factors were primarily analyzed in vitro and in animal models. Only a few studies addressed the analysis of those factors in human aqueous humor, regarding PK by multiplex analysis, so this aspect is discussed in Sect. 4.4.

4.3.9.1 Interleukin 1 Receptor Antagonist

Interleukin-1 receptor antagonist (IL-1RA) competes with IL-1a, as well as IL-1b for the binding sites to IL-1 receptors, and therefore, it is a natural antagonist of IL-1. As corneal epithelial cells produce IL-1RA, the effects mediated by IL-1 are weakened [67]. Therefore, in case of immunological stress, the balance between IL-1 and IL-1RA in the cornea is responsible for the kind of either proinflammatory or immunosuppressive responses [21]. In an animal model of corneal transplantation, IL-1Ra had significantly positive effects in promoting corneal allograft survival [68].

4.3.9.2 Interleukin 4

Interleukin 4 (IL-4) is an anti-inflammatory cytokine secreted by activated T cells, and has various effects, such as the stimulation of activated B- and T-cell proliferation, and the differentiation of CD4+ T cells into Th2-cells. On one hand, this may exert a graft protecting effect, and on the other hand, it may exert an immune reaction-promoting effect in organ transplantation [17]. Furthermore, IL-4 is able to block the induction of corneal angiogenesis, induced by basic fibroblast growth factor [69]. In vivo administration of IL-4 has been successfully used in experimental models of solid organ transplantation to prolong graft survival [70]. However, in a gene therapy approach, it could be shown that overexpression of IL-4 is not sufficient to reduce the rejection rate of corneal allografts in a rat keratoplasty model [71].

4.3.9.3 Interleukin 5

Interleukin 5 is produced by Th2- and mast cells. Its functions are to stimulate B-cell growth and to increase immunoglobulin secretion. It is also a key mediator in eosinophil activation. In an animal model of heart transplantation, it could be shown that IL-5 might prolong allograft survival by down-regulating IL-2 and INF-γ production [72].

4.3.9.4 Interleukin 8

Interleukin-8 (IL-8) is a chemoattractant cytokine produced by a variety of tissue and blood cells. It attracts and activates neutrophils in inflammatory regions, but it has only weak effects on all other immunological cells. Though IL-8 plays a role in the cytokine network, its major pathophysiological role lies in affecting neutrophils [73]. It is unknown whether IL-8 influences the immunological privilege of the anterior ocular segment.

4.3.9.5 Interleukin 12

DCs and phagocytes produce Interleukin 12 (IL-12) in response to pathogens [74]. IL-12 is a pro-inflammatory cytokine that induces the production of IFN-γ, and favors the differentiation of Th1 cells. In rejected corneal allografts of rats, mRNA production of IL-12 was significantly increased [22]. However, in a rat keratoplasty model, anti IL-12 gene therapy could not prolong allograft survival [75].

4.3.9.6 Alpha-Melanocyte-Stimulating Hormone/Calcitonin Gene-Realted Peptide/Thrombospondin/Somatostatin

Furthermore, various other factors are involved in the regulation of the immunological privilege of the anterior chamber beyond the cytokines mentioned above. They might also play important roles in the occurrence and maintenance of endothelial immune reactions. Alpha-melanocyte stimulating hormone (α-MSH) and calcitonin gene-related peptide (CGRP) are able to downregulate innate immunity [76, 77]. These two factors suppress activated macrophages and DCs, and, therefore, also suppress activation of APC, which promote the delayed-type hypersensitivity (DTH)-mediating T cells [78, 79]. Thrombospondin is a potent physiologic regulator of TGF-beta activation [80], and somatostatin [79] has been identified as an important regulator of the ACAID. Thus, all these factors must be taken into consideration for further cytokine analyses of aqueous humor.

> **Summary for the Clinician**
> - Interleukin 1 receptor antagonist is able to antagonize the effects of IL-1a and IL-1b. Therefore, the balance between IL1 and IL1 receptor antagonist may be responsible for the severity of immune reactions.
> - IL-4 may have graft protective effects following PK.
> - IL-5 might prolong allograft survival by down-regulating IL-2 and INF-γ.
> - The role of IL-8 in the context of the ocular immune privilege is unknown.
> - IL-12 favors the differentiation of Th1 cells. However, anti IL-12 gene therapy did not prolong allograft survival in animal models of corneal transplantation.
> - a-MSH and CGRP suppress activation of APC, thrombospondin is a regulator of TGF-b2, and somatostatin is important for the maintenance of the ACAID. However, their functions regarding corneal transplantation are still unclear.

The general characteristics of important cytokines influencing immunological processes in the cornea are described in Table 4.1

Table 4.1 Important cytokines involved in immunological processes of the anterior ocular segment in the context of corneal transplantation (adapted from Torres and Kijlstra (21)). *APC* antigen presenting cells; *MHC* major histocompatibility complex; *AH* aqueous humor; *ACAID* anterior chamber-associated immune deviation; *IR* immune reaction; *PK* penetrating keratoplasty

Cytokine	Source	Stimulant	Target	Main functions		Human PK
				In vitro	Animal models PK	
IL-1b	Macrophages, APC, corneal cells, keratinocytes	Exogenous agents, INF-γ, TNF-α, IL-2, IL-3, IL-1	T cells, B cells, epithelial cells, fibroblasts	Production of IL-2, IL2R, IL-6, IL-8, TNFa, type IV collagen, collagenases	Prevention of ACAID	Results heterogeneous. Might be increased in AH during IR
IL1-RA	Macrophages, corneal cells	IL-1	Cells that produce IL-1	Inhibition of IL-1 functions by competitively binding to the IL-1R	Positive effects on corneal allograft survival. Seems to be increased in cornea during IR	Unknown
IL-2	Th1 cells	IL-1	T cells, B cells, NK cells	Growth factor for T, B, NK cells, production: IL-1, phagocytosis	Not necessary for IR. Seems to be increased in cornea during IR	Results heterogeneous. Might be increased or decreased in AH during IR
IL-3	T cells, NK cells, keratinocytes	Antigen, IgE, parasitic infection	Mast cells, eosinophils, macrophages, basophils, neutrophils	Colony stimulating factor for hematopoietic cells	Unknown	Unknown
IL-4	Th2 cells, mast cells	Antigen	Macrophages, B cells, fibroblasts	Growth factor for T and B cells, antibody 'switching', expression MHC II	Reduction of corneal angiogenesis. Low effect on extended graft survival. Seems to be increased in cornea during IR	Results heterogeneous. Might be increased in AH during IR
IL-5	T cells	Antigen	Eosinophil	Colony stimulating factor for eosinophils	Unknown	Results heterogeneous. Might be increased in AH during IR
IL-6	T cells, macrophages, fibroblasts, corneal cells, vascular endothelium	Endotoxin, IL-1, TNF-α	B cells, hepatocyte	B cell growth factor, antibody production, acute phase proteins	Increased in the cornea during IR	Seems to be increased in AH during IR

(continued)

Table 4.1 (continued)

Cytokine	Source	Stimulant	Target	Main functions — In vitro	Animal models PK	Human PK
IL-8	Macrophages, T cells, corneal cells, fibroblasts, neutrophils, endothelium	IL-1, TNF-α, basophils	Neutrophils, T cells, vascular endothelium	Chemotaxis of T cells, neutrophils, angiogenesis	Unknown	Unknown
IL-10	Th2 cells, macrophages, B cells, keratinocytes	Stressed tissue, antigen	T cells, macrophages	Inhibition of APC by down-regulating MHC II, promoting Th2; inhibiting Th1 cytokine synthesis	Heterogeneous results for IL-10 treatment to prolong allograft survival	Seems to be increased in AH following PK with and without IR
IL-12	Macrophages, APC	Stressed tissue, antigen	T cells	Regulator of Th1 cells	Increased in rejected corneal allografts. Anti IL-12 gene therapy did not improve grafts survival	Results heterogeneous. Might be increased in AH during IR
IL-13	T cells, B cells, mast cells	Antigen	B cells, macrophages	Growth factor for B cells and monocytes	Seems to be increased in cornea during IR	Might be increased in AH during IR
TNF-α	Macrophages, T cells, B cells, keratinocytes	Endotoxin, infectious agents, IL-1	Leukocytes, fibroblasts, vascular endothelium	Activation of T cells, macrophages and neutrophils, MHC expression, IL-1 and IL-6 synthesis, angiogenesis	Up-regulated during allograft rejection	Results heterogeneous. Might be increased in AH during IR
IFN-γ	Th1 cells, macrophages, NK cells	Antigen, IL-12, IL-18	T cells, macrophages	Increased expression of MHC, promoting Th1; inhibiting Th2, macrophage activation	No production in corneal endothelium	Seems to be increased in AH during IR
TGF-β	Virtually all cells	Wounding, inflammation	Immune cells, epithelium, fibroblasts	Induction of pro-inflammatory cytokines, up-regulation of adhesion molecules, ACAID	Maintenance of ACAID. Total levels increased in cornea during IR	Active but not total levels seem to be decreased in AH during IR. Increased in keratoconus patients prior to PK
FAS/FASL	Corneal endothelial and epithelial cells	Antigen in anterior chamber?	T cells	Peripheral lymphocyte homeostasis, apoptosis of Fas+ cells	FasL+ orthografts had decreased rejection rates	More sFasL in AH of patients during IR

4.4 Cytokine Profiles in the Context of Corneal Transplantation

Besides the function of individual cytokines, the interaction within the complex cytokine network in the aqueous humor plays an important role in corneal transplantation by influencing the immunosuppressive climate and the inflammatory response towards acceptance or rejection of corneal allografts.

4.4.1 Cytokine Profiles in Animal Models

In a rat model of allotransplantation, it has been shown that corneal graft rejection is associated with the expression of the Th-1 cytokines IL-2 and INF-γ. The sole surgical trauma induced by PK leads to the expression of IL-1, IL-6, IL-10, as well as the chemokines MCP-1 and MIP-2 [81]. The important effect of IL-1 on corneal allograft rejection has been explained by its effect on Langerhans cell migration in a mouse model [82]. King et al. reported an early cytokine and chemokine response in corneal tissue to the transplantation process in animal experiments (evident in syngeneic and allogeneic grafts) that probably drives angiogenesis, leukocyte recruitment, and affects leukocyte functions. In syngeneic recipients, cytokine levels reduced to pretransplant levels within 2 weeks following corneal grafting. Once an immune response had been generated, allogeneic rejection resulted in the expression of Th-1 cytokines (IL-2, IL-12 p40, IFN-γ), Th2 cytokines (IL-4, IL-6, IL-10, and IL-13), and anti-inflammatory Th3 cytokines (TGF-beta1/2 and IL-1RA) [22].

4.4.2 Cytokine Profiles in Humans

4.4.2.1 Cytokines in the Serum of Patients Following PK

Corneal graft rejection does not only lead to a change of the local cytokine profile in the anterior chamber but also to a systemic cytokine response, as it has been observed that in the serum of patients with a corneal immune reaction, levels of IL-2 receptor [83] and TNF-α [84] are increased.

4.4.2.2 Cytokines in Human Corneas

In human corneal explants from recipients following PK showing inflammatory signs, levels of IL-1 and IL-6 were increased compared to noninflamed corneas from patients with scars, corneal dystrophies, or keratoconus [85].

4.4.2.3 Cytokines in Human Aqueous Humor

When Funding et al. [14] determined 17 different cytokines (IL-1b, IL-2, IL-4, IL-5, IL-6, IL-7, IL-10, IL-12p70, IL-13, IL-17, TNF-α, INF-γ), growth factors (granulocyte-monocyte colony stimulating factor (GM-CSF) and granulocyte colony stimulating factor (G-CSF)) and chemokines (CXCL-8, monocyte chemoattractant protein-1, and macrophage inflammatory protein-1beta) in the aqueous humor of patients with endothelial immune reactions, they found that all these factors were statistically significantly increased compared to patients with cataract or Fuchs' endothelial dystrophy. This contrasts in part with our results of a multiplex bead array analysis of human aqueous humor, as we found only statistically significant differences for IL-10 and INF-γ, but not for IL-1b, IL-2, IL-4, IL-5, IL-8, IL-12, and TNF-α between patients with and without immune reactions and control patients. Concurring with our results, Funding et al. [14] found IL-6 levels to be a thousand times higher in patients with endothelial immune reaction than in control patients. However, we did not observe such statistically significant difference because we noted higher IL-6 levels in our control patients than Funding et al. did in their patients [14]. Another possible reason for the overall differences between our results and the results from Funding et al. might probably be a lack of statistical power from multiple comparisons in our experiments. Although Funding et al. [14] did not correct their statistical analysis for multiple comparisons, their results would not be altered by so doing, due to the very low p-values. It seems unlikely that the use of different multiplex array kits by us and Funding et al. [14] is responsible for the different results, as the underlying analyzing technique was the same. However, another explanation for different cytokines levels might be the way the samples were gained. Funding et al. describe that punctures of the anterior chamber have been performed by different surgeons. In this context, it is not clear whether bleeding occurred or whether the syringe had contact to the iris during the puncture. This could falsify the following cytokine analysis.

> **Summary for the Clinician**
>
> - Corneal graft rejection does not only lead to a change of the local cytokine profile in the anterior chamber but also to a systemic cytokine response.
> - Until now, there are very rare investigations on cytokine profiles in human aqueous humor in the context of PK showing heterogeneous results. Therefore, further studies are necessary to find out whether cytokine profiles in the aqueous humor might allow us to predict the risk of developing endothelial immune reactions following PK.

References

1. Streilein JW. Tissue barriers, immunosuppressive microenvironments, and privileged sites: the eye's point of view. Reg Immunol. 1993;5:253–268.
2. Cousins SW, McCabe MM, Danielpour D, Streilein JW. Identification of transforming growth factor-beta as an immunosuppressive factor in aqueous humor. Invest Ophthalmol Vis Sci. 1991;32:2201–2211.
3. Granstein RD, Staszewski R, Knisely TL, Zeira E, Nazareno R, Latina M, et al. Aqueous humor contains transforming growth factor-beta and a small (less than 3500 daltons) inhibitor of thymocyte proliferation. J Immunol. 1990;144:3021–3027.
4. Jampel HD, Roche N, Stark WJ, Roberts AB. Transforming growth factor-beta in human aqueous humor. Curr Eye Res. 1990;9:963–969.
5. Wahlestedt C, Beding B, Ekman R, Oksala O, Stjernschantz J, Hakanson R. Calcitonin gene-related peptide in the eye: release by sensory nerve stimulation and effects associated with neurogenic inflammation. Regul Pept. 1986;16:107–115.
6. Okamoto S, Streilein JW. Role of inflammatory cytokines in induction of anterior chamber-associated immune deviation. Ocul Immunol Inflamm. 1998;6:1–11.
7. Thavasu PW, Longhurst S, Joel SP, Slevin ML, Balkwill FR. Measuring cytokine levels in blood. Importance of anticoagulants, processing, and storage conditions. J Immunol Methods. 1992;153:115–124.
8. Reinhard T, Bocking A, Pomjanski N, Sundmacher R. Immune cells in the anterior chamber of patients with immune reactions after penetrating keratoplasty. Cornea. 2002;21:56–61.
9. Maier P, Broszinski A, Heizmann U, Boehringer D, Reinhard T. Determination of active TGF-beta 2 in aqueous humor prior to and following cryopreservation. Mol Vis. 2006;12:1477–1482.
10. Carson RT, Vignali DA. Simultaneous quantitation of 15 cytokines using a multiplexed flow cytometric assay. J Immunol Methods. 1999;227:41–52.
11. Virgin HW IV, Wittenberg GF, Bancroft GJ, Unanue ER. Suppression of immune response to *Listeria monocytogenes*: mechanism(s) of immune complex suppression. Infect Immun. 1985;50:343–353.
12. Dinarello CA. Biology of interleukin 1. FASEB J. 1988;2:108–115.
13. Boisjoly HM, Laplante C, Bernatchez SF, Salesse C, Giasson M, Joly MC. Effects of EGF, IL-1 and their combination on in vitro corneal epithelial wound closure and cell chemotaxis. Exp Eye Res. 1993;57:293–300.
14. Funding M, Hansen TK, Gjedsted J, Ehlers N. Simultaneous quantification of 17 immune mediators in aqueous humour from patients with corneal rejection. Acta Ophthalmol Scand. 2006;84:759–765.
15. Stern JB, Smith KA. Interleukin-2 induction of T-cell G1 progression and c-myb expression. Science. 1986;233:203–206.
16. Kawashima H, Prasad SA, Gregerson DS. Corneal endothelial cells inhibit T cell proliferation by blocking IL-2 production. J Immunol. 1994;153:1982–1989.
17. Strom TB, Roy-Chaudhury P, Manfro R, Zheng XX, Nickerson PW, Wood K, et al. The Th1/Th2 paradigm and the allograft response. Curr Opin Immunol. 1996;8:688–693.
18. Steiger J, Nickerson PW, Steurer W, Moscovitch-Lopatin M, Strom TB. IL-2 knockout recipient mice reject islet cell allografts. J Immunol. 1995;155:489–498.
19. Birnbaum F, Jehle T, Schwartzkopff J, Sokolovska Y, Bohringer D, Reis A, et al. Basiliximab following penetrating risk-keratoplasty – a prospective randomized pilot study. Klin Monatsbl Augenheilkd. 2008;225:62–65.
20. Gadient RA, Patterson PH. Leukemia inhibitory factor, Interleukin 6, and other cytokines using the GP130 transducing receptor: roles in inflammation and injury. Stem Cells. 1999;17:127–137.
21. Torres PF, Kijlstra A. The role of cytokines in corneal immunopathology. Ocul Immunol Inflamm. 2001;9:9–24.
22. King WJ, Comer RM, Hudde T, Larkin DF, George AJ. Cytokine and chemokine expression kinetics after corneal transplantation. Transplantation. 2000;70:1225–1233.
23. Funding M, Vorum H, Nexo E, Moestrup SK, Ehlers N, Moller HJ. Soluble CD163 and interleukin-6 are increased in aqueous humour from patients with endothelial rejection of corneal grafts. Acta Ophthalmol Scand. 2005;83:234–239.
24. van Gelderen EB, Van der Lelij A, Volker-Dieben HJ, van der Gaag R, Peek R, Treffers WF. Are cytokine patterns in aqueous humour useful in distinguishing corneal graft rejection from opacification due to herpetic stromal keratitis? Doc Ophthalmol. 1999;99:171–182.
25. Moore KW, de Waal Malefyt R, Coffman RL, O'Garra A. Interleukin-10 and the interleukin-10 receptor. Annu Rev Immunol. 2001;19:683–765.
26. Sulahian TH, Hogger P, Wahner AE, Wardwell K, Goulding NJ, Sorg C, et al. Human monocytes express CD163, which is upregulated by IL-10 and identical to p155. Cytokine. 2000;12:1312–1321.
27. Larkin DF, Alexander RA, Cree IA. Infiltrating inflammatory cell phenotypes and apoptosis in rejected human corneal allografts. Eye. 1997;11(Pt 1):68–74.
28. Torres PF, de Vos AF, Martins B, Kijlstra A. Interleukin 10 treatment does not prolong experimental corneal allograft survival. Ophthalmic Res. 1999;31:297–303.

29. Rosenbaum JT. Cytokines: the good, the bad, and the unknown. Invest Ophthalmol Vis Sci. 1993;34: 2389–2391.
30. David A, Chetritt J, Guillot C, Tesson L, Heslan JM, Cuturi MC, et al. Interleukin-10 produced by recombinant adenovirus prolongs survival of cardiac allografts in rats. Gene Ther. 2000;7:505–510.
31. Klebe S, Sykes PJ, Coster DJ, Krishnan R, Williams KA. Prolongation of sheep corneal allograft survival by ex vivo transfer of the gene encoding interleukin-10. Transplantation. 2001;71:1214–1220.
32. Gong N, Pleyer U, Volk HD, Ritter T. Effects of local and systemic viral interleukin-10 gene transfer on corneal allograft survival. Gene Ther. 2007;14:484–490.
33. Chen WF, Zlotnik A. IL-10: a novel cytotoxic T cell differentiation factor. J Immunol. 1991;147:528–534.
34. Zheng XX, Steele AW, Nickerson PW, Steurer W, Steiger J, Strom TB. Administration of noncytolytic IL-10/Fc in murine models of lipopolysaccharide-induced septic shock and allogeneic islet transplantation. J Immunol. 1995;154: 5590–5600.
35. Nicholls SM, Banerjee S, Figueiredo FC, Crome S, Mistry S, Easty DL, et al. Differences in leukocyte phenotype and interferon-gamma expression in stroma and endothelium during corneal graft rejection. Exp Eye Res. 2006;83: 339–347.
36. Maier P, Broszinski A, Heizmann U, Bohringer D, Reinhard T. Active transforming growth factor-beta2 is increased in the aqueous humor of keratoconus patients. Mol Vis. 2007;13:1198–1202.
37. Rayner SA, King WJ, Comer RM, Isaacs JD, Hale G, George AJ, et al. Local bioactive tumour necrosis factor (TNF) in corneal allotransplantation. Clin Exp Immunol. 2000;122: 109–116.
38. Rayner SA, Larkin DF, George AJ. TNF receptor secretion after ex vivo adenoviral gene transfer to cornea and effect on in vivo graft survival. Invest Ophthalmol Vis Sci. 2001;42:1568–1573.
39. Barton DE, Foellmer BE, Du J, Tamm J, Derynck R, Francke U. Chromosomal mapping of genes for transforming growth factors beta 2 and beta 3 in man and mouse: dispersion of TGF-beta gene family. Oncogene Res. 1988;3: 323–331.
40. Connor TB Jr, Roberts AB, Sporn MB, Danielpour D, Dart LL, Michels RG, et al. Correlation of fibrosis and transforming growth factor-beta type 2 levels in the eye. J Clin Invest. 1989;83:1661–1666.
41. Gupta A, Monroy D, Ji Z, Yoshino K, Huang A, Pflugfelder SC. Transforming growth factor beta-1 and beta-2 in human tear fluid. Curr Eye Res. 1996;15:605–614.
42. Khalil N. TGF-beta: from latent to active. Microbes Infect. 1999;1:1255–1263.
43. Knisely TL, Bleicher PA, Vibbard CA, Granstein RD. Production of latent transforming growth factor-beta and other inhibitory factors by cultured murine iris and ciliary body cells. Curr Eye Res. 1991;10:761–771.
44. Peress NS, Perillo E. TGF-beta 2 and TGF-beta 3 immunoreactivity within the ciliary epithelium [corrected]. Invest Ophthalmol Vis Sci. 1994;35:453–457.
45. Sano Y, Okamoto S, Streilein JW. Induction of donor-specific ACAID can prolong orthotopic corneal allograft survival in "high-risk" eyes. Curr Eye Res. 1997;16: 1171–1174.
46. Sporn MB, Roberts AB, Wakefield LM, de Crombrugghe B. Some recent advances in the chemistry and biology of transforming growth factor-beta. J Cell Biol. 1987;105: 1039–1045.
47. Tripathi RC, Chan WF, Li J, Tripathi BJ. Trabecular cells express the TGF-beta 2 gene and secrete the cytokine. Exp Eye Res. 1994;58:523–528.
48. Wilson SE, Lloyd SA. Epidermal growth factor and its receptor, basic fibroblast growth factor, transforming growth factor beta-1, and interleukin-1 alpha messenger RNA production in human corneal endothelial cells. Invest Ophthalmol Vis Sci. 1991;32:2747–2756.
49. Zamiri P, Masli S, Kitaichi N, Taylor AW, Streilein JW. Thrombospondin plays a vital role in the immune privilege of the eye. Invest Ophthalmol Vis Sci. 2005;46: 908–919.
50. Neurohr C, Nishimura SL, Sheppard D. Activation of transforming growth factor-beta by the integrin alphavbeta8 delays epithelial wound closure. Am J Respir Cell Mol Biol. 2006;35:252–259.
51. Saika S. TGFbeta pathobiology in the eye. Lab Invest. 2006;86:106–115.
52. Pasquale LR, Dorman-Pease ME, Lutty GA, Quigley HA, Jampel HD. Immunolocalization of TGF-beta 1, TGF-beta 2, and TGF-beta 3 in the anterior segment of the human eye. Invest Ophthalmol Vis Sci. 1993;34:23–30.
53. Ohta K, Wiggert B, Taylor AW, Streilein JW. Effects of experimental ocular inflammation on ocular immune privilege. Invest Ophthalmol Vis Sci. 1999;40: 2010–2018.
54. Ohta K, Yamagami S, Taylor AW, Streilein JW. IL-6 antagonizes TGF-beta and abolishes immune privilege in eyes with endotoxin-induced uveitis. Invest Ophthalmol Vis Sci. 2000;41:2591–2599.
55. Reinhard T, Bonig H, Mayweg S, Bohringer D, Gobel U, Sundmacher R. Soluble Fas ligand and transforming growth factor beta2 in the aqueous humor of patients with endothelial immune reactions after penetrating keratoplasty. Arch Ophthalmol. 2002;120:1630–1635.
56. Streilein JW. Unraveling immune privilege. Science. 1995;270:1158–1159.

57. Maier P, Broszinski A, Heizmann U, Reinhard T. Decreased active TGF-beta2 levels in the aqueous humour during immune reactions following penetrating keratoplasty. Eye. 2008;22:569–575.
58. Kuchle M, Cursiefen C, Nguyen NX, Langenbucher A, Seitz B, Wenkel H, et al. Risk factors for corneal allograft rejection: intermediate results of a prospective normal-risk keratoplasty study. Graefes Arch Clin Exp Ophthalmol. 2002;240:580–584.
59. Smiddy WE, Stark WJ, Young E, Klein PE, Bias WD, Maumenee AE. Clinical and immunological results of corneal allograft rejection. Ophthalmic Surg. 1986;17:644–649.
60. Nagata S, Golstein P. The Fas death factor. Science. 1995;267:1449–1456.
61. Griffith TS, Brunner T, Fletcher SM, Green DR, Ferguson TA. Fas ligand-induced apoptosis as a mechanism of immune privilege. Science. 1995;270:1189–1192.
62. Tanaka M, Suda T, Takahashi T, Nagata S. Expression of the functional soluble form of human fas ligand in activated lymphocytes. EMBO J. 1995;14:1129–1135.
63. Hohlbaum AM, Moe S, Marshak-Rothstein A. Opposing effects of transmembrane and soluble Fas ligand expression on inflammation and tumor cell survival. J Exp Med. 2000;191:1209–1220.
64. Ferguson TA. The molecular basis of anterior associated immune deviation (ACAID). Ocul Immunol Inflamm. 1997;5:213–215.
65. Stuart PM, Griffith TS, Usui N, Pepose J, Yu X, Ferguson TA. CD95 ligand (FasL)-induced apoptosis is necessary for corneal allograft survival. J Clin Invest. 1997;99:396–402.
66. Sugita S, Taguchi C, Takase H, Sagawa K, Sueda J, Fukushi K, et al. Soluble Fas ligand and soluble Fas in ocular fluid of patients with uveitis. Br J Ophthalmol. 2000;84:1130–1134.
67. Hemo I, BenEzra D, Maftzir G, Birkenfeld V. Angiogenesis and interleukins. Ocular circulation and neovascularization. Doc Ophthalmol Proc Ser. 1987;50:505–509.
68. Dana MR, Yamada J, Streilein JW. Topical interleukin 1 receptor antagonist promotes corneal transplant survival. Transplantation. 1997;63:1501–1507.
69. Volpert OV, Fong T, Koch AE, Peterson JD, Waltenbaugh C, Tepper RI, et al. Inhibition of angiogenesis by interleukin 4. J Exp Med. 1998;188:1039–1046.
70. He XY, Chen J, Verma N, Plain K, Tran G, Hall BM. Treatment with interleukin-4 prolongs allogeneic neonatal heart graft survival by inducing T helper 2 responses. Transplantation. 1998;65:1145–1152.
71. Pleyer U, Bertelmann E, Rieck P, Hartmann C, Volk HD, Ritter T. Survival of corneal allografts following adenovirus-mediated gene transfer of interleukin-4. Graefes Arch Clin Exp Ophthalmol. 2000;238:531–536.
72. He XY, Verma N, Chen J, Robinson C, Boyd R, Hall BM. IL-5 prolongs allograft survival by downregulating IL-2 and IFN-gamma cytokines. Transplant Proc. 2001;33:703–704.
73. Bickel M. The role of interleukin-8 in inflammation and mechanisms of regulation. J Periodontol. 1993;64:456–460.
74. Trinchieri G. Interleukin-12 and the regulation of innate resistance and adaptive immunity. Nat Rev Immunol. 2003;3:133–146.
75. Ritter T, Yang J, Dannowski H, Vogt K, Volk HD, Pleyer U. Effects of interleukin-12p40 gene transfer on rat corneal allograft survival. Transpl Immunol. 2007;18:101–107.
76. Buchanan KL, Murphy JW. Kinetics of cellular infiltration and cytokine production during the efferent phase of a delayed-type hypersensitivity reaction. Immunology. 1997;90:189–197.
77. Star RA, Rajora N, Huang J, Stock RC, Catania A, Lipton JM. Evidence of autocrine modulation of macrophage nitric oxide synthase by alpha-melanocyte-stimulating hormone. Proc Natl Acad Sci U S A. 1995;92:8016–8020.
78. Taylor AW, Streilein JW, Cousins SW. Identification of alpha-melanocyte stimulating hormone as a potential immunosuppressive factor in aqueous humor. Curr Eye Res. 1992;11:1199–1206.
79. Taylor AW, Yee DG. Somatostatin is an immunosuppressive factor in aqueous humor. Invest Ophthalmol Vis Sci. 2003;44:2644–2649.
80. Schultz-Cherry S, Murphy-Ullrich JE. Thrombospondin causes activation of latent transforming growth factor-beta secreted by endothelial cells by a novel mechanism. J Cell Biol. 1993;122:923–932.
81. Torres PF, De Vos AF, van der Gaag R, Martins B, Kijlstra A. Cytokine mRNA expression during experimental corneal allograft rejection. Exp Eye Res. 1996;63:453–461.
82. Dana MR, Dai R, Zhu S, Yamada J, Streilein JW. Interleukin-1 receptor antagonist suppresses Langerhans cell activity and promotes ocular immune privilege. Invest Ophthalmol Vis Sci. 1998;39:70–77.
83. Foster CS, Wu HK, Merchant A. Systemic (serum) soluble interleukin-2 receptor levels in corneal transplant recipients. Doc Ophthalmol. 1993;83:83–89.
84. Pleyer U, Milani JK, Ruckert D, Rieck P, Mondino BJ. Determinations of serum tumor necrosis factor alpha in corneal allografts. Ocul Immunol Inflamm. 1997;5:149–155.
85. Becker J, Salla S, Dohmen U, Redbrake C, Reim M. Explorative study of interleukin levels in the human cornea. Graefes Arch Clin Exp Ophthalmol. 1995;233:766–771.

Chapter 5

Limbal Stem Cell Transplantation: Surgical Techniques and Results

Alex J. Shortt, Stephen J. Tuft, Julie T. Daniels

Core Messages

- The ocular surface is composed of two functionally specialized epithelia that are both essential to maintain the surface integrity of the eye and the optical transparency of the cornea.
- Ocular surface failure is thought to result from destruction of limbal epithelial stem cells (LESCs).
- Penetrating keratoplasty (PKP) is seldom a successful treatment for surface failure because the limbal stem cells are not replaced, and thus the epithelial surface over the PKP will again ultimately fail.
- Ocular surface reconstruction (OSR) is the restoration of the normal function of the ocular surface by surgical transplantation of limbal epithelial stem cells.
- Available options for limbal stem cell transplantation include conjunctival limbal autograft transplantation (CLAU), living-related conjunctival limbal allograft transplantation (lr-CLAL), keratolimbal allograft transplantation (KLAL), and ex vivo expansion and transplantation of cultured limbal stem cells.

5.1 Introduction

5.1.1 The Corneal Epithelium

The ocular surface is covered by the corneal and conjunctival epithelia. Both epithelia are structurally distinct, and numerous specializations in the corneal epithelium are essential for maintaining structural integrity and optical transparency. For example, the glycocalyx of the microvilli and microplicae of the apical surface is formed by the transmembrane mucins (MUC) type 1, 2, and 4 that interact with the secreted mucins in the tear film to anchor the tear film to the corneal surface. This complex arrangement lowers the surface tension of the tear film and facilitates tear film spreading and wetting of the corneal surface. The corneal epithelium is transparent because it contains sparse numbers of cytoplasmic organelles such as mitochondria, Golgi apparatus, and endoplasmic reticulum [1, 2]. The numerous basal hemidesmosomes anchor the multilayered epithelial sheet to the stroma, which allows it to resist shearing forces from the eyelids or trauma [3, 4]. Tight junctions (zona occludens) between the superficial epithelial cells obliterate the intercellular space, and this forms a barrier to the passage of fluid or solutes through the epithelium, which prevents fluid entry and stromal oedema, as well as providing a barrier to the entry of pathogens [5]. Corneal epithelial cells also play a crucial role in maintaining the avascularity of the cornea as a whole by secreting soluble VEGF receptor-1 (sVEGFR-1; also known as sflt-1) that binds and inactivates VEGF-A, and thus inhibits the growth of vessels in to the cornea [6].

5.1.2 The Limbus and Corneal Epithelial Homeostasis

The corneal limbus is the transitional region between the cornea and sclera. Although this zone anatomically includes both Schlemm's canal and the trabecular meshwork on its inner aspect, the term usually refers only to the superficial portion composed of the epithelium, underlying connective tissue, and the deeper corneoscleral collagen lamellae (Fig. 5.1).

Like all stratified squamous epithelia, the corneal epithelium is continuously regenerated. Cells are shed from the corneal surface into the tear film, and cells moving upwards from the basal layers of the epithelium and centrally from the limbus replace these cells. Thoft and Friend proposed the "XYZ hypothesis" to explain how

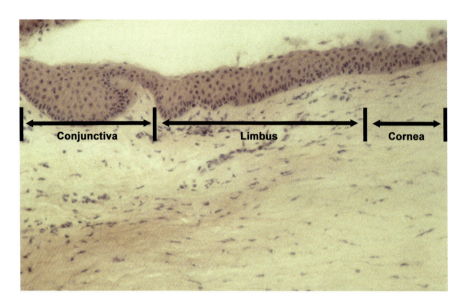

Fig. 5.1 *The corneal limbus.* Photomicrograph of a radially orientated cross section through the human limbus stained with haematoxylin and eosin. The locations of the *cornea, limbus and conjunctiva* are indicated. The conjunctiva is elevated above the plane of the cornea by artifact (magnification *40)

proliferation of basal corneal epithelial cells (X) and centripetal migration of cells (Y) offsets the loss of squames into the tear film (Z) (Fig. 5.2) [7].

However, Thoft and Friend's original XYZ hypothesis only partially explains corneal epithelial renewal over the lifetime of the cornea. The basal corneal epithelial cells are incapable of continuous replication and enter senescence after several cell divisions [8]. It has long been thought that the basal corneal epithelial cells themselves are constantly replenished by the daughter cells of slowly dividing LESCs located more peripherally in the basal layer of the epithelium of the limbus [9–15]. Interestingly, a recent report has suggested the presence of stem cells in the central corneal epithelium of the mouse; however, the results have yet to be verified in the adult human cornea [16].

The prevailing view of LESC proliferation is that one division of each LESC generates a daughter TAC that migrates centrally across the cornea while the original stem cell remains within its niche in the basal epithelium of the limbus. The TACs then divide rapidly in the basal corneal epithelial layer and move anteriorly as they differentiate into post mitotic cells (PMCs) that form the wing-cell layer of the corneal epithelium. The wing cells then become terminally differentiated cells (TDCs) that form the flattened superficial squamous external layer of the corneal epithelium [17]. The result of this migration and differentiation is that the corneal epithelium is renewed every 7–10 days in this manner [18, 19]. Despite

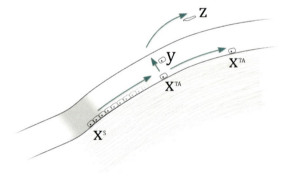

Fig. 5.2 *The XZY hypothesis.* The turnover of the corneal epithelial cell mass is the result of three independent phenomena. X represents a combination of proliferation and centripetal migration of the basal epithelial cells. Xs represents the asymmetric division of limbal epithelial stem cells to generate one daughter cell that remains in the limbus as a stem cell and a second daughter cell which migrates out of the limbus into the basal corneal epithelium and becomes a transient amplifying cell (TAC) (X^{TA}). The X^{TA} vector arises through a combination of proliferation and centripetal migration of the basal TACs. As the basal epithelial cells divide they give rise to suprabasal cells that form the stratified layers of the cornea giving rise to the Y vector. Z represents the shedding of squamous epithelial cells from the surface of cornea into the tear film. Corneal epithelial maintenance can thus be defined by the equation $X+Y=Z$, which simply states that if corneal epithelium is to be maintained, cell loss must be balanced by cell replacement [7]

the abundant evidence that LESCs are located at the corneal limbus, the key structural features and the functional mechanisms that operate within the LESC niche are unknown.

> **Summary for the Clinician**
> - The ocular surface is composed of two structurally distinct epithelia, both of which have features essential for maintaining the integrity and optical transparency of the cornea.
> - The corneal epithelium is continually regenerated from LESCs that are located in the basal layer of the corneal limbus.

5.2 Corneal LESC Deficiency

The LESCs appear to represent a finite body of cells that cannot be replaced naturally. A state of corneal limbal stem cell deficiency (LSCD) occurs if the number of LESCs is depleted below a critical threshold by trauma or disease. The LSCD can be sectorial or total. It is characterized by conjunctivalization of the cornea, a pathological process whereby conjunctival epithelial cells from the peripheral to the limbus migrate onto the corneal surface to replace the normal corneal epithelium [20, 21].

This pathologic state can be reproduced in rabbits by surgically excising the limbal epithelium [17]. In the experimental and clinical situations, corneas with LSCD show poor epithelialization (persistent epithelial defects or recurrent erosions), chronic stromal inflammation (keratitis), corneal vascularization, and conjunctival epithelial overgrowth of the stroma (Fig. 5.3). As a result patients with LSCD can experience pain or irritation, photophobia, and decreased vision from opacity and irregular astigmatism [22]. Clinically, the presence of LSCD may be accompanied by the loss of the limbal palisades (of Vogt) on slit-lamp examination [23], and by late fluorescein staining as a result of poor epithelial barrier function [18, 24].

5.2.1 Diagnosis and Classification of Corneal LESC Deficiency

The presence of a conjunctival phenotype on the cornea (conjunctival overgrowth, conjunctivalization) is central to the diagnosis of LSCD [9, 15, 20, 22]. Clinical signs that support this diagnosis are epithelial haze, superficial and subepithelial vascularization, late fluorescein staining,

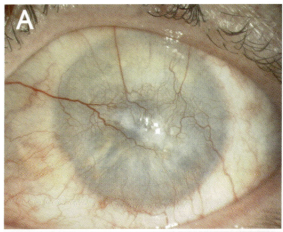

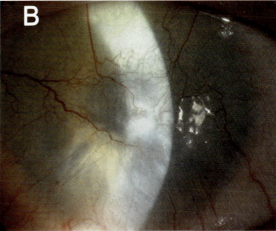

Fig. 5.3 Clinical photographs of a human cornea with limbal stem cell deficiency (LSCD). (**a**) Diffuse illumination. (**b**) Slit beam illumination. The clinical features are of stromal scarring secondary to chronic stromal inflammation, corneal vascularization, and conjunctival epithelial overgrowth of the cornea

epithelial breakdown and persistent epithelial defects, stromal inflammation, and loss of the limbal palisades of Vogt [9, 18, 21–24]. The clinical diagnosis should be confirmed using Impression cytology. Specimens can be stained with periodic acid Schiff stain to identify goblet cells, or monoclonal antibodies to cytokeratin 3 (CK3) and cytokeratin19 (CK19) to confirm a conjunctival phenotype (CK3−/CK19+) [20, 23, 25, 26]. Identification of goblet cells on the surface of the cornea is useful in making the diagnosis of LSCD. In advanced disease, especially those where keratinisation of the epithelium occurs (Steven's Johnson, ocular pemphigoid, Lyell syndrome), conjunctival goblet cells may be completely absent and, therefore, will not be detectable on impression cytology. Therefore, the presence of goblet cells on the surface of the cornea is not mandatory for making a diagnosis of LSCD.

LSCD may be classified as partial or total [9]. In partial deficiency, there is localized deficiency of LESCs in a region of limbus but an intact population of LESCs in other areas. This results in sectoral ingrowth of conjunctival epithelium from focal areas of SC deficiency (columnar keratopathy) and a mosaic pattern of stain with impression cytology [20, 27, 28]. In total stem cell deficiency there is functional loss of the entire LESC population and conjunctivalization of the entire cornea [20, 22, 27, 28].

Patients with LSCD can also be classified according to the presumed principal etiology of their disease with the primary site of injury at the LESCs themselves, their supporting niche, or a combination of both (Table 5.1). In some patients there is an identifiable event that has caused ocular surface injury with direct damage to the LESCs such as chemical or thermal burn, Stevens-Johnson syndrome/toxic epidermal necrolysis, multiple surgeries or cryotherapy, medications (iatrogenic), contact lens wear, severe microbial infection, radiation, and antimetabolites including 5-fluorouracil and mitomycin C [10, 27–34]. A second category is characterized by a gradual loss of the LESC population without a known or identifiable precipitating factor, and in this group a loss of the limbal stromal niche may be the primary disease mechanism. This group contains conditions such as aniridia, neoplasia, autoimmune polyglandular syndrome (APS1), peripheral ulcerative corneal disease, neurotrophic keratopathy, as well as idiopathic limbal deficiency [20, 23, 35–37].

Summary for the Clinician

- Corneal LSCD is characterized by "conjunctivalization" of the cornea, with epithelial haze, late fluorescein staining, subepithelial vascularization, persistent or recurrent epithelial defects, stromal inflammation and loss of the limbal palisades of Vogt.
- The clinical diagnosis may be confirmed by impression cytology. There are typically goblet cells and a conjunctival phenotype with negative expression for monoclonal antibodies to cytokeratin 3 (CK3−) but positive expression for cytokeratin19 (CK19+).
- LSCD may be the result of congenital or acquired disease, and corneal involvement may be partial or total.

Table 5.1 Classification of the etiology of limbal epithelial stem cell deficiency based on presumed site of damage to the LECSs or their niche

Clinical disease	Destructive loss of LESCs	Altered stromal niche
Hereditary		
Anirida	✓?	✓?
Autoimmune polyglandular syndrome (APS1)	✓	
Ectrodactyly-ectodermal dysplasia clefting (EEC syndrome)	✓	
Acquired		
Chemical or thermal burn	✓	✓
Stevens-Johnson syndrome, toxic epidermal necrolysis, ocular cicatricial pemphigoid (OCP)	✓	
Multiple surgeries or cryotherapies to limbus	✓	✓
Contact lens-induced keratopathy	✓	
Severe microbial infection extending to limbus	✓	✓
Antimetabolite uses (5-FU or mitomycin C)	✓	✓
Radiation	✓	✓
Chronic limbitis (vernal, atopy, phlyctenular)		✓
Peripheral ulcerative keratitis (Mooren's ulcer)		✓
Neurotrophic keratopathy	✓	
Chronic bullous keratopathy	✓	
Pterygium		✓
Idiopathic	✓?	✓?

LESC limbal epithelial stem cell; *5-FU* 5-fluorouracil

5.3 Management of Patients with Limbal Stem Cell Deficiency

5.3.1 Conservative Options

The conservative options for managing patients with LSCD are the use of intensive nonpreserved lubrication, bandage contact lenses, and autologous serum eye drops. Only the latter is supported by evidence in the literature [38–40]. Conservative treatment usually provides temporary remission but the condition tends to deteriorate over time.

5.3.2 Surgical Options for Partial Limbal Stem Cell Deficiency

For partial LSCD, it has been demonstrated that in the acute phase following injury repeated debridement of migrating conjunctival epithelium, known as sequential sector conjunctival epitheliectomy (SSCE), can reduce or prevent conjunctival ingrowth [41]. The use of an amniotic membrane graft as an inlay to promote corneal epithelial migration over the area of LSCD has also been reported to be successful [33, 42–44] (reviewed by Fernandes et al. [45], Tosi et al. [46] and Dua et al. [47]).

5.3.3 Surgical Options for Total Limbal Stem Cell Deficiency

For total LSCD, one of a group of surgical procedures collectively called ocular surface reconstruction (OSR) is required to restore a corneal phenotype. The need for such procedures is most obvious in patients with bilateral blinding ocular surface diseases such as Stevens Johnson syndrome (SJS), ocular cicatricial pemphigoid (OCP), and severe chemical/ thermal burns. The shared pathway to disease in these patients is dysfunction and destruction of the LESCs. A standard penetrating keratoplasty (PKP), which does not transfer stem cells, is unlikely to restore a stable ocular surface in such patients, and a systematic approach is needed. The process draws on a wide range of medical and surgical options that aim to improve the quality and quantity of tears, remove the abnormal corneal and conjunctival epithelium and associated fibrovascular tissue, and then replace it with either transplanted autologous or allogeneic cells. Clinically, the process involves a sequential three-step approach.

Correct any dry eye disease and lid abnormality that is contributing to ocular surface failure

This includes correction of meibomian gland dysfunction, punctal occlusion, and the frequent application of preservative-free artificial tears or autologous serum. Corneal exposure, trichiasis, and entropion should be corrected. Symblepharon and restriction of eye movement should also be repaired by fornix reconstruction using amniotic or buccal mucous membrane, and this should be completed before corneal surface reconstruction is attempted.

Remove the conjunctival epithelium from the cornea and restore a normal stromal environment

Abnormal conjunctival epithelium and subepithelial fibrous tissue must be debrided. This can be done mechanically and the combined tissue can often be peeled off the cornea. For total LSCD, it is also usual to perform a peritomy and resection of the conjunctival epithelium for up to 4 mm from the surgical limbus. Hemostasis is essential and mitomycin C may be applied over the exposed sclera to reduce recurrence of scarring and subepithelial fibroblastic proliferation. Lamellar or PKP may also be performed at this stage if it is thought there is visually significant stromal opacity.

Transplant corneal LESCs to reestablish an intact and transparent epithelium

When LSCD is total, a population of autologous or allogeneic LESCs must be transplanted if a stable corneal epithelial phenotype is to be regained [9–12, 15, 22, 27, 28, 48–54]. A variety of techniques have been developed to transplant limbal stem cells. The terminology and nomenclature used are those proposed by Holland et al. [28], and the procedures that will be discussed are: conjunctival limbal autograft (CLAU), living-related conjunctival limbal allograft (lr-CLAL), keratolimbal allograft (KLAL), and ex vivo expansion and transplantation of cultured LESCs. The first to be introduced, and the most widely employed, are techniques in which blocks of tissue containing stroma and overlying epithelium were transferred such as (KLAL) [49, 55–57], (CLAU), and (lr-CLAL) [27, 32, 58, 59]. An oversized and eccentric PKP that includes part of the limbus have also been employed [60–62].

> **Summary for the Clinician**
>
> - Conservative treatment of LSCD may provide temporary relief but can eventually fail as the natural history of LSCD has tended toward gradual deterioration over time.
> - Partial LSCD may be treated surgically with SSCE or an amniotic membrane graft inlay.
> - Total LSCD requires OSR, which is a multistep process of treating dry eye disease and correcting lid abnormalities to restore a normal stromal environment. This is followed by removal of the abnormal conjunctival epithelial covering of the cornea and transplantation of corneal LESCs.

5.4 Surgical Techniques for Transplanting Corneal Limbal Stem Cells

5.4.1 Conjunctival Limbal Autograft (CLAU)

First reported by Kenyon and Tseng in 1989 [63], CLAU rapidly became popular for the treatment of unilateral limbal deficiency. CLAU involves the transfer of autologous limbal tissue from the unaffected fellow eye to the stem cell deficient eye. For total unilateral LSCD it still may be the procedure of choice [34, 63]. The surgical procedure is shown in Fig. 5.4.

After chemical burns, severe inflammation and ischemia drastically reduces the chance of success of CLAU in the acute stage [63, 64]. A more appropriate initial approach in this setting is the use of a temporary amniotic membrane overlay patch to suppress inflammation, encourage epithelial wound healing, and prevent adhesions and symblepharon [45–47].

A significant percentage of the limbus is transferred for an autograft, and partial stem cell deficiency in a previously normal eye has been described following limbal biopsy for CLAU [22, 25]. The use of an amniotic membrane graft to cover the defect in the donor eye may promote proliferation of the remaining LESCs and reduce this risk.

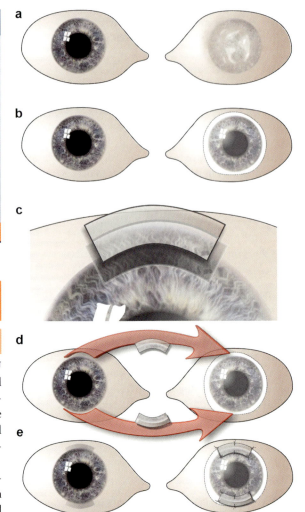

Fig. 5.4 Surgical procedure for performing a conjunctival-limbal autograft: (**a**) The eye on the *left hand side* of the image is normal. The eye on the *right* has total limbal epithelial stem cell deficiency. (**b**) The conjunctival pannus is removed from the corneal surface of the *right eye* by performing a peritomy followed by superficial keratectomy with blunt dissection. (**c**) Two conjunctival-limbal grafts are dissected from the healthy eye by superficial lamellar keratectomy at the 6 and 12 o'clock positions. (**d**) Each spans 6–7 mm limbal arc length and consists of 5 mm of conjunctiva and limbus with 1 mm of clear cornea. (**e**) These two free grafts are transferred and secured to the recipient eye at the corresponding anatomic sites using interrupted 10-0 nylon or Vicryl sutures to the limbus and 8-0 Vicryl sutures to the sclera

5.4.2 Living-Related Conjunctival Limbal Allograft Transplant (lr-CLAL)

When there is bilateral total LSCD, allogeneic limbus is the only potential source of LESCs. When a conjunctival-limbal graft is taken from a living related donor and transplanted to the recipient's stem cell deficient eye it is called living-related conjuctival-limbal allograft transplantation (lr-CLAL). The surgical technique of lr-CLAL is otherwise identical to CLAU. Amniotic membrane can be used similarly to eliminate the concern of removing LESCs from the healthy donor eye and to augment the effect of CLAU in the recipient eye.

Nevertheless, unless the donor and the recipient are perfectly matched, there is a risk of rejection of a lr-CLAL and systemic immunosuppressionis required [59, 65].

5.4.2.1 Clinical Outcomes of CLAU and lr-CLAL

Reports of these procedures have generally been favorable. Kenyon and Tseng [63] reported a successful outcome in 95% of CLAU procedures with a mean follow up of 24 months (range 6–45 months, $n > 26$). Jenkins et al. [66] reported a 60% success rate for CLAU at a mean follow-up of 24 months (range 12–36 months, $n > 5$). Santos et al. [32] reported a combination of CLAU and lr-ClAL, with an overall combined survival rate of 40% after 1 year and 33% after 2 years, with a cumulative survival of 33% after a mean follow-up interval of 33 months ($n > 33$). Kwitko et al. [67] reported 91.6% survival in their series of lr-CLAL at a mean follow-up of 17.2 months (range 5–29 months, $n > 12$). Rao et al. [65] reported a survival for lr-CLAL of 77.8% with a mean follow-up of 17.2 months (range 3–33 months, $n > 9$), and Daya et al. [59] reported a lr-CLAL survival of 80% with mean follow-up of 26.2 months (range 17–43 months, $n > 10$).

5.4.3 Keratolimbal Allograft Transplant

The third option for transplanting LESCs is to perform a KLAL using tissue from cadaveric donors. This surgical technique may restore the corneal phenotype in patients with bilateral LSCD or, less commonly, in patients with unilateral LSCD who do not wish to jeopardize the healthy eye with any surgery. The surgical procedure of KLAL is schematically depicted in Fig. 5.5. It should be noted that if the stroma is clear a PKP or lamellar keratoplasty (LK) is unnecessary. Some authors recommend that a PKP, if it is necessary, is best delayed for 3 or 4 months when the eye is less inflamed because there is less chance of rejection and the graft survival rate improves [44, 49, 57].

Because the tissue transplanted in KLAL is allogeneic, systemic immunosuppression is required in the same regimen as after lr-CLAL. Despite continuous oral administration of cyclosporin A (CSA) for 5 years, Tsubota et al. [68] reported the long-term success rate of KLAL as 51% at 3 years ($n > 43$), Solomon et al. [56] reported a 44.6% success rate at 5 years ($n > 39$), while Ilari and Daya [57] reported a 21.2% success rate at 5 years of follow-up ($n > 23$). Therefore, despite systemic

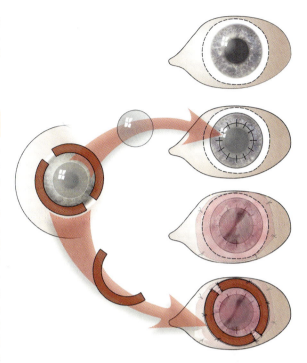

Fig. 5.5 Surgical procedure of keratolimbal allograft (KLAL). A peritomy is performed on the recipient eye and the fibrovascular pannus is removed. The residual corneal stromal bed may be clear. A piece of amniotic membrane is placed over the cornea with the basement membrane side external and secured around the limbus with interrupted 8-0 vicryl sutures to the scleral tissue. The central corneal button of the donor cornea is removed by trephine, the residual corneo-limbal rim is trimmed, and the underlying stroma is thinned to create a smooth and thin corneal–scleral limbal rim. This rim of tissue that contains the limbus is then laid onto the recipient cornea and secured with interrupted 10-0 nylon sutures. In order to promote corneal epithelial healing, another amniotic membrane is placed over the cornea as a patch and secured to the sclera with a running 10-0 nylon suture that remains in position for 1 or 2 weeks. Alternatively, a bandage contact lens or temporary tarsorrhaphy can be considered

immunosuppression, allograft rejection is still the most important factor limiting the success of KLAL. Signs of allograft rejection include telangiectasia and engorged limbal blood vessels, epithelial rejection lines and epithelial breakdown, and severe limbal inflammation. One reason for the poor long-term prognosis is chronic inflammation from ongoing ocular surface disease, which may enhance sensitization, leading to allograft rejection. Amniotic membrane transplantation (as a corneal inlay) has been used to augment the success of KLAL based on the fact that it may help suppress inflammation and restore the damaged limbal stromal environment [44, 69].

5.4.4 Ex Vivo Expansion and Transplantation of Cultured Limbal Stem Cells

The most recent development for transplanting LESCs is ex vivo expansion of LESCs (for review see Shortt et al. 2007 [70]). This technique is based on the pioneering work in skin of Rheinwald and Green [71–74]. Figure 5.6 illustrates how the procedure is performed.

The protocols used to cultivate cells for transplantation vary widely. Some studies used an "explant culture system" in which a small limbal biopsy is placed directly onto an amniotic membrane and the limbal epithelial cells then migrate out of the biopsy and proliferate to form an epithelial sheet [52, 54, 75–83]. The amniotic membrane substrate is then purported to act as a surrogate stem cell niche environment [84, 85]. An alternative technique is a "suspension culture system" in which limbal epithelial cells are first released from the limbal biopsy following enzyme treatment and a suspension of individual cells is seeded either onto amniotic membrane or onto a layer of growth-arrested 3T3 feeder cells [53, 86–90]. A carrier substrate such as fibrin may also be used to transfer the cells to the eye [53]. Although laboratory studies suggest that the suspension culture system is a more efficient method of isolating LESCs for culture [91, 92], there is no evidence of superiority in terms of clinical outcome. Similarly, although a feeder layer of embryonic mouse 3T3 fibroblasts in a co-culture system has been shown help maintain an undifferentiated epithelial phenotype [8], it is unclear whether this results in a better clinical outcome.

The use of ex vivo expansion techniques in humans was first described by Pellegrini et al. in 1997 [86]. Since then, seventeen further reports of the use of this technology to treat patients have been published [52–54, 75–83, 87–90, 93]. Four further studies have also reported the transplantation of ex vivo cultured autologous oral mucosal epithelial cells to treat LSCD [94–97]. We recently reviewed all clinical reports of these treatments and found the success rate from 33–100% with a mean of 77% [70].

The ex vivo expansion technique has theoretical advantages over conventional limbal transplantation methods. Compared with CLAU and lr-CLAL, the size of the limbal biopsy that is required is substantially smaller, although more than one biopsy may be required to obtain a successful explant or cell culture. This minimizes the risk of precipitating stem cell failure in the donor eye and provides the option for a second biopsy if necessary. Another theoretical advantage over KLAL and lr-CLAL is a potentially reduced risk of allograft rejection due to the absence of antigen-presenting macrophages and Langerhan's cells in ex vivo cultured LEC grafts.

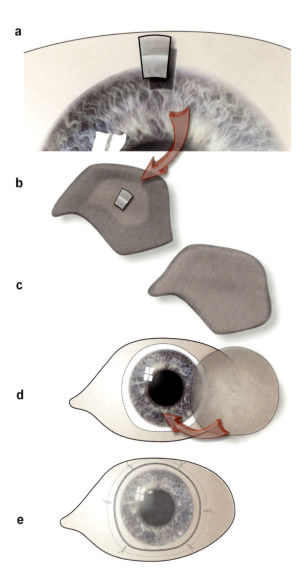

Fig. 5.6 Schematic drawing of ex vivo expansion of limbal SC (SC). A limbal biopsy measuring 2×2 mm is performed on the donor eye (**a**). This biopsy is then placed on amniotic membrane, allowed to adhere and then submerged in a culture medium (**b**). Limbal epithelial cells migrate out of the biopsy onto the amnion, and after 2–3 weeks the epithelial outgrowth measures 2–3 cm in diameter (**c**). After the fibrovascular pannus is removed from the recipient eye the explant is placed on the cornea (**d**) and sutured to the sclera (**e**)

5.4.5 Regulations Governing the Clinical Use of Ex vivo Cultured Tissue

As cell-based therapy has become more widely employed, the laboratory process of graft production has rightly come under scrutiny and the regulatory requirements have grown significantly. It is no longer appropriate or ethical to culture cells in an informal manner in a research laboratory if they are destined for human transplantation. Groups providing cellular therapies in the European Union (EU) have to comply with EU law, which requires that grafts are only produced by accredited tissue banks under the defined conditions of good manufacturing practice (GMP). The tissue bank facilities and processes must also be regularly inspected by the relevant authority. The supervision of tissue banking in the United States of America is more complex. There are currently no regulations governing this procedure, but the FDA has proposed new regulations requiring registration of all tissue banks, expanded screening and testing, and the introduction of practices similar to GMP. The level of regulatory compliance in most previously published series is not stated [52–54, 75–82, 86–89]. It is not known whether compliance with these regulations will affect the ability to perform the difficult and sensitive process of cell culture, and, hence, whether compliance will affect clinical outcomes.

5.4.6 Evidence of the Presence of Stem Cells in Ex vivo Cultures and Grafts

The evidence of stem cells in the transplanted cell population is based upon the following observations; functional assays of the colony forming ability of transplanted cells (only stem cells can give rise to large colonies in culture [8, 71], immunohistological analysis of grafts, and evidence of donor cell survival. Schwab et al. estimated that between 2–9% of cells in ex vivo expanded limbal epithelial cultures demonstrated the colony forming characteristics of stem cells [88]. The basal cells of ex vivo cultured LEC sheets also express cytokeratin 19 (CK19), β1 integrin, and p63 [91], which are characteristics of a limbal rather than a corneal phenotype. However, this does not prove that these basal cells are stem cells. Indeed, LESCs probably only account for <9% of the total limbal epithelial population in vivo, and unless a selection process is performed during isolation, it is likely that stem cells will account for a relatively small percentage of the cells present on grafts [98–100]. Further investigation of this variable has not been possible to date as there is no definitive marker of LESCs.

5.4.7 Assessing Outcomes Following LESC Transplantation

A recent review found that the methods used to diagnose LESC deficiency and determine success of ex vivo cultured LESC therapy vary widely and are often poorly defined [70]. Rama et al. [53] devised a scoring system based on clinical observations and impression cytology to grade the severity of LSCD. These features were assessed and scored before and after treatment, and statistical analysis of the differences was performed. This provided an objective assessment of treatment success. Koizumi et al. [52] and Daya et al. [89] also defined success as improvement in a set of clinical parameters used to assess LSCD. Although other studies have described an improvement in clinical parameters of LSCD, they do not explicitly state which parameters were used [54, 76–83, 86–88, 90]. In general, these studies lacked objectivity as there was no pre and post treatment comparison. Outcome data for visual acuity was reported in all studies, and information on the subjective improvement in pain and discomfort were reported in four studies, although no formal method of assessment was employed [53, 82, 86, 89].

Our group recently described the use of impression cytology and confocal microscopy as defined clinical outcome measures to determine success in restoring a corneal epithelial phenotype [93]. Using this approach we were able to objectively demonstrate and partially quantify changes in the corneal phenotype postoperatively. The correlation between impression cytology and corneal confocal microscopy was excellent, and demonstrates the potential for this technology.

5.4.8 Evidence for Donor Cell Survival Following Ex Vivo Cultured LESC Transplantation

There is a lack of evidence to support the long-term survival and proliferation of transplanted ex vivo cultured LESC. Rama et al. reported the results of impression cytology after transplantation [53]. They examined CK3 and CK12 (markers of epithelial cells) expression in cells obtained by impression cytology at 12–27 months after treatment. When the findings were scored according to a defined grading system the cytokeratin profile after treatment was more consistent with a normal corneal phenotype than preoperatively. Pellegrini et al. performed corneal biopsies on two patients at 19 and 24 months after treatment and demonstrated a normal corneal epithelial phenotype with absence of without goblet cells and with a normal pattern of CK3 expression [86]. Similarly, patients that have undergone PKP following ex vivo cultured LEC transplantation provide an insight into the biology of this therapy [53, 77, 79, 86, 89, 101]. Histology of excised central corneal buttons consistently demonstrates the presence of a multilayered epithelium with a similar phenotype to limbal epithelium. Whilst this data confirms the restoration of a functioning corneal epithelium following treatment in a previously stem cell deficient cornea, it is not direct evidence that transplanted limbal stem cells have survived.

In the search for direct evidence of cell survival, Daya et al. used polymerase chain reaction (PCR) genotyping to determine the origin of the cells populating the ocular surface postoperatively [88]. DNA was extracted from the patient's blood, from the donor corneoscleral rim used to establish cell cultures, and from the amniotic membrane used in each operation. These were compared with the DNA extracted from corneal epithelial cells obtained by impression cytology from the corneas of seven patients after transplantation. Donor DNA was detected from only two of seven eyes. One of these samples was positive for allogeneic donor DNA at 2 months but negative at 22 months, the second was positive at 7 months but negative at 9 months. Samples from the other five patients were negative for donor DNA when tested between 1 and 7 months postoperatively [89]. The epithelia from three further patients who had a subsequent PKP were examined using the same technique. The DNA genotype of epithelial cells on the ocular surface matched that of the host and not that of the allogeneic donor. This data suggests that the epithelium on the ocular surface in the majority of patients had a host DNA genotype, and that although donor cells may persist for 7–9 months they are ultimately replaced by host cells. If this is the case, the clinical effect of ex vivo cultured LESC transplantation may rely on the provision of a new niche for the regeneration of the host stem cell population rather than providing a new population of LESCs that can continue to function indefinitely. More recent data from this group suggests that transplanted allogeneic cells may not last more than 28 weeks [102].

5.4.9 Role of Tissue Matching in Transplantation of Allogeneic Tissue or Cells

When allogeneic limbal stem cells are transplanted, tissue matching strategies may be considered in an attempt to improve outcomes. There is no direct evidence that tissue matching improves outcome when performing lr-CLAU, KLAL or transplantation of ex vivo cultured LESC. However, in cases where eccentric PKP was performed to treat stem cell deficiency, grafts with 0–1 mismatches (HLA A, B, DR loci) were significantly more likely to be clear 5 years postoperatively. Furthermore, successful clinical outcomes correlated with the detection of allogeneic donor DNA on the ocular surface, indicating the survival of transplanted cells [61].

5.4.10 Alternative Sources of Autologous Stem Cells

The use of oral mucosa epithelium as a source of cells to treat bilateral LSCD has potential advantages. Because the cells are autologous, there is no risk of immune-mediated rejection, and thus immuosuppression is not required. Other potential advantages are that oral mucosa is thought to be at a lower stage of differentiation than epidermal keratinocytes [17, 103], they divide rapidly, and they can be maintained in culture for prolonged periods without keratinization [104]. Cytokeratin 3 (CK3) is similarly expressed by both corneal epithelium [17] and oral mucosa [103, 105], suggesting that gene expression is similar. A theoretical disadvantage of the use of oral mucosa to treat autoimmune diseases such as OCP is that the oral and ocular mucosa may both secrete a common basement membrane target antigen [104]. In the latter case, epithelial stem cells derived from the hair follicle may have potential for therapeutic application on the corneal surface. A recent paper described a method for altering the phenotype of hair follicle-derived epithelial cells to that of a limbal epithelial cell-like phentoype using conditioned medium collected from limbal fibroblasts [106].

5.4.11 Issues Surrounding Ex Vivo Cultured LESC Transplantation that Require Further Investigation

Ex vivo expansion and transplantation of limbal epithelium has been performed by several separate groups in a number of countries. It has been used to treat a variety of ocular surface disorders that are thought to be the result of limbal SC failure. Despite a substantial number of experimental models of this technique, and an ever-growing body of laboratory data on limbal epithelial SC biology, the scientific understanding of this procedure is poor. Some key questions still need to be answered. The exact proportion of SCs present in ex vivo cultured LEC sheets is unclear and needs to be determined. The behavior of LESCs following transplantation also needs to be elucidated. It has been proposed that the success of this treatment relies on the reintegration of exogenous cultured limbal SCs into the ocular surface, and that these cells function to continuously replenish the corneal epithelium [9–11, 15]. However, it may be that the composite amniotic membrane and ex vivo cultured LESC graft act as a biological bandage that provides an opportunity or stimulus for the patient's own endogenous LESC population to regenerate. In the case of total LSCD, this process could theoretically include the recruitment of precursor cells from the bone marrow. This is supported by evidence that cells derived from bone marrow SCs can be found in the normal scleral stroma [107] and also following scleral injury [108], and that that transplantation of cultured bone marrow SCs on amniotic membrane can reconstruct the corneal epithelium following chemical injury in rats [109].

It is interesting that despite the different methodologies employed, the success rate and outcomes of ex vivo expansion and transplantation of limbal epithelium are remarkably similar. It could therefore be inferred that as long as viable LESCs are transferred, the method that is used to achieve this is relatively unimportant. On the other hand, the inability to identify transplanted cells on the cornea of patients more than 9 months after treatment may indicate that long-term survival of transplanted cells is not essential, and that other mechanisms are responsible for the improvement of the epithelial phenotype. Elucidation of key factors that control the environment of the LESC niche could allow these conditions to be replicated in-vitro to make the process of culturing LESCs more efficient, and permit optimization of the ocular surface for receipt of transplanted LESCs. Unfortunately, our ability to answer some of the questions is hampered by the lack of a definite molecular marker of LESCs and the inability to track living cells after transplantation. Progress in this area has recently been reviewed by Chee et al. [110]. Recent data suggests that deltaN P63 [111, 112] and ABCG2 [98–100] are the leading candidates for such a marker.

Summary for the Clinician

- There is no single solution to treating total LSCD.
- The available surgical techniques for transplanting corneal limbal stem cells are CLAU, lr-CLAL, KLAL, and ex vivo expansion and transplantation of cultured LESCs.
- Ex vivo expansion and transplantation of cultured LESCs is a novel cell therapy. There is evidence that stem cells are present in ex vivo cultures and early grafts, but poor evidence is available for the long-term survival of these cells after transplantation.
- There is a need to develop more objective methods of assessing outcomes following LESC transplantation.
- Oral mucosa is an alternative stem cell source for OSR.
- There are many issues regarding the mechanism and scientific understanding of ex vivo cultured LESC transplantation that require further investigation

5.5 Conclusion

The treatment of corneal LSCD is complex. There is no simple treatment option, but the clinician must choose from the array of options based on a review of each case. The advent of cell-based technology has added to the tools available to treat these patients; however, this technology is still in its infancy and its long-term efficacy still remains to be proven. The scientific basis of this therapy required further research.

References

1. Snell RA, Lemp MA (eds) (1998). Clinical anatomy of the eye 2nd edn. Blackwell Science, MA, U.S.A, pp 132–213
2. Tsubota K, Tseng SC (2002) Nordlund ML. In: Holland EJ, Mannis MJ (eds) Ocular surface disease, 1st edn. Springer, New York
3. Gipson IK (1992) Adhesive mechanisms of the corneal epithelium. Acta Ophthalmol Suppl (202):13–17
4. Gipson IK, Spurr-Michaud SJ, Tisdale AS (1988) Hemidesmosomes and anchoring fibril collagen appear synchronously during development and wound healing. Dev Biol 126:253–262
5. Klyce SD, Crosson CE (1985) Transport processes across the rabbit corneal epithelium: a review. Curr Eye Res 4: 323–331
6. Ambati BK, Nozaki M, Singh N et al (2006) Corneal avascularity is due to soluble VEGF receptor-1. Nature 443: 993–997
7. Thoft RA, Friend J (1983) The X, Y, Z hypothesis of corneal epithelial maintenance. Invest Ophthalmol Vis Sci 24: 1442–1443
8. Pellegrini G, Golisano O, Paterna P et al (1999) Location and clonal analysis of stem cells and their differentiated progeny in the human ocular surface. J Cell Biol 145: 769–782
9. Dua HS, Azuara-Blanco A (2000) Limbal stem cells of the corneal epithelium. Surv Ophthalmol 44:415–425
10. Dua HS, Saini JS, Azuara-Blanco A et al (2000) Limbal stem cell deficiency: concept, aetiology, clinical presentation, diagnosis and management. Indian J Ophthalmol 48: 83–92
11. Daniels JT, Dart JK, Tuft SJ et al (2001) Corneal stem cells in review. Wound Repair Regen 9:483–494
12. Lavker RM, Sun TT (2003) Epithelial stem cells: the eye provides a vision. Eye 17:937–942
13. Cotsarelis G, Cheng SZ, Dong G et al (1989) Existence of slow-cycling limbal epithelial basal cells that can be preferentially stimulated to proliferate: implications on epithelial stem cells. Cell 57:201–209

14. Ramaesh K, Dhillon B (2003) Ex vivo expansion of corneal limbal epithelial/stem cells for corneal surface reconstruction. Eur J Ophthalmol 13:515–524
15. Tseng SC (1989) Concept and application of limbal stem cells. Eye 3(Pt 2):141–157
16. Majo F, Rochat A, Nicolas M et al (2008) Oligopotent stem cells are distributed throughout the mammalian ocular surface. Nature 456:250–254
17. Schermer A, Galvin S, Sun TT (1986) Differentiation-related expression of a major 64 K corneal keratin in vivo and in culture suggests limbal location of corneal epithelial stem cells. J Cell Biol 103:49–62
18. Dua HS, Gomes JA, Singh A (1994) Corneal epithelial wound healing. Br J Ophthalmol 78:401–408
19. Hanna C, O'Brien JE (1960) Cell production and migration in the epithelial layer of the cornea. Arch Ophthalmol 64:536–539
20. Puangsricharern V, Tseng SC (1995) Cytologic evidence of corneal diseases with limbal stem cell deficiency. Ophthalmology 102:1476–1485
21. Huang AJ, Tseng SC (1991) Corneal epithelial wound healing in the absence of limbal epithelium. Invest Ophthalmol Vis Sci 32:96–105
22. Tseng SCG, Espana EM (2005) Di Pascuale MA. In: Tasman W, Jaeger EA (eds) Duane's clinical ophthalmology on CD-ROM, 2005th edn. Lippincott Williams and Wilkins, Baltimore, PA
23. Nishida K, Kinoshita S, Ohashi Y et al (1995) Ocular surface abnormalities in aniridia. Am J Ophthalmol 120: 368–375
24. Huang AJ, Tseng SC, Kenyon KR (1990) Alteration of epithelial paracellular permeability during corneal epithelial wound healing. Invest Ophthalmol Vis Sci 31:429–435
25. Calonge M, Diebold Y, Saez V et al (2004) Impression cytology of the ocular surface: a review. Exp Eye Res 78: 457–472
26. Dart J (1997) Impression cytology of the ocular surface–research tool or routine clinical investigation? Br J Ophthalmol 81:930
27. Holland EJ (1996) Epithelial transplantation for the management of severe ocular surface disease. Trans Am Ophthalmol Soc 94:677–743
28. Holland EJ, Schwartz GS (1996) The evolution of epithelial transplantation for severe ocular surface disease and a proposed classification system. Cornea 15:549–556
29. Clinch TE, Goins KM, Cobo LM (1992) Treatment of contact lens-related ocular surface disorders with autologous conjunctival transplantation. Ophthalmology 99:634–638
30. Fujishima H, Shimazaki J, Tsubota K (1996) Temporary corneal stem cell dysfunction after radiation therapy. Br J Ophthalmol 80:911–914
31. Espana EM, Di Pascuale MA, He H et al (2004) Characterization of corneal pannus removed from patients with total limbal stem cell deficiency. Invest Ophthalmol Vis Sci 45: 2961–2966
32. Santos MS, Gomes JA, Hofling-Lima AL et al (2005) Survival analysis of conjunctival limbal grafts and amniotic membrane transplantation in eyes with total limbal stem cell deficiency. Am J Ophthalmol 140:223–230
33. Gomes JA, Santos MS, Ventura AS et al (2003) Amniotic membrane with living related corneal limbal/conjunctival allograft for ocular surface reconstruction in Stevens-Johnson syndrome. Arch Ophthalmol 121:1369–1374
34. Dua HS, Azuara-Blanco A (2000) Autologous limbal transplantation in patients with unilateral corneal stem cell deficiency. Br J Ophthalmol 84:273–278
35. Espana EM, Raju VK, Tseng SC (2002) Focal limbal stem cell deficiency corresponding to an iris coloboma. Br J Ophthalmol 86:1451–1452
36. Espana EM, Grueterich M, Romano AC et al (2002) Idiopathic limbal stem cell deficiency. Ophthalmology 109: 2004–2010
37. Gass JD (1962) The syndrome of keratoconjunctivitis, superficial moniliasis, idiopathic hypoparathyroidism and Addison's disease. Am J Ophthalmol 54:660–674
38. Geerling G, Maclennan S, Hartwig D (2004) Autologous serum eye drops for ocular surface disorders. Br J Ophthalmol 88:1467–1474
39. Poon AC, Geerling G, Dart JK et al (2001) Autologous serum eyedrops for dry eyes and epithelial defects: clinical and in vitro toxicity studies. Br J Ophthalmol 85: 1188–1197
40. Young AL, Cheng AC, Ng HK et al (2004) The use of autologous serum tears in persistent corneal epithelial defects. Eye 18:609–614
41. Dua HS (1998) The conjunctiva in corneal epithelial wound healing. Br J Ophthalmol 82:1407–1411
42. Anderson DF, Ellies P, Pires RT et al (2001) Amniotic membrane transplantation for partial limbal stem cell deficiency. Br J Ophthalmol 85:567–575
43. Pires RT, Chokshi A, Tseng SC (2000) Amniotic membrane transplantation or conjunctival limbal autograft for limbal stem cell deficiency induced by 5-fluorouracil in glaucoma surgeries. Cornea 19:284–287
44. Tseng SC, Prabhasawat P, Barton K et al (1998) Amniotic membrane transplantation with or without limbal allografts for corneal surface reconstruction in patients with limbal stem cell deficiency. Arch Ophthalmol 116:431–441
45. Fernandes M, Sridhar MS, Sangwan VS et al (2005) Amniotic membrane transplantation for ocular surface reconstruction. Cornea 24:643–653
46. Tosi GM, Massaro-Giordano M, Caporossi A et al (2005) Amniotic membrane transplantation in ocular surface disorders. J Cell Physiol 202:849–851
47. Dua HS, Gomes JA, King AJ et al (2004) The amniotic membrane in ophthalmology. Surv Ophthalmol 49:51–77

48. Dua HS, Joseph A, Shanmuganathan VA et al (2003) Stem cell differentiation and the effects of deficiency. Eye 17: 877–885
49. Espana EM, Di PM, Grueterich M et al (2004) Keratolimbal allograft in corneal reconstruction. Eye 18:406–417
50. Dua HS, Shanmuganathan VA, Powell-Richards AO et al (2005) Limbal epithelial crypts: a novel anatomical structure and a putative limbal stem cell niche. Br J Ophthalmol 89:529–532
51. Kinoshita S, Adachi W, Sotozono C et al (2001) Characteristics of the human ocular surface epithelium. Prog Retin Eye Res 20:639–673
52. Koizumi N, Inatomi T, Suzuki T et al (2001) Cultivated corneal epithelial stem cell transplantation in ocular surface disorders. Ophthalmology 108:1569–1574
53. Rama P, Bonini S, Lambiase A et al (2001) Autologous fibrin-cultured limbal stem cells permanently restore the corneal surface of patients with total limbal stem cell deficiency. Transplantation 72:1478–1485
54. Tsai RJ, Li LM, Chen JK (2000) Reconstruction of damaged corneas by transplantation of autologous limbal epithelial cells. N Engl J Med 343:86–93
55. Holland EJ, Djalilian AR, Schwartz GS (2003) Management of aniridic keratopathy with keratolimbal allograft: a limbal stem cell transplantation technique. Ophthalmology 110:125–130
56. Solomon A, Ellies P, Anderson DF et al (2002) Long-term outcome of keratolimbal allograft with or without penetrating keratoplasty for total limbal stem cell deficiency. Ophthalmology 109:1159–1166
57. Ilari L, Daya SM (2002) Long-term outcomes of keratolimbal allograft for the treatment of severe ocular surface disorders. Ophthalmology 109:1278–1284
58. Tsubota K, Shimmura S, Shinozaki N et al (2002) Clinical application of living-related conjunctival-limbal allograft. Am J Ophthalmol 133:134–135
59. Daya SM, Ilari FA (2001) Living related conjunctival limbal allograft for the treatment of stem cell deficiency. Ophthalmology 108:126–133
60. Reinhard T, Sundmacher R, Spelsberg H et al (1999) Homologous penetrating central limbo-keratoplasty (HPCLK) in bilateral limbal stem cell insufficiency. Acta Ophthalmol Scand 77:663–667
61. Reinhard T, Spelsberg H, Henke L et al (2004) Long-term results of allogeneic penetrating limbo-keratoplasty in total limbal stem cell deficiency. Ophthalmology 111:775–782
62. Spelsberg H, Reinhard T, Henke L et al (2004) Penetrating limbo-keratoplasty for granular and lattice corneal dystrophy: survival of donor limbal stem cells and intermediate-term clinical results. Ophthalmology 111:1528–1533
63. Kenyon KR, Tseng SC (1989) Limbal autograft transplantation for ocular surface disorders. Ophthalmology 96: 709–722
64. Ronk JF, Ruiz-Esmenjaud S, Osorio M et al (1994) Limbal conjunctival autograft in a subacute alkaline corneal burn. Cornea 13:465–468
65. Rao SK, Rajagopal R, Sitalakshmi G et al (1999) Limbal allografting from related live donors for corneal surface reconstruction. Ophthalmology 106:822–828
66. Jenkins C, Tuft S, Liu C et al (1993) Limbal transplantation in the management of chronic contact-lens-associated epitheliopathy. Eye 7(Pt 5):629–633
67. Kwitko S, Marinho D, Barcaro S et al (1995) Allograft conjunctival transplantation for bilateral ocular surface disorders. Ophthalmology 102:1020–1025
68. Tsubota K, Satake Y, Kaido M et al (1999) Treatment of severe ocular-surface disorders with corneal epithelial stem-cell transplantation. N Engl J Med 340:1697–1703
69. Tsubota K, Satake Y, Ohyama M et al (1996) Surgical reconstruction of the ocular surface in advanced ocular cicatricial pemphigoid and Stevens-Johnson syndrome. Am J Ophthalmol 122:38–52
70. Shortt AJ, Secker GA, Notara MD et al (2007) Transplantation of ex vivo cultured limbal epithelial stem cells: a review of techniques and clinical results. Surv Ophthalmol 52:483–502
71. Barrandon Y, Green H (1987) Three clonal types of keratinocyte with different capacities for multiplication. Proc Natl Acad Sci USA 84:2302–2306
72. Green H, Rheinwald JG, Sun TT (1977) Properties of an epithelial cell type in culture: the epidermal keratinocyte and its dependence on products of the fibroblast. Prog Clin Biol Res 17:493–500
73. Rheinwald JG (1980) Serial cultivation of normal human epidermal keratinocytes. Methods Cell Biol 21A:229–254
74. Rheinwald JG, Green H (1975) Serial cultivation of strains of human epidermal keratinocytes: the formation of keratinizing colonies from single cells. Cell 6:331–343
75. Koizumi N, Inatomi T, Suzuki T et al (2001) Cultivated corneal epithelial transplantation for ocular surface reconstruction in acute phase of Stevens-Johnson syndrome. Arch Ophthalmol 119:298–300
76. Shimazaki J, Aiba M, Goto E et al (2002) Transplantation of human limbal epithelium cultivated on amniotic membrane for the treatment of severe ocular surface disorders. Ophthalmology 109:1285–1290
77. Grueterich M, Espana EM, Touhami A et al (2002) Phenotypic study of a case with successful transplantation of ex vivo expanded human limbal epithelium for unilateral total limbal stem cell deficiency. Ophthalmology 109: 1547–1552
78. Nakamura T, Koizumi N, Tsuzuki M et al (2003) Successful regrafting of cultivated corneal epithelium using amniotic membrane as a carrier in severe ocular surface disease. Cornea 22:70–71

79. Sangwan VS, Vemuganti GK, Singh S et al (2003) Successful reconstruction of damaged ocular outer surface in humans using limbal and conjuctival stem cell culture methods. Biosci Rep 23:169–174
80. Sangwan VS, Vemuganti GK, Iftekhar G et al (2003) Use of autologous cultured limbal and conjunctival epithelium in a patient with severe bilateral ocular surface disease induced by acid injury: a case report of unique application. Cornea 22:478–481
81. Nakamura T, Inatomi T, Sotozono C et al (2004) Successful primary culture and autologous transplantation of corneal limbal epithelial cells from minimal biopsy for unilateral severe ocular surface disease. Acta Ophthalmol Scand 82:468–471
82. Sangwan VS, Murthy SI, Vemuganti GK et al (2005) Cultivated corneal epithelial transplantation for severe ocular surface disease in vernal keratoconjunctivitis. Cornea 24:426–430
83. Sangwan VS, Matalia HP, Vemuganti GK et al (2006) Clinical outcome of autologous cultivated limbal epithelium transplantation. Indian J Ophthalmol 54:29–34
84. Grueterich M, Espana E, Tseng SC (2002) Connexin 43 expression and proliferation of human limbal epithelium on intact and denuded amniotic membrane. Invest Ophthalmol Vis Sci 43:63–71
85. Grueterich M, Espana EM, Tseng SC (2003) Ex vivo expansion of limbal epithelial stem cells: amniotic membrane serving as a stem cell niche. Surv Ophthalmol 48:631–646
86. Pellegrini G, Traverso CE, Franzi AT et al (1997) Long-term restoration of damaged corneal surfaces with autologous cultivated corneal epithelium. Lancet 349:990–993
87. Schwab IR (1999) Cultured corneal epithelia for ocular surface disease. Trans Am Ophthalmol Soc 97:891–986
88. Schwab IR, Reyes M, Isseroff RR (2000) Successful transplantation of bioengineered tissue replacements in patients with ocular surface disease. Cornea 19:421–426
89. Daya SM, Watson A, Sharpe JR et al (2005) Outcomes and DNA analysis of ex vivo expanded stem cell allograft for ocular surface reconstruction. Ophthalmology 112:470–477
90. Nakamura T, Inatomi T, Sotozono C et al (2006) Transplantation of autologous serum-derived cultivated corneal epithelial equivalents for the treatment of severe ocular surface disease. Ophthalmology 113:1765–1772
91. Kim HS, Jun Song X, de Paiva CS et al (2004) Phenotypic characterization of human corneal epithelial cells expanded ex vivo from limbal explant and single cell cultures. Exp Eye Res 79:41–49
92. Zhang X, Sun H, Tang X et al (2005) Comparison of cell-suspension and explant culture of rabbit limbal epithelial cells. Exp Eye Res 80:227–233
93. Shortt AJ, Secker GA, Rajan MS et al (2008) Ex vivo expansion and transplantation of limbal epithelial stem cells. Ophthalmology 115(11):1989–1997
94. Nakamura T, Inatomi T, Sotozono C et al (2004) Transplantation of cultivated autologous oral mucosal epithelial cells in patients with severe ocular surface disorders. Br J Ophthalmol 88:1280–1284
95. Nishida K, Yamato M, Hayashida Y et al (2004) Corneal reconstruction with tissue-engineered cell sheets composed of autologous oral mucosal epithelium. N Engl J Med 351:1187–1196
96. Inatomi T, Nakamura T, Koizumi N et al (2006) Midterm results on ocular surface reconstruction using cultivated autologous oral mucosal epithelial transplantation. Am J Ophthalmol 141:267–275
97. Inatomi T, Nakamura T, Kojyo M et al (2006) Ocular surface reconstruction with combination of cultivated autologous oral mucosal epithelial transplantation and penetrating keratoplasty. Am J Ophthalmol 142(5):757–764
98. de Paiva CS, Chen Z, Corrales RM et al (2005) ABCG2 transporter identifies a population of clonogenic human limbal epithelial cells. Stem Cells 23:63–73
99. Watanabe K, Nishida K, Yamato M et al (2004) Human limbal epithelium contains side population cells expressing the ATP-binding cassette transporter ABCG2. FEBS Lett 565:6–10
100. Budak MT, Alpdogan OS, Zhou M et al (2005) Ocular surface epithelia contain ABCG2-dependent side population cells exhibiting features associated with stem cells. J Cell Sci 118:1715–1724
101. Sangwan VS, Matalia HP, Vemuganti GK et al (2005) Early results of penetrating keratoplasty after cultivated limbal epithelium transplantation. Arch Ophthalmol 123:334–340
102. Sharpe JR, Daya SM, Dimitriadi M et al (2007) Survival of cultured allogeneic limbal epithelial cells following corneal repair. Tissue Eng 13:123–132
103. Collin C, Ouhayoun JP, Grund C et al (1992) Suprabasal marker proteins distinguishing keratinizing squamous epithelia: cytokeratin 2 polypeptides of oral masticatory epithelium and epidermis are different. Differentiation 51:137–148
104. Hata K, Kagami H, Ueda M et al (1995) The characteristics of cultured mucosal cell sheet as a material for grafting; comparison with cultured epidermal cell sheet. Ann Plast Surg 34:530–538
105. Juhl M, Reibel J, Stoltze K (1989) Immunohistochemical distribution of keratin proteins in clinically healthy human gingival epithelia. Scand J Dent Res 97:159–170
106. Blazejewska EA, Schlotzer-Schrehardt U, Zenkel M et al (2009) Corneal limbal microenvironment can induce transdifferentiation of hair follicle stem cells into corneal epithelial-like cells. Stem Cells 27:642–652

107. Nakamura T, Ishikawa F, Sonoda KH et al (2005) Characterization and distribution of bone marrow-derived cells in mouse cornea. Invest Ophthalmol Vis Sci 46: 497–503
108. Ozerdem U, Alitalo K, Salven P et al (2005) Contribution of bone marrow-derived pericyte precursor cells to corneal vasculogenesis. Invest Ophthalmol Vis Sci 46: 3502–3506
109. Ma Y, Xu Y, Xiao Z et al (2006) Reconstruction of chemically burned rat corneal surface by bone marrow-derived human mesenchymal stem cells. Stem Cells 24:315–321
110. Chee KY, Kicic A, Wiffen SJ (2006) Limbal stem cells: the search for a marker. Clin Experiment Ophthalmol 34: 64–73
111. Di IE, Barbaro V, Ruzza A et al (2005) Isoforms of DeltaNp63 and the migration of ocular limbal cells in human corneal regeneration. Proc Natl Acad Sci USA 102: 9523–9528
112. Pellegrini G, Dellambra E, Golisano O et al (2001) p63 identifies keratinocyte stem cells. Proc Natl Acad Sci USA 98:3156–3161

Chapter 6

Cell Cycle Control and Replication in Corneal Endothelium

Nancy C. Joyce

Core Messages

- Excessive loss of endothelial cells causes loss of the barrier function of the corneal endothelium, resulting in bullous keratopathy, permanent corneal clouding, and loss of visual acuity.
- In vivo repair of the endothelium following cell loss occurs by cell enlargement and migration, rather than by cell division.
- Human corneal endothelial cells (HCEC) do not divide in vivo, because they are inhibited in G1-phase of the cell cycle; however, they retain proliferative capacity.
- The cell cycle is divided into multiple phases. After mitogenic stimulation, cells enter G1-phase to prepare cells for DNA duplication, which occurs in S-phase. Cells then move into G2-phase to prepare cells for division, which occurs in M-phase.
- Movement of cells from G1- to S-phase can be prevented by the activity of the cyclin-dependent kinase inhibitors, p27Kip1, p21Cip1, and p16INK4a. These inhibitors prevent activation of the transcription factor, E2F, which is required for S-phase entry.
- Several factors contribute to inhibition of the proliferation of HCEC in vivo, including formation of strong cell–cell contacts (contact inhibition), lack of autocrine or paracrine growth factor stimulation, and the suppressive effect of transforming growth factor-beta2. This inhibition appears to be mediated, in large part, by p27Kip1.
- Although HCEC retain the ability to divide, their capacity to proliferate decreases with increasing age. This decrease is characterized by an age-related reduction in the rate of cell cycle entry and in the relative number of dividing cells. Evidence strongly suggests that this age-related decrease is the result of an up-regulation of the expression and activity of p21Cip1 and p16INK4a, but not of p27Kip1.
- HCEC can be induced to divide by overcoming or bypassing G1-phase inhibition using molecular biological approaches. The most promising approach so far is ectopic expression of the transcription factor, E2F2, which increases endothelial cell proliferation in ex vivo corneas from both young (<30 years old) and older donors (>50 years old).
- Proliferative capacity and the expression of senescence characteristics are also affected by endothelial topography. Cells within the central 6.0 mm diameter of the endothelium in corneas from older donors exhibit the lowest proliferative capacity and contain the highest percentage of senescent cells.
- The age- and topographically related decrease in proliferative capacity observed in HCEC is not due to the presence of critically short telomeres, but appears to result from sub-lethal oxidative nuclear DNA damage.
- Research has led to a new hypothesis regarding the molecular basis for the age- and topographically related decrease in proliferative capacity. This hypothesis states that, with increasing age, oxidative stress increases in HCEC due to their high metabolic activity and due to chronic light exposure. This results in a gradual increase in oxidative nuclear DNA damage, which leads to a decreased ability to divide, mediated by the G1-phase inhibitors, p21Cip1, and p16INK4a.
- This new hypothesis provides the basis for further exploration of the molecular mechanisms underlying the age- and topographically related decrease in proliferative capacity of HCEC. This exploration could lead to the development of methods to prevent or reverse the effects of oxidative stress on these cells, thereby increasing their ability to divide in order to repair the endothelial monolayer and prevent the devastating effect on vision of the loss of endothelial barrier function.

6.1 Relationship of Endothelial Barrier Function to Corneal Transparency

The corneal endothelium is the single layer of flattened cells located at the posterior of the cornea, forming a boundary between the cornea and fluid aqueous humor. In young individuals, the endothelium consists of polygonal cells, 4–6 μm thick with a diameter of approximately 20 μm [1]. The basal aspect of the cells rests on Descemet's membrane, which is the thick extracellular matrix secreted by the endothelium. The apical aspect is bathed by aqueous humor. The lateral plasma membranes of endothelial cells are remarkable for their extensive interdigitation with neighboring cells [2]. Actin filaments are located at the periphery of the cells, forming a circumferential band that contributes to maintenance of cell shape [3]. Focal, rather than belt-like, tight junctions are located on the apical-most aspect of the lateral membranes [4]. These junctions form a semi-permeable ("leaky") barrier between cells [5]. Proteins associated with tight junctions that have been identified in corneal endothelial cells include zonula occludins-1 (ZO-1) [4] and junction adhesion molecule-A (JAM-A) [6]. The tight junction protein, occludin, has been detected in cultured human corneal endothelial cells (HCEC) [7], but was not detected in HCEC in ex vivo corneas by immunostaining [4]. This discrepancy may be due to the techniques or specific antibodies used to detect occludin in the studies. Adhesion junctions are located basally with respect to the tight junctions. These junctions mediate close contact between the lateral plasma membranes of adjacent cells and the underlying actin cytoskeleton, thereby strengthening cell–cell contacts [4]. Adhesion junctions are comprised of several proteins, including cadherins and catenins. Gap junctions form communicating channels between cells, and are located on the lateral membranes basal to the tight junctions [8]. Connexin-43 is a major gap junction protein expressed in corneal endothelium [9]. Junctional complexes formed between endothelial cells are calcium-sensitive [10], and break down if the calcium concentration is decreased below a threshold level.

A major function of the endothelium is to maintain corneal transparency by regulating corneal hydration. Since healthy cornea is avascular, much of the nutrition of corneal cells is supplied by the aqueous humor. The "leaky" junctions formed between cells permit water and nutrients to enter the stroma [11], while, at the same time, these junctions form a sufficiently tight barrier to prevent the bulk flow of fluid into the cornea. This inward fluid flow is counterbalanced by the activity of ionic "pump" proteins, located in the plasma membrane of HCEC [12]. Na^+/K^+-ATPase and bicarbonate-dependent Mg^{2+}-ATPase are among the proteins that form the endothelial ionic "pump." These pump proteins promote transport of excess fluid from within the corneal stroma back to the aqueous humor. The water channel protein, aquaporin-1 (AQP1), is an integral membrane protein expressed on the plasma membrane of corneal endothelial cells [13]. In mice lacking AQP1, recovery of corneal transparency and thickness after hypotonic swelling is markedly delayed, suggesting that AQP1 plays a role in fluid movement [14]; however, the details of its role in regulating fluid flow remain to be elucidated.

The delicate fluid balance provided by the endothelial barrier and "pump" functions is dependent on maintenance of the integrity of the endothelial monolayer [12]. To maintain monolayer integrity, endothelial cell density (ECD: # cells/mm^2) must remain above a critical number—usually 400–500 cells/mm^2. If the density of endothelial cells is too low, barrier function is lost and more fluid enters the cornea than can be removed through the activity of the ionic "pumps." Loss of endothelial barrier function results in corneal edema and the development of bullous keratopathy, a painful blistering disease characterized by permanent corneal clouding and loss of visual acuity.

Summary for the Clinician

- The major function of the corneal endothelium is to maintain corneal clarity through its barrier and ionic "pump" functions.
- The barrier function of the endothelium is based on the formation of "leaky" tight junctions between cells that permit movement of fluid and nutrients from the aqueous humor into the corneal stroma, but prohibit bulk fluid flow.
- The ionic "pump" function rests in ATP-ase molecules within the plasma membrane. The activity of these ionic "pumps" counterbalances inward fluid flow by promoting movement of excess fluid from the stroma back to the aqueous humor.
- Loss of endothelial cells can compromise the integrity of the endothelium, resulting in corneal edema, bullous keratopathy, corneal clouding, and loss of visual acuity.

6.2 Corneal Endothelial Cell Loss and Repair Mechanisms

6.2.1 Causes of Cell Loss

The decrease in ECD that occurs with age does not normally have a negative effect on the function of the endothelial monolayer. However, endothelial cell loss can be accelerated beyond that observed with increasing age, and it is this loss that can lead to endothelial dysfunction. A significant decrease in ECD can occur for a number of reasons, including accidental or surgical trauma, previous penetrating or endothelial keratoplasty, metabolic stress resulting from systemic or ocular disease, such as diabetes or glaucoma, and endothelial dystrophies.

6.2.2 Repair of the Endothelial Monolayer

Corneal endothelium in humans has a limited capacity for repair. The decrease in ECD observed in vivo as the result of aging or trauma strongly suggests that cell division either does not occur at all or is not efficient enough to replace cells and restore the monolayer to its original density. Microscopic studies clearly indicate that, when a small number of cells die, healthy cells nearest the resulting denuded area respond by flattening and membrane ruffling. Once cells have made contact with their neighbors, this activity stops and mature cell–cell contacts are reformed [15]. In response to larger wounds, cells surrounding the wound and several rows back from the wound area enlarge, flatten, and often shift position as a group to cover the wound [16]. This type of repair is termed "spreading." Individual cells at the wound margin will also migrate into the wound bed, helping to repopulate the area of injury [17]. The overall result of these wound-healing mechanisms is an increase in the overall cell size (polymegathism) and an alteration in cell shape from hexagonal to polygonal to pleomorphic, depending on the extent of the injury [15]. Cell enlargement and the alteration from a hexagonal to more rounded shape can stress cell–cell junctions, thereby compromising monolayer integrity and the ability of the endothelium to retain its barrier function.

> **Summary for the Clinician**
> - Corneal endothelial cells can be lost due to accidental or surgical trauma, previous corneal transplantation, metabolic stress, or dystrophies.
> - Repair of the endothelial monolayer occurs by cell enlargement and migration, rather than by cell division.

6.3 Are Human Corneal Endothelial Cells Able to Divide?

Currently, the loss of corneal clarity caused by the failure of the endothelial barrier is restored by full-thickness corneal transplantation or, more recently, by endothelial keratoplasty. Although keratoplasty has been a successful treatment to restore visual acuity following loss of endothelial integrity, there is a growing interest in determining whether corneal endothelial cells can be induced to divide to increase cell numbers either directly in vivo, or for the preparation of bioengineered endothelium as a means of providing new treatments to maintain or restore monolayer integrity and normal barrier function.

6.3.1 Proliferative Status In Vivo

Several methods have been used to determine whether HCEC retain proliferative capacity. Early specular microscopic studies conducted by Laing, et al. [18] on the endothelium of a corneal graft following a rejection reaction revealed the presence in the endothelium of apparent mitotic figures, suggesting that, at least in some cases, proliferative capacity is retained in vivo. This laboratory conducted studies to determine the cell cycle status of HCEC in vivo [19, 20]. Ex vivo corneas were used to reflect as closely as possible the in vivo condition of normal endothelium. Corneas were obtained with appropriate maintenance of donor confidentiality and selected for study using strict exclusion criteria [21]. The cell cycle status of corneal endothelial cells was determined by observing the relative staining intensity and subcellular localization of a battery of key cell cycle proteins in transverse corneal sections using immunofluorescence microscopy. Together, the results strongly suggest that, under normal conditions, HCEC in vivo are arrested in G1-phase of the cell cycle (see information below regarding the cell cycle).

6.3.2 Evidence that HCEC Retain Proliferative Capacity

A number of studies have been conducted to determine whether HCEC are capable of cell division. One study from this laboratory [22] used an ex vivo corneal wound model in which a portion of the endothelium was removed by gentle mechanical abrasion. Wounded corneas were then incubated in the presence of mitogens. At various times after wounding, cells were immunostained for Ki67, a recognized marker for actively cycling cells.

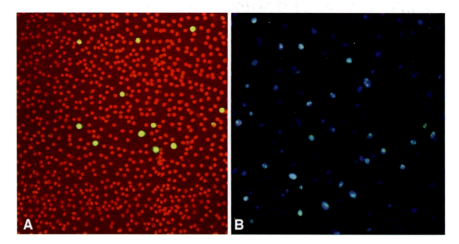

Fig. 6.1 Evidence that HCEC retain proliferative capacity. Confocal fluorescence microscopic image in (**a**) is of the endothelium in an ex vivo cornea from a 66-year-old donor. The endothelium was treated with EDTA to release cell–cell contacts, incubated in mitogen-containing culture medium for 30 h, and then immunostained for Ki67. The image in (**b**) shows subconfluent HCEC cultured from the cornea of a 16-year-old donor and immunostained for Ki67. Cells were stained for Ki67 (*green*) and then counterstained with either propidium iodide (*red*) or DAPI (*blue*) to show all nuclei. Original magnifications: A = 20×; B = 16×

Observation of the staining patterns and counting of Ki67-positive cells clearly indicated that cells at the wound edge and within the wound area were able to proliferate. In another study [23], the endothelium of ex vivo corneas was treated with ethylenediaminetetraacetic acid (EDTA), a calcium–magnesium chelator, to release cell–cell contacts, then incubated in the presence of mitogens, and immunostained for Ki67. Fluorescence confocal microscopic analysis revealed that cells were able to both enter and complete the cell cycle. There is also ample evidence from this and other laboratories that HCEC are able to divide when cultured under appropriate stimulatory conditions [24–26]. Figure 6.1 presents images of Ki67-positive cells in the endothelium of an ex vivo cornea and in a subconfluent culture of HCECs. Altogether, there is sufficient evidence demonstrating that, although HCEC are inhibited in G1-phase of the cell cycle and do not normally divide in vivo, they retain the ability to proliferate.

Summary for the Clinician

- Corneal endothelial cells in vivo do not normally divide, because they are arrested in G1-phase of the cell cycle.
- Under appropriate stimulatory conditions, HCECs will divide, indicating that they retain proliferative capacity.

6.4 The Cell Cycle

To gain a better understanding of the molecular basis underlying the in vivo inhibition of HCEC proliferation and to explore methods to take advantage of the capacity of these cells to divide, it became necessary to gain a better understanding of how the cell cycle is regulated. The cell cycle is divided into multiple phases, each consisting of a highly regulated series of molecular events that lead to cell division. Below is a discussion of important events that are involved in cell cycle progression and in the negative regulation of G1-phase of the cycle.

6.4.1 Positive Regulation of the Cell Cycle

A diagram of the major phases of the cell cycle is presented in Fig. 6.2a. Quiescent, nondividing cells are normally in G0-phase—a "resting" state in which cell cycle protein synthesis is very low and DNA is present in an unduplicated (2N) form. Exposure of cells to appropriate mitogens induces a signaling cascade that leads to entry into G1-phase of the cell cycle. This important phase prepares cells for DNA duplication, which occurs in S-phase. Central to the temporal control of movement from G1- into S-phase is regulation of the activity of the E2F transcription factor, which activates genes required for DNA synthesis [27]. In quiescent cells, the retinoblastoma tumor suppressor, pRb, tightly binds E2F, preventing its activation. In order to negatively regulate E2F activity, pRb must be in a hypophosphorylated state. This low state of pRb phosphorylation is

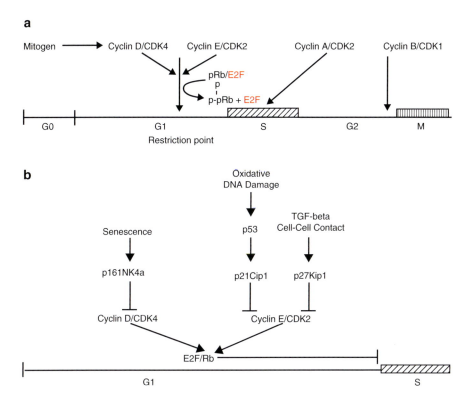

Fig. 6.2 Diagrams illustrating positive regulation of the cell cycle (**a**) and negative regulation of G1-phase of the cell cycle (**b**)

maintained, in part, by the activity of the cyclin-dependent kinase inhibitors (CKIs), p27Kip1, p21Cip1, and p16INK4a. These inhibitors prevent the formation/activation of the cyclin-dependent kinase (CDK) complexes, cyclin D/CDK4, and cyclin E/CDK2. Upon mitogenic stimulation, the cellular level of p27Kip1, p21Cip1, and p16INK4a is decreased due to transcriptional inhibition and/or due to increased degradation by the ubiquitin-proteasome pathway. At about the same time, synthesis of the positive G1-phase regulatory protein, cyclin D, is induced [28]. Cyclin D then binds to CDK4, forming an active kinase complex. pRb is the specific substrate of cyclin D/CDK4 kinase activity. Hyperphosphorylation of pRb by this complex alters the pRb-E2F interaction, promoting activation of E2F, leading to S-phase entry. Cyclin E is synthesized late in G1-phase upon E2F activation. Cyclin E binding to CDK2 helps activate this kinase complex during late G1- and early S-phase. Cyclin E/CDK2 kinase activity, in part, promotes continued hyperphosphorylation of pRb. Thus, a complex positive autoregulatory circuit is formed, promoting movement into S-phase, independent of mitogenic stimulation. Prior to entry into S-phase, cells must pass a "restriction point" in which all molecular conditions must be favorable for DNA duplication. If conditions are not favorable, cells will remain arrested in G1-phase until all molecular criteria for DNA synthesis are met. In S-phase, DNA is duplicated under highly controlled conditions. Effective DNA duplication moves DNA from the 2N to a 4N state. Cyclin A synthesis begins in late G1-phase. Cyclin A binds to CDK2, and the activity of this complex helps down-regulate E2F activity by facilitating its degradation, thus promoting forward progression from S- to G2-phase. Cyclin B synthesis is activated at the end of S-phase. In G2-phase, cyclin B binds to and activates the kinase activity of CDK1. Cyclin B/CDK1 activity promotes molecular changes, such as chromosome condensation, nuclear membrane disassembly, and microtubule reorganization, which prepare the cell for M-phase (mitosis), in which cells undergo division, forming two daughter cells, each of which contains 2N DNA.

6.4.2 Negative Regulation of G1-Phase of the Cell Cycle

An overview of negative regulation of G1-phase is presented in Fig. 6.2b. As mentioned above, the kinase activity of the G1-phase cyclin/CDK complexes is inhibited by CKIs. There are two families of CKIs. The "INK" family includes p16INK4a, which specifically binds to free CDK4, and prevents binding of cyclin D to CDK4 to form an active complex [29]. p16INK4a also competes with cyclin D for binding to CDK4 in existing complexes, thus dissociating the complex. Inhibition of cyclin D/CDK4 kinase activity by p16INK4a prevents the initial downstream hyperphosphorylation of pRb that is required for E2F activation and S-phase entry. Metabolic changes that occur during the development of cellular senescence lead to up-regulation of p16INK4a and subsequent G1-phase arrest. The "Cip/Kip" family includes p21Cip1 and p27Kip1 [30, 31]. Both these inhibitors bind G1-phase cyclin/CDK complexes, inhibiting their kinase activity. In the presence of p16INK4a, the "Cip/Kip" proteins mainly bind and inhibit the activity of cyclin E/CDK2 complexes. Synthesis of p21Cip1 (also known as Waf1 or Sdi1) is induced by the transcription factor, p53, which can be activated by a number of microenvironmental factors, including oxidative DNA damage [32]. The cellular level of p27Kip1 is increased in response to TGF-beta binding to specific cellular receptors and in response to the formation of mature cell–cell contacts [31]. The inhibitory function of all the G1-phase CKIs is extremely important, because it prevents unscheduled entry into S-phase and inappropriate DNA synthesis.

6.5 Potential Causes for Inhibition of HCEC Proliferation In Vivo

In order to evaluate the proliferative capacity of endothelial cells, it is important to understand the reasons why a cell type that retains the ability to divide does not do so, even after significant cell loss. Several factors appear to contribute to the inhibition of division of these physiologically important, but fragile cells. Among these are contact inhibition, lack of significant paracrine or autocrine growth factor stimulation, and the suppressive effect of transforming growth factor-beta. Each of these will be discussed in more detail below.

6.5.1 Cell–Cell Contacts Inhibit Division

As discussed above, corneal endothelium contains focal tight junctions, as well as adhesion and gap junctions. Together, these junctions contribute to the stability of the endothelial monolayer and to its barrier function. In many cell types, the formation of mature cell–cell contacts, particularly those mediated by the cadherin-based adhesion junctions, induces a series of molecular events that result in the inhibition of cell division. This effect of junction formation is frequently called "contact inhibition." In contact-inhibited cells, resistance to cell cycle entry is maintained even when cells are exposed to serum or positive growth factors. Studies in a number of cell types indicate that the G1-phase inhibitor, p27Kip1, plays an important role in mediating cell cycle arrest in contact inhibited cells [31]. A series of studies was conducted in this laboratory to determine whether contact inhibition plays a role in the inhibition of endothelial cell division that normally takes place during corneal development [33]. Neonatal rats were used for these studies, because maturation of the corneal endothelium takes place after birth, facilitating tissue sampling. At several time-points after birth, corneas were removed and the relative expression and subcellular localization of specific cell cycle proteins was determined. Results indicated that the time at which endothelial cell division ceased, as indicated by loss of staining for bromodeoxyuridine (BrdU), correlated with the time that mature cell–cell contacts were formed. This timing also correlated with an increase in the expression of p27Kip1 protein, implicating a role for this CKI in mediating contact inhibition in corneal endothelium. Of importance is the fact that the time at which p21Cip1 was expressed did not correlate with the cessation of division during corneal development, suggesting that this CKI does not play a significant role in contact inhibition in these cells.

> **Summary for the Clinician**
> - The cell cycle is divided into multiple phases, each consisting of a highly regulated series of molecular events that lead to cell division.
> - After mitogenic stimulation, cells enter G1-phase of the cell cycle, which prepares for DNA duplication that occurs in S-phase. After DNA has been duplicated, cells move into G2-phase to prepare cells for actual division into two daughter cells, which occurs in M-phase (mitosis).
> - A key step in the movement of cells from G1- to S-phase is inactivation of the retinoblastoma protein, pRb, resulting in the release and the subsequent activity of the transcription factor, E2F.
> - Movement of cells from G1- to S-phase can be prevented by the activity of the CKIs, p27Kip1, p21Cip1, and p16INK4a, which prevent the inactivation of pRb.

(The expression of p16INK4a was not tested in these studies.) In confluent, contact-inhibited cultures of rat corneal endothelial cells, the protein level of p27Kip1 was found by Western blot analysis to be 20-fold higher than in subconfluent cultures; however, when confluent cultures were treated with EDTA to release cell–cell contacts, the level of p27Kip1 was greatly reduced, providing additional evidence for a role for p27Kip1 in mediating contact inhibition in rat corneal endothelium [34]. A role for cell–cell contacts in the inhibition of proliferation has also been demonstrated for human corneal endothelium in situ and in culture. As described above, in ex vivo human corneas, mechanical wounding of the endothelium [22] or release of cell–cell contacts by treatment with EDTA [23] is sufficient to promote cell division, if the endothelium is exposed to mitogens. Although much information is still needed, accumulating data strongly suggest that the formation and maintenance of cell–cell contacts contributes to the inhibition of cell division observed in corneal endothelium in vivo, and that the CKI, p27Kip1, helps mediate this inhibition.

6.5.2 Endothelium In Vivo Lacks Effective Paracrine or Autocrine Growth Factor Stimulation

It appears that contact inhibition is a major mechanism responsible for cell cycle arrest in corneal endothelium in vivo as long as a critical cell density is maintained. Importantly, cell division also does not occur to any significant extent in corneas in which the endothelial density has decreased below a critical number—a condition in which contact inhibition per se may no longer effectively prevent cell division. This suggests that there are other factors that contribute to the inhibition of cell division in vivo [35]. Although growth factors are present in aqueous humor, associated with Descemet's membrane, and also synthesized by endothelial cells themselves, they may not be present in sufficient concentration or bind effectively enough to cellular receptors to induce and sustain a positive mitogenic signal. Several positive growth factors have been detected within aqueous humor from normal eyes. These include acidic-fibroblast growth factor (FGF), basic-FGF, platelet-derived growth factor (PDGF), and hepatocyte growth factor/scatter factor. Relative levels of these growth factors within aqueous humor appear to be low, and may vary from individual to individual. Levels of certain growth factors may change significantly in response to inflammation, tissue injury, disease, or other ocular insults. Descemet's membrane has been found to bind both acidic- and basic-FGF [36]. In addition to the potential paracrine effect of growth factors in aqueous humor or associated with Descemet's membrane, corneal endothelial cells themselves synthesize and express several growth factors and their receptors, including epidermal growth factor, acidic- and basic-FGF, transforming growth factor-alpha and -beta [37]. Thus, although there is the potential for both paracrine and autocrine growth factor stimulation of corneal endothelial cells in vivo, stimulation of significant cell division does not normally occur.

6.5.3 TGF-Beta2 Has a Suppressive Effect on S-phase Entry

Besides the presence in aqueous humor of several positive growth factors, there is also the potential for negative regulation by factors, such as transforming growth factor-beta2 (TGF-beta2). TGF-beta2 is present mainly in latent form in aqueous humor; however, corneal endothelial cells have been shown to express proteins, such as thrombospondin, which are able to activate TGF-beta [38]. HCEC express mRNA and protein for TGF-beta receptors I, II, and III—all of which are needed for optimal TGF-beta-induced signal transduction [39]. Tritiated-thymidine incorporation studies, as well as semi-quantitative analysis of BrdU incorporation in cultured rabbit [40] and rat corneal endothelial cells [41] indicate that exogenously added TGF-beta2 or activated TGF-beta2 from aqueous humor suppress S-phase entry, thereby suppressing cell division. In other cell types, TGF-beta helps mediate cell cycle arrest by suppressing ubiquitin-proteasome-mediated degradation of p27Kip1, thereby maintaining relatively high levels of this inhibitor. This CDK has also been implicated as a mediator of TGF-beta-induced suppression of corneal endothelial proliferation. In rabbit corneal endothelial cells, TGF-beta2 down-regulates the expression of CDK4 and also prevents nuclear export of p27Kip1 for degradation, thus maintaining a high level of this inhibitory protein [42]. Interestingly, recent evidence suggests that the TGF-beta2 suppressive effect may be due to its stimulation of the synthesis and secretion of prostaglandin E2, which is capable of inhibiting corneal endothelial cell proliferation in a dose-dependent manner [43]. Additional studies are needed to more specifically delineate the cell cycle mechanisms that mediate this inhibitory effect.

> **Summary for the Clinician**
>
> - Several factors contribute to the inhibition of the proliferation of HCEC in vivo, including formation of strong cell–cell contacts (contact inhibition), lack of autocrine or paracrine growth factor stimulation, and the suppressive effect of transforming growth factor-beta2.
> - In vivo G1-phase inhibition of HCEC appears to be mediated, in large part, by the CKI, p27Kip1.

6.6 Proliferative Capacity of HCEC Differs with Donor Age

A number of studies provide strong evidence that HCEC retain the capacity to undergo cell division, although they do not normally divide in vivo. The factors described above appear to contribute to the inhibition of proliferation in vivo. Further study has identified additional factors that affect the relative proliferative capacity of HCEC. One of these factors is donor age. Baum, et al. [24] first described age-related differences in the proliferation of cultured HCEC. In their studies, endothelial cells from donors who were less than 20 years old grew well in culture, whereas, cells from older donors were either difficult to grow or did not grow at all. Results of those early studies have been confirmed and expanded by studies conducted in this laboratory using two different models. The ex vivo corneal wound model described above has provided an opportunity to directly compare the kinetics of cell cycle traverse in HCEC from young (<30 years old) and older donors (>50 years old) [22]. Semi-quantitative analysis of Ki67-positive cells in the wound area revealed a significant decrease in the rate of cell cycle entry and in the relative number of dividing cells in corneas from older compared with younger donors. These age-related differences in proliferative response are illustrated by the graph in Fig. 6.3a. Using a cultured cell model [26, 44], the same number of HCEC isolated from young and older donors were plated at subconfluent density and incubated in mitogen-containing medium. At various times after plating, cells were removed from the tissue culture plate and directly counted. As shown in the graph in Fig. 6.3b, very similar age-related differences in proliferative response were observed in cultured cells as were observed using the ex vivo wound model. Calculation of population doubling time from the log phase of growth indicates that the average doubling time for HCEC cultured from older donors was 90.25 h compared with 46.25 h for cells cultured from young donors [45]. This age-related difference in relative proliferative capacity is also demonstrated by an increase in cell size and a decrease in cell density when HCEC cultured from older donors reach confluence [26]. Comparison of the density of confluent HCEC cultured from young and older donors showed that, in cultures from young donors, cell density averaged 2000 cells/mm^2, while cultures of HCEC from older donors averaged 754.6 cells/mm^2, indicating a statistically significant difference ($p < 0.0001$) between the two [45]. Taken together, studies indicate that, under very similar growth-promoting conditions, there is a difference in relative proliferative capacity based on donor age. The fact that the behavior of cultured HCEC closely mimics cells in situ in terms of their relative proliferative capacity makes cultured HCEC an excellent model to explore the regulation of the corneal endothelial cell cycle.

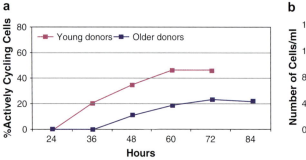
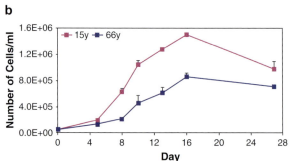

Fig. 6.3 Growth curves demonstrating similar age-related differences in proliferative capacity using an ex vivo corneal wound model (**a**) and a tissue culture model (**b**) as described in the text. Graph in (**a**) presents the average percent of actively cycling cells in the wound area from at least three corneas per age group. Graph in (**b**) presents representative cell counts obtained from HCEC cultured from a 15-year-old and a 66-year-old donor at various times after plating in the presence of mitogens. Adapted from Joyce [44]

6.6.1 Analysis of pRb Hyperphosphorylation

Because the proliferative capacity of HCEC was found to differ with donor age, studies were conducted to examine more closely the molecular mechanisms that underlie that difference. As indicated above, growth factor stimulation leads to the hyperphosphorylation of pRb by specific G1-phase cyclin/CDK complexes. This results in the release and activation of E2F and leads to the downstream expression of proteins required for S-phase entry. Western blot studies of cultured HCEC [46] were conducted to determine whether there is a difference in the level or rate of pRb hyperphosporylation following mitogenic stimulation that would contribute to the observed age-related difference in growth capacity. Semiquantitative analysis of the blots using an antibody that recognizes total pRb protein indicated that the overall expression of pRb was very similar in HCEC, regardless of donor age. Subconfluent cells from the same donors as were used to test total pRb expression were plated at low density and maintained for 24 h in basal medium with no mitogens to induce mitotic quiescence. Mitogens were then added and samples were taken for Western blot analysis at 0, 24, 48, and 72 h after mitogenic stimulation. Hyperphosphorylated pRb was detected using an antibody that specifically recognizes the pRb Ser 807/811 phosphorylation site. Results indicate that pRb was hyperphosphorylated in HCEC from both age groups. In cells from younger donors, pRb hyperphosphorylation increased to maximum levels within the first 24 h, and the level remained high over the 72-h course of the experiment. Importantly, HCEC from older donors exhibited a significantly lower ($p = 0.0077$) basal level of hyperphosphorylation compared with younger cells, and maximum levels of hyperphosphorylation were not reached until 48 h after exposure to mitogens. These results indicate that the kinetics of pRb hyperphosphorylation, a major step in G1-phase leading to E2F activation and S-phase entry, differ in an age-dependent manner, and suggest the existence of age-related differences in the negative regulation of G1-phase in these cells.

6.6.2 Analysis of Replication Competence

Formation of origin-recognition complexes on DNA is required for S-phase entry. These complexes associate with DNA during G1-phase, and are present at sites on chromatin that are at or near future sites of initiation of DNA replication. Binding of these complexes makes chromatin competent (licensed) for replication [47]. Minichromosome maintenance-2 (MCM2) protein is a member of the origin-recognition complex. It is synthesized during G1-phase, binds to specific DNA sites with other components of the origin-recognition complex, and then dissociates from DNA during S-phase. Expression of MCM2 is considered to be a reliable marker to identify replication-competent cells [48]. Studies were conducted using the ex vivo cornea wound model to compare the relative number of replication-competent HCEC in corneas obtained from young and older donors [49]. The endothelium was wounded, incubated in mitogens, immunostained for MCM2 at various times after plating, and positive cells quantified in a manner similar to that described above. Figure 6.4 presents results showing that more HCEC from young donors become competent to replicate. In addition, the relative time at which cells become competent to replicate occurs sooner after mitogenic stimulation in HCEC from young compared with older donors.

6.6.3 Analysis of CKI Protein Expression

The kinetics of pRb hyperphosphorylation in cultured HCEC were similar to those obtained using an ex vivo corneal wound model to examine replication competence. In both cases, fewer HCEC from older donors responded to mitogenic stimulation, and the response was slower than observed in cells from young donors. Overall, the kinetics of the response to mitogens observed in these studies are strikingly similar to the kinetics of cell growth discussed above. Together, these data provide strong evidence that HCEC from older donors are slower

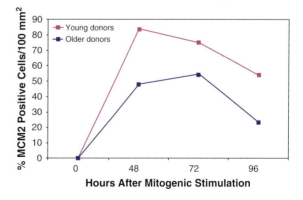

Fig. 6.4 Graph demonstrating an age-related difference in replication competence in HCEC. An ex vivo corneal wound model was used to test for replication competence by immunostaining for MCM2 in HCEC from young and older donors. Graph presents the percent of MCM2-positive cells observed per 100 mm^2 of endothelial wound. Adapted from Mimura [49]

to respond to growth factor stimulation, and exhibit an overall reduced proliferative capacity compared with HCEC from young donors. Since p27Kip1, p21Cip1, and p16INK4a are important negative regulators of G1-phase of the cell cycle, studies were conducted to determine whether differences in the relative expression of these proteins could be responsible, at least in part, for the age-related difference in proliferative capacity [46]. Results from Western blots comparing the relative expression of these three CKIs in primary cultures of HCEC from young and older donors are shown in Fig. 6.5. These results indicate that the relative expression of p27Kip1 does not differ significantly between age groups; however, the expression of both p16INK4a and p21Cip1 was significantly higher in HCEC cultured from older donors.

Together, the results from the studies described above strongly suggest that the CKI, p27Kip1, plays an important role in mediating contact inhibition in corneal endothelium. The similarity in expression of this inhibitor in both age groups suggests that the inhibitory activity of p27Kip1 does not differ with age or significantly contribute to the age-related difference in relative proliferative capacity observed in HCEC. On the other hand, the significant increase in protein levels of both p21Cip1 and p16INK4a in HCEC from older donors provides evidence that both these CKIs help mediate the observed age-related decrease in proliferative capacity. Importantly, a similar profile of CKI expression has been observed in studies of age-related changes in other cell types [50]. Overall, the data provides evidence that the negative regulation of G1-phase induced by the p53/p21Cip1 and p16INK4a/pRb pathways contribute to the age-related decrease in proliferative capacity observed in HCEC.

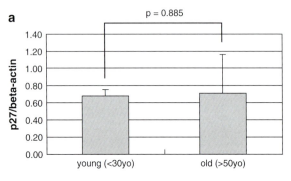
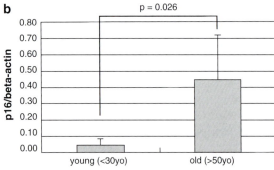
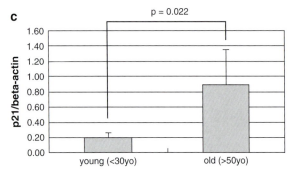

Fig. 6.5 Semi-quantitative analysis of Western blots demonstrating age-related differences in the expression of G1-phase inhibitors in primary cultures of HCEC. Results indicate no significant age-related difference in the relative expression of p27Kip1; however, both p16INK4a and p21Cip1 expression was significantly increased in HCEC cultured from older donors. Adapted from Enomoto et al. [46]. The Association for Research in Vision and Ophthalmology is the original copyright holder

Summary for the Clinician

- Although HCEC retain the ability to divide, their capacity to proliferate decreases with increasing age.
- This decrease has been observed in ex vivo corneal endothelial wounds and in culture.
- The age-related decrease in proliferative capacity is characterized by a decrease in the rate of cell cycle entry and in the relative number of dividing cells.
- Evidence strongly suggests that this age-related decrease in proliferative capacity is the result of an up-regulation in the expression and activity of p21Cip1 and p16INK4a.

6.7 Efforts to Stimulate Corneal Endothelial Proliferation by Interfering with G1-phase Inhibition

The studies described above provide evidence that HCEC retain the ability to proliferate, although they are inhibited in G1-phase of the cell cycle in vivo. Several studies have tested whether HCEC can be induced to divide by overcoming or bypassing this G1-phase inhibition. These are described below.

6.7.1 Overcoming G1-phase Inhibition

The human papilloma virus type 16 oncoproteins, E6 and E7, and the SV40 large-T antigen oncoprotein specifically interfere with the inhibitory activity of the retinoblastoma (pRb) and p53 tumor suppressor proteins, thus overcoming G1-phase inhibition and promoting cell cycle progression. Studies have demonstrated that ectopic expression of either E6/E7 [51] or the SV40 large-T antigen [52] in cultured HCEC results in multiple rounds of cell division, indicating that overcoming G1-phase inhibition promotes proliferation. Another possible method to promote cell cycle progression in HCEC is to overcome G1-phase inhibition by lowering the level of one or more CKIs and thereby removing the constraint to S-phase entry. Studies have been conducted to determine whether treatment of HCEC with p27Kip1 siRNA would promote proliferation, since this CKI appears to play an important role in contact inhibition of these cells [53]. Interestingly, p27Kip1 siRNA treatment successfully decreased expression of p27Kip1 protein in confluent HCEC cultured from both young and older donors; however, this reduced expression only promoted a significant ($p \leq 0.05$) increase in cell numbers in HCEC cultured from young donors. This finding provides evidence that treatment of HCEC with siRNA for CKIs can be effective. The fact that p27Kip1 siRNA treatment only promoted proliferation in HCEC from young donors provides additional evidence that the CKIs, p21Cip1, and p16INK4a, play an important role in G1-phase inhibition in cells from older donors. Studies are currently being conducted in this laboratory to test the effectiveness of p21Cip1 and/or p16INK4a siRNA treatment in promoting proliferation in HCEC cultured from older donors.

6.7.2 Bypassing G1-phase Inhibition

Studies from this laboratory [54] have also attempted to induce proliferation by bypassing G1-phase inhibition and ectopically expressing E2F2, one of the isoforms of E2F that is responsible for activating genes necessary for S-phase entry [55]. For these studies, the endothelium of ex vivo corneas from both young and older donors was transfected with an adenoviral vector containing the full-length gene for E2F2. Ectopic expression of E2F2 was able to induce S-phase entry, as determined by immunostaining for BrdU. The effect of E2F2 expression on cell division was demonstrated by a significant increase ($p \leq 0.05$) in endothelial cell density compared with vector controls. Together, these studies indicate that it is possible to stimulate division in HCEC by overcoming or bypassing G1-phase inhibition.

> **Summary for the Clinician**
>
> - HCEC can be induced to divide by overcoming or bypassing G1-phase inhibition.
> - G1-phase inhibition can be overcome by negating the effect of the CKIs, p27Kip1, p21Cip1, and p16INK4a, through ectopic expression of the viral oncogenes E6/E7 or the SV40-large-T antigen.
> - The inhibitory effect of p27Kip1 can be overcome in HCEC from young donors (<30 years old) by treatment of cells with p27Kip1 small interfering RNA (siRNA), resulting in an increase in cell division. This treatment does not increase cell division in HCEC from older donors (>50 years old), suggesting that p21Cip1 and p16INK4a increase the negative proliferative pressure with increasing donor age.
> - G1-phase inhibition can be bypassed, and cell division can be increased in the endothelium of both young and older donors by ectopic expression of the transcription factor, E2F2.

6.8 Endothelial Topography Affects the Proliferative Capacity of HCEC

Morphologic studies by Amman, et al. [56] have provided evidence that the relative density of HCEC in vivo differs with endothelial topography. These studies demonstrated that, regardless of donor age, the relative density of endothelial cells in the paracentral (2.7 mm from the center) and peripheral regions (4.7 mm from the center) was significantly higher than in central endothelium. The relative density of cells in each region decreased with increasing donor age; however, cells in central endothelium always exhibited the lowest density. Interestingly, topographic differences in proliferative capacity and in the distribution of senescent cells have also been observed in the endothelium.

6.8.1 Differences in Proliferative Capacity

Studies conducted by Bednarz, et al. [57] found that HCEC cultured from the central 6.5 mm diameter of the endothelium have a morphology similar to that of cells in vivo and exhibit no mitogenic activity. In contrast, cells cultured from the 6.5 to 9.0 mm peripheral rim appeared to have looser cell–cell contacts and exhibited greater mitogenic activity. Together, results suggested that the proliferative capacity of HCEC differs based not only on donor age, but also on their in vivo location. Studies conducted in this laboratory [49] have further explored this idea. To determine whether there is a relationship between proliferative capacity and endothelial topography, the endothelium was divided into two areas for study. The 6.0 mm diameter central area was designated as "central" endothelium, while the 6.0–9.5 mm rim was designated as "peripheral" endothelium. Experiments were conducted using an ex vivo corneal wound model to determine whether there are topographically related differences in relative proliferative capacity in the endothelium. In these studies, a wound was made in the endothelium of corneal quarters. This wound extended from the center to the peripheral rim. Corneas were then incubated in mitogen-containing medium and, at 12-h intervals, were immunostained for MCM2 to identify replication-competent cells. The relative percent of MCM2-positive cells was then determined. Results for the first 72 h after wounding showed that the competence of HCECs to replicate was consistently lower in central endothelium compared with the peripheral rim in both age-groups. Interestingly, the relative percent of replication-competent cells was significantly lower (average p-value 36–72 h after wounding was $p=0.0017$; range: $p=0.0012$–0.0127) in the central area of older donors compared with young donors.

6.8.2 Differences in Senescence Characteristics

Characteristics of senescent cells include decreased saturation density, slower cell cycle kinetics, stable arrest with a 2N DNA content, and increased expression of p21Cip1 and p16INK4a protein [58, 59]. Senescent cells also stain for senescence-associated beta-galactosidase (SA-B-Gal), a recognized marker of cellular senescence [60]. Since HCEC from older donors exhibit a number of these characteristics, studies were conducted to further identify senescent cells within the endothelial population [49]. The presence of senescent cells was investigated by staining the endothelium of ex vivo corneas for SA-B-Gal. SA-B-Gal is not a specific form of beta-galactosidase, but staining for the "senescence" form can be detected at pH 6.0 rather than the normal pH 4.0 [60]. Scoring of the endothelium for the relative intensity of SA-B-Gal staining showed few to no senescent cells in either the central or peripheral area in corneas from young donors. In corneas from older donors, SA-B-Gal staining was detectable at low to moderate levels in the periphery, but moderate to intense levels in cells within the central area, indicating a greater percentage of senescent cells in central endothelium of older donors.

The structural basis for the topographical changes observed in HCEC from older donors remains to be identified. Age-related changes similar to those found in HCEC have been described in other ocular cells that lie within the light-path, including retinal pigment epithelial cells (RPE) [61] and lens epithelial cells [62]. Interestingly, RPE cells exhibit a topographical difference in growth potential, similar to that found in HCEC, in that cells from the macula exhibit reduced proliferative capacity compared with cells from the peripheral equatorial region [63]. Thus, it is possible that similar mechanisms are responsible for decreased proliferative capacity in cells that are located within the light path.

> **Summary for the Clinician**
> - Proliferative capacity and the expression of senescence characteristics are also affected by endothelial topography.
> - Cells within the central 6.0 mm diameter of the endothelium in corneas from older donors exhibit the lowest proliferative capacity and contain the greatest percentage of senescent cells.

6.9 Identification of Mechanisms Responsible for Decreased Proliferative Capacity

Together, the accumulated data strongly suggest that there is both an age-related and topographical difference in the relative proliferative capacity of corneal endothelial cells, and that this difference is related to cellular senescence. Researchers in the field have identified two forms of cellular senescence: replicative senescence and stress-induced premature senescence. Replicative senescence results from the successive shortening of telomeres that occurs during DNA replication [64]. Once telomeres have eroded to a critically short length, the senescence program is activated and cells become irreversibly inhibited from dividing. Stress-induced premature senescence is caused by exposure of cells to certain environmental stresses [65]. Stress-induced premature senescence is considered to be "premature" because cells lose the ability to proliferate prior to telomere exhaustion. Thus, in this form of senescence, cells retain proliferative potential based on telomere length, but stop dividing due to inhibitory mechanisms activated by stress-induced damage pathways. Studies have been conducted to identify the form of "senescence" that is responsible for the age- and topographically-related decrease in proliferative capacity in HCEC.

6.9.1 Are Critically Short Telomeres Responsible for Decreased Proliferative Capacity?

Egan, et al. [66] measured telomere restriction fragment (TRF) lengths in HCEC isolated from donors aged 5 weeks to 84 years, and found that the mean TRF length was 12.2 kb, regardless of donor age. This length is sufficient to support several additional rounds of cell division prior to the formation of critically short telomeres. This laboratory confirmed and extended these findings using a peptide nucleic acid/fluorescein isothiocyanate (PNA/FITC) probe that specifically binds to telomere repeats [67]. The intensity of telomere staining in ex vivo corneas and in HCEC freshly isolated from donor corneas showed no statistical age-related or topographic difference indicative of a difference in telomere length. Together, these data strongly suggest that HCEC retain the potential to divide based on telomere length, and that the observed decrease in proliferative capacity is NOT due to "replicative senescence."

6.9.2 Is Sub-lethal Oxidative DNA Damage Responsible for Decreased Proliferative Capacity?

Stress-induced premature senescence can be induced by sub-lethal oxidative stress, which occurs when the concentration of reactive oxygen species (ROS) exceeds antioxidant defenses [68]. ROS are normal intracellular by-products of metabolism, and the rate of ROS production is determined by the metabolic rate of the cell [69]. ROS are generated in mitochondria, peroxisomes, and microsomes. Of these, mitochondria appear to generate the greatest amount of ROS. Light, particularly in the UV wavelengths, is an environmental source that generates ROS by the physical activation of oxygen [70]. Chronic low levels or acute high levels of oxidative stress can cause damage to cellular constituents, including lipids, proteins, and DNA. Although both mitochondrial DNA (mtDNA) and nuclear DNA are targets of oxidative damage, the nuclear genome is considered to be the most vulnerable, because it normally contains only two copies of DNA, while mtDNA is present in several thousand copies per cell [71]. Oxidation of guanine to form 8-hydroxy-2′-deoxyguanosine (8-OHdG) acts as a marker of oxidized DNA and accumulates with age [69, 72]. When DNA is damaged, cells initiate a response that is appropriate for the extent of the damage. This response can include DNA repair, activation of checkpoint pathways that lead to cell cycle delay, entry into senescence, or induction of apoptosis. Stress-induced DNA damage inhibits proliferation and induces cellular senescence through activation of specific checkpoint pathways [68, 73]. The DNA damage response appears to be actively maintained in senescent cells, suggesting that DNA damage signals persist and cell cycle inhibition is maintained as long as DNA has not been appropriately repaired [74].

Corneal endothelium is metabolically very active and lies directly in the light-path, making it potentially vulnerable to oxidative stress and subsequent DNA damage. As such, studies were recently conducted to determine whether there is a relationship between oxidative stress, oxidative DNA damage, and reduced proliferative capacity in HCEC [21]. DNA damage was first quantified by a competitive ELISA assay using an antibody directed against 8-OHdG. Total DNA was purified from HCEC that had been directly isolated from the central and peripheral endothelium of young and older donors. The average concentration of 8-OHdG per nanogram of DNA was found to be higher in cells isolated from older donors, and this difference was mainly contributed by a statistically significant ($p = 0.0031$) increase in oxidative DNA damage within the central endothelium. Since DNA is present in both mitochondria and nuclei, immunostaining for 8-OHdG was used to determine the location of oxidized DNA damage in the endothelium of ex vivo corneas. Within the peripheral area, the majority of 8-OHdG staining was found in a punctate pattern within the cytoplasm. Similar localization and staining intensity was observed in the peripheral area from both young and older donors, strongly suggesting that, in this area of the endothelium, oxidative DNA damage is localized mainly within mitochondria. As shown by the images in Fig. 6.6, localization and intensity of 8-OHdG differed in central endothelium in an age-dependent manner. In corneas from young donors, only a light staining was visible in nuclei, and the majority of stain was localized in the cytoplasm in a pattern very similar to that observed in the periphery. Interestingly, intense 8-OHdG staining was found in the nuclei of cells within the central endothelium of older donors. Observation of a number of samples from older donors indicated that there was a difference in the relative number of cells within the central area, exhibiting intense nuclear 8-OHdG staining, and suggesting that the relative extent of oxidative DNA damage differed from cell to cell and from donor to donor. Overall, the 8-OHdG staining patterns indicate that there is a greater amount of oxidative nuclear DNA damage in HCEC within the central area in older donors, but that the extent of the damage can differ.

To test whether there is a relationship between oxidative stress and proliferative capacity in HCEC, a study

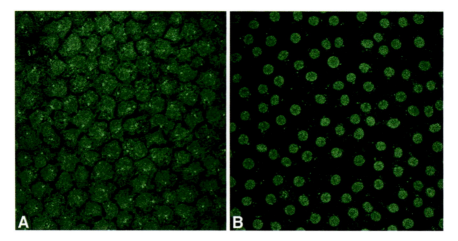

Fig. 6.6 Representative confocal fluorescence micrographs illustrating 8-OHdG staining patterns in central endothelium of a 27-year-old (**a**) and 71-year-old donor (**b**). Note the light punctate staining of the cytoplasm in (**a**) and the intense nuclear staining in (**b**). Original magnification: 40X, zoom 2

was conducted in which subconfluent HCEC cultured from young donors were exposed to low concentrations of hydrogen peroxide (H_2O_2), a known oxidative stressor. Cells were then tested for their ability to divide using a protocol that was based on a study designed to determine the effect of oxidative stress on the proliferation of human diploid fibroblasts [75]. As shown in the graph in Fig. 6.7, HCEC not exposed to H_2O_2 and cells exposed to a low concentration (25 μM) of H_2O_2 showed similar robust growth curves. With increasing concentrations of H_2O_2, the growth of HCEC was reduced. Importantly, the growth kinetics of these cells from young donors closely resembled those observed in HCEC from older donors (compare with Fig. 6.3a, b). Together, these results provide strong evidence for the existence of a relationship between oxidative stress, oxidative nuclear DNA damage, and reduced proliferative capacity in HCEC.

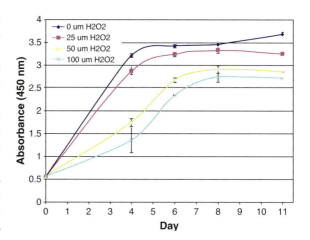

Fig. 6.7 Graph demonstrating a dose-dependent effect of H_2O_2-induced oxidative stress on the growth of HCEC from a 26-year-old donor. Cell numbers were determined over a period of 11 days using a WST-8 spectrophotometric assay. This graph presents cell numbers as a function of absorbance at 450 mm. Note the decrease in both growth rate and saturation density upon exposure of young HCEC to 50 or 100 μM H_2O_2. Reprinted with permission from: Joyce et al. [21]. The Association for Research in Vision and Ophthalmology is the original copyright holder

Summary for the Clinician

- Decreased proliferative capacity in HCEC is not due to the presence of critically short telomeres, a hallmark of "replicative senescence."
- The age- and topographically related decrease in the ability of HCEC to proliferate appears to be due to a form of "stress-induced premature senescence" caused by sub-lethal oxidative nuclear DNA damage.

6.10 Future Directions

Over the last several years, the study of cell cycle control and replication in corneal endothelium has progressed significantly. The data indicate that HCEC are normally inhibited in G1-phase of the cell cycle, due, at least in part, to the activity of the CKIs, p27Kip1, p21Cip1, and p16INK4a. Data also suggest that p27Kip1 is mainly involved in contact inhibition, while p21Cip1 and p16INK4a expression and activity are mainly dependent on environmental factors. Correlation of the age-related reduction in proliferative capacity with the age-related increase in p21Cip1 and p16INK4a expression is important, because it has focused studies toward the identification of molecular mechanisms that may be responsible for these changes. The finding that HCEC do not possess critically short telomeres, regardless of donor age, strongly suggests that the age-related reduction in proliferative capacity is due to a form of stress-induced premature senescence. The fact that replication competence is reduced and SA-B-Gal staining is increased in the central endothelium of older donors is significant, because it has provided a potential link between age, oxidative stress, and reduced proliferative capacity. This relationship was demonstrated in studies in which the kinetics of cell cycle progression in HCEC from young donors were altered compared to those in older donors by exposure of young cells to H_2O_2-induced oxidative stress.

Together, results of these studies have led to the following hypothesis: Throughout life, the corneal endothelium does not normally replicate and is inhibited in G1-phase of the cell cycle as the result of contact inhibition and other anti-proliferative environmental conditions. In young individuals, G1-phase inhibition of HCEC is mediated mainly by the CKI, p27kip1; however, these cells retain a high capacity to proliferate. With increasing age, oxidative stress increases in HCEC due to their high metabolic activity and chronic exposure to light. This accumulated stress results in a gradual increase in oxidative nuclear DNA damage, particularly in central endothelium. This damage induces a signaling cascade that results in apoptosis in highly damaged cells, and in increased expression of p21Cip1 with a subsequent decrease in proliferative capacity. This accumulated damage, together with other unidentified factors, results in up-regulation of the expression of p16INK4a, which provides additional inhibitory pressure and further reduces proliferative capacity. Clearly, additional studies are needed to support this hypothesis, but it provides a framework with which to consider the regenerative capacity of corneal endothelial cells.

As mentioned above, there is growing interest in developing new treatments for the loss of clear vision that accompanies loss of corneal endothelial barrier function. In order to successfully develop such treatments, it is important to move forward with studies to overcome or bypass G1-phase inhibition in vivo and to explore culture methods to prepare bioengineered endothelium, since several methods are promising and can take advantage of the proliferative capacity retained by endothelial cells. At the same time, there is the intriguing possibility that further exploration into the molecular mechanisms underlying the age- and topographically related reduction in proliferative capacity would yield information that could prevent or reverse the effects of oxidative stress on these cells, thereby increasing the ability to these fragile cells to divide.

Summary for the Clinician

- The new data presented here and future proof of this new hypothesis should provide the basis for further exploration of the molecular mechanisms underlying the age- and topographically related decrease in proliferative capacity of HCEC.
- This exploration could lead to the development of methods to prevent or reverse the effects of oxidative stress on HCEC.
- These new methods would increase the ability of HCEC to divide to actively repair the endothelial monolayer and prevent the devastating effect of the loss of endothelial barrier function on vision.

References

1. Waring GO 3rd, Bourne WM, Edelhauser HF et al (1982) The corneal endothelium: normal and pathologic structure and function. Ophthalmology 89:531–590
2. Kreutziger GO (1976) Lateral membrane morphology and gap junction structure in rabbit corneal endothelium. Exp Eye Res 23:285–293
3. Barry PA, Petroll WM, Andrews PM et al (1995) The spatial organization of corneal endothelial cytoskeletal proteins and their relationship to the apical junctional complex. Invest Ophthalmol Vis Sci 36:1115–1124
4. Petroll WM, Hsu JK, Bean J et al (1999) The spatial organization of apical junctional complex-associated proteins in feline and human corneal endothelium. Curr Eye Res 18:10–19
5. Ottersen OP, Vegge T (1977) Ultrastructure and distribution of intercellular junctions in corneal endothelium. Acta Ophthalmol (Copenh) 55:69–78
6. Mandell KJ, Berglin L, Severson EA et al (2007) Expression of JAM-A in the human corneal endothelium and retinal pigment epithelium: localization and evidence for role in barrier function. Invest Ophthalmol Vis Sci 48:3928–3936
7. Valtink M, Gruschwitz R, Funk RH et al (2008) Two clonal cell lines of immortalized human corneal endothelial cells

show either differentiated or precursor cell characteristics. Cells Tissues Organs 187:286–294
8. Leuenberger PM (1973) Lanthanum hydroxide tracer studies on rat corneal endothelium. Exp Eye Res 15:85–91
9. Williams K, Watsky M (2002) Gap junctional communication in the human corneal endothelium and epithelium. Curr Eye Res 25:29–36
10. Kaye GI, Mishima S, Cole JD et al (1968) Studies on the cornea. VII. Effects of perfusion with a Ca^{++}-free medium on the endothelium. Invest Ophthalmol Vis Sci 7:53–66
11. Stiemke MM, McCartney MC, Cantu-Crouch D et al (1991) Maturation of the corneal endothelial tight junction. Invest Ophthalmol Vis Sci 32:2757–2765
12. Maurice DM (1972) The location of the fluid pump in the cornea. J Physiol 221:43–54
13. Hamann S, Zeuthen T, La Cour M et al (1998) Aquaporins in complex tissues: distribution of aquaporins 1–5 in human and rat eye. Am J Physiol 274:C1332–C1345
14. Thiagarajah JR, Verkman AS (2002) Aquaporin deletion in mice reduces corneal water permeability and delays restoration of transparency after swelling. J Biol Chem 277:19139–19144
15. Laing RA, Sandstrom MM, Berrospi AR et al (1976) Changes in the corneal endothelium as a function of age. Exp Eye Res 22:587–594
16. Honda H, Ogita Y, Higuchi S et al (1982) Cell movements in a living mammalian tissue: long-term observation of individual cells in wounded corneal endothelial of cats. J Morphol 174:25–39
17. Matsuda M, Sawa M, Edelhauser HF et al (1985) Cellular migration and morphology in corneal endothelial wound repair. Invest Ophthalmol Vis Sci 26:443–449
18. Laing RA, Neubauer L, Oak SS et al (1984) Evidence of mitosis in the adult corneal endothelium. Ophthalmology 91:1129–1134
19. Joyce NC, Meklir B, Joyce SJ et al (1996) Cell cycle protein expression and proliferative status in human corneal cells. Invest Ophthalmol Vis Sci 37:645–655
20. Joyce NC, Navon SE, Roy S et al (1996) Expression of cell cycle-associated proteins in human and rabbit corneal endothelium in situ. Invest Ophthalmol Vis Sci 37:1566–1575
21. Joyce NC, Zhu CC, Harris DL (2009) Relationship between oxidative stress, DNA damage, and proliferative capacity in human corneal endothelium. Invest Ophthalmol Vis Sci 50(5):2116–2122
22. Senoo T, Joyce NC (2000) Cell cycle kinetics in corneal endothelium from old and young donors. Invest Ophthalmol Vis Sci 41:660–667
23. Senoo T, Obara Y, Joyce NC (2000) EDTA: a promoter of proliferation in human corneal endothelium. Invest Ophthalmol Vis Sci 41:2930–2935
24. Baum JL, Niedra R, Davis C et al (1979) Mass culture of human corneal endothelial cells. Arch Ophthalmol 97:1136–1140
25. Chen KH, Azar D, Joyce NC (2001) Transplantation of adult human corneal endothelium ex vivo. Cornea 20:731–737
26. Zhu CC, Joyce NC (2004) Proliferative response of corneal endothelial cells from young and older donors. Invest Ophthalmol Vis Sci 45:1743–1751
27. Leone G, DeGregori J, Jakoi L et al (1999) Collaborative role of E2F transcriptional activity and G1 cyclin dependent kinase activity in the induction of S phase. Proc Natl Acad Sci USA 96:6626–6631
28. Sherr CJ (1993) Mammalian G1 cyclins. Cell 73:1059–1065
29. Serrano M, Hannon GJ, Beach D (1993) A new regulatory motif in cell-cycle control causing specific inhibition of cyclin D/CDK4. Nature 366:704–707
30. Harper JW, Adami GF, Wei N et al (1993) The p21 Cdk-interacting protein Cip1 is a potent inhibitor of G1-cyclin-dependent kinases. Cell 75:805–816
31. Polyak K, Kato JY, Solomon MJ et al (1994) P27Kip1, a cyclin-Cdk inhibitor, links transforming growth factor-β and contact inhibition to cell cycle arrest. Genes Dev 8:9–22
32. Helton ES, Chen X (2007) p53 modulation of the DNA damage response. J Cell Biochem 100:883–896
33. Joyce NC, Harris DL, Zieske JD (1998) Mitotic inhibition of corneal endothelium in neonatal rats. Invest Ophthalmol Vis Sci 39:2572–2583
34. Joyce NC, Harris DL, Mello DM (2002) Mechanisms of mitotic inhibition in corneal endothelium: contact inhibition and TGF-β2. Invest Ophthalmol Vis Sci 43:2152–2159
35. Joyce NC (2003) Proliferative capacity of corneal endothelium. Prog Retin Eye Res 22:359–389
36. Gospodarowicz D, Delgado D, Vlodavsky I (1980) Permissive effect of the extracellular matrix on cell proliferation in vitro. Proc Natl Acad Sci USA 77:4094–4098
37. Wilson SE, Schultz GF, Chegini N et al (1994) Epidermal growth factor, transforming growth factor alpha, transforming growth factor beta, acidic fibroblast growth factor, basic fibroblast growth factor, and interleukin-1 proteins in the cornea. Exp Eye Res 59:63–71
38. Schultz-Cherry S, Lawler J, Murphy-Ullrich JE (1994) The type 1 repeats of thrombospondin 1 activate latent transforming growth factor-beta. J Biol Chem 269:26783–26788
39. Joyce NC, Zieske JD (1997) Transforming growth factor-beta receptor expression in human cornea. Invest Ophthalmol Vis Sci 38:1922–1928

40. Harris DL, Joyce NC (1999) Transforming growth factor-beta suppresses proliferation of rabbit corneal endothelial cells in vitro. J Interferon Cytokine Res 19:327–334
41. Chen KH, Harris DL, Joyce NC (1999) TGF-beta2 in aqueous humor suppresses S-phase entry in cultured corneal endothelial cells. Invest Ophthalmol Vis Sci 40:2513–2519
42. Kim TY, Kim WI, Smith RE et al (2001) Role of p27(Kip1) in cAMP- and TGF-beta2-mediated antiproliferation in rabbit corneal endothelial cells. Invest Ophthalmol Vis Sci 42:3142–3149
43. Chen KH, Hsu WM, Chiang CC et al (2003) Transforming growth factor-beta2 inhibition of corneal endothelial proliferation mediated by prostaglandin. Curr Eye Res 26: 363–370
44. Joyce NC (2005) Cell cycle status in human corneal endothelium. Exp Eye Res 81:629–638
45. Joyce NC, Zhu CC (2004) Human corneal endothelial cell proliferation: potential for use in regenerative medicine. Cornea 23:S8–S19
46. Enomoto K, Mimura T, Harris DL et al (2006) Age-related differences in cyclin-dependent kinase inhibitor expression and retinoblastoma hyperphosphorylation in human corneal endothelial cells. Invest Ophthalmol Vis Sci 47:4330–4340
47. Stoeber K, Tlsty TD, Happerfield I et al (2001) DNA replication licensing and human cell proliferation. J Cell Sci 114:2027–2041
48. Wharton SB, Chan KK, Anderson JR et al (2001) Replicative Mcm2 protein as a novel proliferation marker in oligodendrogliomas and its relationship to Ki67 labelling index, histological grade and prognosis. Neuropathol Appl Neurobiol 27:305–313
49. Mimura T, Joyce NC (2006) Replication competence and senescence in central and peripheral human corneal endothelium. Invest Ophthalmol Vis Sci 47:1387–1396
50. Quereda V, Martinalbo J, Dubus P et al (2007) Genetic cooperation between p21Cip1 and INK4 inhibitors in cellular senescence and tumor suppression. Oncogene 26: 7665–7674
51. Wilson SE, Weng J, Blair S et al (1995) Expression of E6/E7 or SV40 large T antigen-coding oncogenes in human corneal endothelial cells indicates regulated high-proliferative capacity. Invest Ophthalmol Vis Sci 36:32–40
52. Wilson SE, Lloyd SA, He YG et al (1993) Extended life of human corneal endothelial cells transfected with the SV40 large T antigen. Invest Ophthalmol Vis Sci 34:2112–2123
53. Kikuchi M, Zhu C, Senoo T et al (2006) p27kip1 siRNA induces proliferation in corneal endothelial cells from young, but not older donors. Invest Ophthalmol Vis Sci 47:4803–4809
54. McAlister JC, Joyce NC, Harris DL et al (2005) Induction of replication in human corneal endothelial cells by E2F2 transcription factor cDNA transfer. Invest Ophthalmol Vis Sci 46:3597–3603
55. DeGregori J, Leone G, Miron A et al (1997) Distinct roles for E2F proteins in cell growth control and apoptosis. Proc Natl Acad Sci USA 94:7245–7250
56. Amann J, Holley GP, Lee SB et al (2003) Increased endothelial cell density in the paracentral and peripheral regions of the human cornea. Am J Ophthalmol 135:584–590
57. Bednarz J, Rodokanaki-von Schrenck A, Engelmann K (1998) Different characteristics of endothelial cells from central and peripheral human cornea in primary culture and after subculture. In Vitro Cell Dev Biol Anim 34:149–153
58. Campisi J (1996) Replicative senescence: an old lives' tale? Cell 84:497–500
59. Cristofalo VJ (1988) Cellular biomarkers of aging. Exp Gerontol 23:297–305
60. Dimri GP, Lee X, Basile G et al (1995) A biomarker that identifies senescent human cells in culture and in aging skin in vivo. Proc Natl Acad Sci USA 92:9363–9367
61. Hjelmeland LM, Cristofalo VJ, Funk W et al (1999) Senescence of the retinal pigment epithelium. Mol Vis 5:33
62. Chylack LT Jr (1984) Mechanisms of senile cataract formation. Ophthalmology 91:596–602
63. Burke JM, Soref C (1988) Topographical variation in growth in cultured bovine retinal pigment epithelium. Invest Ophthalmol Vis Sci 29:1784–1788
64. Wright WE, Shay JW (1992) Telomere positional effects and the regulation of cellular senescence. Trends Genet 8:193–197
65. Ben-Porath I, Weinberg RA (2005) The signals and pathways activating cellular senescence. Int J Biochem Cell Biol 37:961–976
66. Egan CA, Savre-Train I, Shay JW et al (1998) Analysis of telomere lengths in human corneal endothelial cells from donors of different ages. Invest Ophthalmol Vis Sci 39:648–653
67. Konomi K, Joyce NC (2007) Age and topographical comparison of telomere lengths in human corneal endothelial cells. Mol Vis 13:1251–1258
68. Toussaint O, Medrano EE, von Zglinicki T (2000) Cellular and molecular mechanisms of stress-induced premature senescence (SIPS) of human diploid fibroblasts and melanocytes. Exp Gerontol 35:927–945
69. Melov S (2000) Mitochondrial oxidative stress: physiologic consequences and potential for a role in aging. Ann NY Acad Sci 908:219–225
70. Van der Zee J, Krootjes BBH, Chignell CF et al (1993) Hydroxyl radical generation by a light-dependent Fenton reaction. Free Radic Biol Med 14:105–113

71. Lombard DB, Chua KF, Mostoslavsky R et al (2005) DNA repair, genome stability, and aging. Cell 120:497–512
72. Beckman KB, Ames BN (1997) Oxidative decay of DNA. J Biol Chem 272:19633–19636
73. Von Zglinicki T, Saretzki G, Ladhoff J et al (2005) Human cell senescence as a DNA damage response. Mech Ageing Dev 126:111–117
74. Lou Z, Chen J (2006) Cellular senescence and DNA repair. Exp Cell Res 312:2641–2646
75. Chen JH, Stoeber K, Kinsgbury S et al (2004) Loss of proliferative capacity and induction of senescence in oxidatively stressed human fibroblasts. J Biol Chem 279: 49439–49446

Chapter 7

Current State of the Art of Fitting Gas-Permeable (GP) Contact Lenses

Silke Lohrengel, Dieter Muckenhirn

Core Messages

- The range of indications for GPs has increased greatly in recent years.
- New technical developments in corneal measuring techniques, rational and reproducible oscillating contact lens (CL) manufacturing techniques, and modern automatic CL fitting modules on new generation corneal topographer systems allow more fittings in less time with the same or better quality and accuracy.
- When fitting CL in patients with KC, the three-point touch method, or bridging of the apex with central oblong geometries are recommended in both spherical and toric lenses.
- New keratoplasty techniques do not make visual rehabilitation with CL redundant. GP in various designs (primarily toric and quadrant differentiated) are the solution of choice.

7.1 Corneal Topography and Automatic Fitting Programs

When selecting and fitting the back surface of a GP, it is important to be as well informed as possible about the cornea's contours. The current state-of-the-art technique for acquiring such knowledge is video corneal topography (VCT) [1, 2].

Some corneal topographers offer a selection of lens designs from various manufacturers, and thus the possibility to simulate a GP's sit and fluo-image [3–7]. Automatic fitting programs allow us to choose, for extremely variable corneal shapes, from all the lens types now being manufactured, and to simulate their fit, thus enabling us to identify the ideal lens for every corneal contour.

The programs are easy to use. After the measurements have been taken, the data relevant to fitting are fed into the automatic fitting program. The software evaluates the data, and then produces an "ideal" lens geometry model corresponding to the input data. A suggestion is then made regarding the fit. Rotation-symmetric, multicurved lenses are usually required for spherical corneas with slight eccentricity, aspherical lenses for corneas with increased eccentricity, and for toric corneas, the appropriate toric lenses with radius differences corresponding to the corneal torus.

The same applies to the keratoconus (KC), whereby KC lenses are recommended according to the stage of the disease. Lenses with oblong or reverse geometry are recommended for postoperative corneas whose periphery is steeper than the center. Lenses tailor-made according to varying quadrants can be fitted on complex corneas such as those having undergone keratoplasty (PK). It is important that all the possible GP designs be available and that each particular lens suggestion be individually processed.

Summary for the Clinician

- Manifold representation and analytical methods of the corneal surface up to diagnosis and classification of the KC and/or other corneal irregularities with VCT
- Automatic fitting programs make a realistic fluo-image simulation possible, offering a practical solution for nearly all conditions with the result of fewer or no diagnostic lenses

7.2 Fitting CLs

Corneal lenses with a total diameter smaller than that of the cornea are in much wider use than scleral lenses. However, scleral lenses have been attracting more attention recently for patients with complex corneal conditions. They are indicated when an irregular corneal topography cannot be fitted with any other type of lens (including quadrant-differentiated GPs). They are also indicated for patients as therapeutic CL for various tearing-related dysfunctions, when they function as tear reservoirs [8].

All CLs, whether GP or soft, should fit so that wearing them is as comfortable as possible. Well-fitting CLs should fulfill the following requirements:

- They should only disturb the corneal metabolism to the extent that no permanent damage to, or changes in, the cornea can occur.
- They should fit so well on the cornea that the patient has no or only minimal foreign-body sensation in the eyes.
- They should prevent any and all corneal deformations.
- They should fulfill these criteria for many years.

These criteria can only be fulfilled when corneal topography, lens design, and fitting technique are closely coordinated. This is best achieved using the alignment fitting technique [9, 10]. This method is based on the selection of a back surface whose central area parallels the corneal profile, and whose peripheral area of the CL has a slightly higher eccentricity than the cornea. This permits the broadest possible distribution of pressure, good lens mobility, and unhindered tear exchange at the same time.

Every cornea has a natural surface that cannot be compared with a technical surface, which is why the alignment fitting technique can only be employed with certain restrictions.

When presented with high central toricity, the alignment fit is adapted with the flatter meridian while the steeper meridian is fitted with two thirds of the difference in the radii. This procedure causes the lens to tip slightly during blinking, which encourages the exchange of tears while facilitating vertical lens movement.

Irregular corneal topographies challenge us with completely different conditions. Still, the alignment fitting method's fundamentals should be adhered to as far as possible when dealing with them as well. With quadrant-differentiated lenses, the CL specialist can achieve a fit accommodating the corneal topography that both improves the site of the lens and enhances wearing comfort.

> **Summary for the Clinician**
>
> - Alignment fitting technique provides the broadest possible distribution of pressure, good lens mobility, and unhindered tear exchange at the same time
> - The rate of peripheral corneal flattening affects significantly the GP fitting relationship. Thus, the eccentricity is the key to choosing the best CL geometry.
> - Corneal lenses are usually the lens of choice, even for irregular corneas. Scleral or miniscleral lenses are a temporary solution, or indicated for patients with tearing-related dysfunctions.

7.3 The Keratoconus

The keratoconus (KC) is well known as a bilateral, asymmetric, and progressive disease of the eye that involves stromal thinning and a corneal bulge [11]. Nowadays, thanks to modern topographical systems, the disease is being diagnosed earlier and more often than previously – its incidence is 50–230:100,000 [12], and its etiology remains unknown. There are thus numerous theories, and eye rubbing is considered a cause (or at least responsible for the condition's progression). Another is the effect of CL and their fit on keratoconic eyes [13–18]. The belief that a flat-fitting CL can have a therapeutic effect has been disproven convincingly. Rather than being a form of therapy, it is the only form of correction prior to keratoplasty with which to improve visual acuity (VA).

7.3.1 KC Peculiarities in Conjunction with CL

7.3.1.1 Corneal Sensitivity and Maximum Resilience

The corneal sensitivity of KC patients is 2.5 times greater than that of a normal cornea, and the KC cornea is also softer. Moreover, KC patients wearing GPs had more inflammatory cells in their lacrimal fluid than did a group of myopics with whom they were compared [19]. Their risk of infection is therefore higher, and special attention must be paid to achieving good GP mobility and sufficient tear exchange.

7.3.1.2 Corneal Contour-KC Stage-KC Type

The following key characteristics of the KC cornea are important for the fitting technique, GP geometry and centering:

- relatively steeper central radius compared to the normal eye
- eccentricity (of ≥0.7) that usually exceeds that of a normal eye
- position and steep inclination of the apex
- regular astigmatic sections and
- condition (i.e., scarring, subepithelial hyperplasia)

7.3.2 Forms of Correction

When a KC is being fitted with a GP, the goal is always to improve VA in comparison to uncorrected or spectacle-corrected vision. As about 50% of KC patients rub their eyes excessively, it is not clear whether rubbing, or in the same context GP wear, exacerbates the disease. Glasses remain the preferred form of correction when VA is adequate.

7.3.2.1 Soft Lenses

Soft lenses only function in patients with regular astigmatism, not the irregular type. Even thick soft lenses cannot correct aberrations substantially better than glasses [20]. They are thus only an alternative to glasses in patients with anisometropias in need of correction. Maximum priority must be given to good mobility and use of a highly oxygen-permeable material so as to prevent vascularization. The newest generation of up to 0.4 mm central, thick soft lenses is not recommended due to insufficient oxygen permeability even with the highest oxygen-permeable materials.

7.3.2.2 GP Contact Lenses

Of all the available forms of correction, it is rigid lenses that are worn by 65–90% of all KC CL wearers [18, 21, 22]. They possess the best vision-improving characteristics and provide the KC patient with the best VA. Moreover, irregular astigmatism is corrected by the lacrimal lens that is formed, which improves aberrations caused by KC most effectively as well [23].

7.3.2.3 Piggyback

The wishful thinking behind this form of correction is the combining of the comfort of a soft lens with the corrective benefits of GP lenses. A drawback is the handling and cleaning of both systems – a considerable inconvenience. Furthermore, oxygen permeability is significantly reduced. The piggyback system, rather like training wheels, makes sense for beginners who find RGP lenses too uncomfortable initially but then "graduate" to them later [21].

7.3.2.4 Hybrid Lenses

The problem with these CLs, which have a rigid center and soft rim, is that their parameters are too few and not varied enough, and they have a very low DK value in the periphery. Sticking CL and vascularization are often the result, making this form of correction inadvisable.

> **Summary for the Clinician**
>
> - RGP are the best and most common treatment for KC.

7.3.3 Fitting Techniques

The GP lens is the CL of choice for patients with KC [11, 13, 14, 18, 20–22, 24]. Below is a list of the main fitting methods employed.

7.3.3.1 The Reshape and Splint Method

With the reshape and splint method the CL for a patient with KC is designed to be flat in the center and sometimes even in the periphery, which causes increased pressure on the apex. VA is ultimately better than that with a parallel-fitted GP [14], although potential damage to the cornea is a drawback. The reshape and splint technique may raise the risk of apical abrasion, staining, and scarring, while the disease's progression is not interrupted, as used to be believed. The reshape and splint technique in association with increased apical load is not generally recommended for patients with KC [11, 13, 18, 20–22, 24].

7.3.3.2 The Three-Point Touch Method

The current fitting method of choice is the three-point touch method, which involves gentle touching of the apex and the distribution of the main source of pressure over the midperiphery [25]. On a cross-sectional view, the lens seems to be resting on three points. Without using a VCT, the clinician

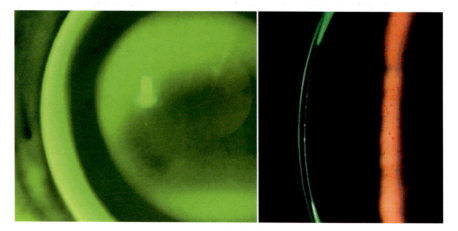

Fig. 7.1 Optical section for tear-layer thickness control

chooses the central GP radius measuring 0.1 mm steeper than the cornea's horizontal radius. It is important to use a flexibly formable GP geometry with good edge lift so as to do justice to the gradually flattening corneal contour. There is a good compromise between VA and corneal integrity. The only limitation is that in cases of progressive KC, this method can quickly degenerate into a precipitous reshape and splint method with its familiar drawbacks. The optical section with the slit lamp is the best control of tear-layer thickness (Fig. 7.1). Frequent follow-ups are required.

7.3.3.3 The Apical Clearance Method

Here, the apex is relieved of pressure while pressure from the GP is transferred over to the midperiphery with good edge lift and pooling. This fitting technique is necessary in the presence of central scarring or hyperplasias. VA is worsened because of the steeper GP radii together with a pressure relieved apex. To improve VA while maintaining the sagittal depth (thus improving the condition of the apex), it is recommended that the peripheral multicurved and central oblong GP geometry be used. They seem to rectify the KC eye's aberrations and thus to at least maintain, or even improve, VA [25, 26]. This typification of GP geometry may become the standard fitting method of the future, bringing patients apical relief without vision loss – as long as peripheral edge lift is maintained (Lohrengel (2008) Individual fit of KC lenses. VDC; Widmer (2008) What are we doing with the apex? Berner KC symposium, unpublished presentations) (Fig. 7.2).

7.3.3.4 Scleral Fitting Method

In patients with KC Type-C or pellucid marginal degeneration – that is, the apex lies very deep – it could be necessary to fit a miniscleral lens to distribute lens pressure on the sclera. We can only recommend this fitting of miniscleral lenses over corneal lenses in exceptional cases because of poorer tear exchange.

7.3.4 GP Fitting Following Cross Linking

The cornea's radii and its geometry can change due to crosslinking, which is why a new GP fitting session is necessary after this treatment. Subjective tolerability is often reduced because these patients have heightened sensitivity. An apex-relieving fit = apical clearance fitting method is usually advisable (Ecke (2008) GP fitting after crosslinking, Berner KC symposium (presentation), unpublished).

> **Summary for the Clinician**
> - Whether the three-point touch or apical clearance method is used depends on the cornea's epithelial condition in conjunction with the patient's potential VA and good comfort. An alignment fit is optimal, but usually achievable only in very mild cases of KC. From there, aim is the three-point touch method or an apical clearance fit, usually with corneal lenses.
> - Best control of apical clearance is the optical section with the slit lamp (Fig. 7.1).
> - Whether spherical, toric, or quadrant-differentiated KC back surfaces are used depends on whether the KC patient has regular or irregular corneal astigmatism, as well as the peripheral surface gradient.
> - Good peripheral edge lift and pooling is imperative to achieve subjective wearing comfort and adequate tear exchange.

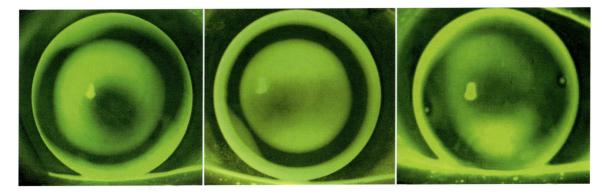

Fig. 7.2 Three-point touch method (KAKC-F); apical clearance (KAKC-F Pro 2), three-point touch method with a toric KAKC-F

7.4 CL Fitting Following Penetrating Keratoplasty

The most common diseases that lead to penetrating keratoplasty (PK) and subsequent CL fitting are KC (63%), Fuchs' endothelial dystrophy (18%) and trauma (7.4%). All the other categories such as bullous keratopathy, caustic injury, other types of dystrophy, herpes, etc., only amount each to 1–3% (retrospective data over 5 years, Eye Hospital, University Freiburg). These CL data differ from common indications for PK, especially on country-specific differences [27, 28].

7.4.1 Indications for CLs Following PK

Regardless of the underlying disease or surgical technique CLs, CLs are fit for optical or therapeutic reasons. Optical reasons [29–33] are irregular astigmatism in 62.9% of patients, and severe regular astigmatism making glasses inappropriate, as well as spheric (57.1%) and astigmatic (54.3%) anisometropias (multiple answers were permitted). Any visual deficiency that can be corrected with glasses consisting of the magnification of an image by 5% can be better corrected with CL. Whether soft or GP lenses are required depends on the cornea's irregularities. Only regular astigmatism can be corrected with soft CLs. Soft lenses allow for only minimally better VA than glasses, whereas GP lenses compensate for the cornea's irregularities and thus overall imaging defects via the tear film [20]. An average of 30% of transplanted patients wear GP lenses and enjoy complete visual rehabilitation [34]. What plays a key role in determining patient motivation to wear CL is the underlying disease, a history of allergy, maximum VA with glasses, and their own VA expectations. Many patients with a VA of more than 20/40 but low visual demand prefer to wear glasses, even if CL provided better vision. Patients with PK after KC are usually the most highly motivated, thanks to their positive experience with CL prior to surgery. Tolerance problems with CL are most common in patients with a history of allergy. Advice concerning lens care and what solutions to use is more important for them because they generate more lens deposits.

Soft CLs that are highly oxygen-permeable or very large and flat (total diameter ≈17.5, central radius ≈9 mm) are used therapeutically [32] to accelerate epithelial healing.

7.4.2 Indications for CLs Following PK in Comparison with Newer Surgical Techniques

Newer surgical techniques such as PK with Intrastromal Ring or Femtolaser and Descemet Stripping Automated Endothelial Keratoplasty (DSAEK) and Deep Anterior Lamellar Keratoplasty (DALK) For CL specialists it is worth noting how new techniques change the corneal surface and thus the typical indications for CL (i.e., irregular or high astigmatism, anisometropia, and high-order aberrations) just like they also change visual stability and the time it takes to achieve it. That visual results correlate with the surgeon and his skill is a statement common in all recent publications. What remains controversial is the degree of astigmatism and visual outcome following different surgical techniques [28, 35, 36]. Results in Freiburg revealed average postoperative astigmatism following traditional PK, which did not differ from that associated with PK with an intrastromal ring [37] or deep anterior lamellar keratoplasty (DALK). Apparently high-order aberrations tend to increase in association with DALK [36], which would make CL continuation to be necessary. In those patients in whom a descemet stripping automated endothelial keratoplasty (DSAEK) is indicated, this new surgical procedure leads to less astigmatism and faster visual rehabilitation than when PK alone is carried out [28, 37, 38]. In those cases, CL fitting mostly proves to be unnecessary. For KC patients, who represent the majority of CL wearers following PK, PK with the Femtolaser is of particular interest. Further investigation will demonstrate whether astigmatism can be reduced and what effects the procedure has on total visual rehabilitation.

7.4.3 PK Peculiarities in Conjunction with CLs

7.4.3.1 Corneal Sensitivity, Fitting Quality, and Frequent Follow-Ups

The corneas of patients who have undergone PK are much less sensitive long after surgery. Even after 7 years, only 18% of PK patients have regained normal corneal sensitivity, whereas 40% have no central sensitivity [39, 40]. This obviously means that the fitter must take special care to monitor the fit, since most patients cannot feel when something is wrong. Frequent follow-ups are a must.

7.4.3.2 The Endothelium and Choice of GP Materials

It is advisable to use a hyper oxygen-permeable material (DK 81-140) because the postPK cornea suffers from a chronic loss of endothelial cells [41–44] and it does not become dehydrated so rapidly. When deciding which material is most appropriate, it is not enough to consider its oxygen permeability (DK) value alone, rather, the DK value must be converted over the average thickness (DK/L) of the lens for each refraction as shown in Table 7.1.

Materials with columns in red do not possess adequate oxygen permeability for daily wear. Only materials and lens power in black do not hinder endothelial function.

7.4.3.3 Immune Reactions

Immune reactions occur in about 25% of normal-risk PK after 5 years [45], whereas prognosis of high-risk cases is significantly worse (history of ocular herpes simplex virus keratitis: 60%, increased risk of graft rejection as the only risk factor: 35%, glaucoma: 30%, and limbal stem cell insufficiency: 56%. These immune reactions do not seem to be triggered by GP wear (retrospective study over 4 years) [31] as long as no vascularization or loose sutures occur [30]. After 7 years, there was no effect on endothelial cell density compared to a group without GP. [46].

7.4.4 When to Fit?

The highest priority regarding when to fit must be given to improving the patient's VA, particularly, when the other eye is also seriously impaired. In such cases, fitting can be initiated after 6 weeks (with sutures in place) as long as the postoperative course has been good and follow-up frequent. VA improves significantly after 3 months, as do contrast and stereo vision [29, 30]. Therefore, it might be preferable to start fitting 3 months postoperatively.

The ideal fitting time, however, is 6 months following surgery [29, 47, 48], since by then the corneal surface is more stable (corticosteroid ointment or eyedrops have been discontinued, and healing has progressed).

Table 7.1 DK/L of GP materials with averaged thickness according to lens power

GP power		−12.00 dpt	−6.00 dpt	−3.00 dpt	0.00 dpt	+3.00 dpt	+6.00 dpt	+12.00 dpt
Average thickness (mm)		0.258	0.213	0.207	0.227	0.211	0.239	0.295
Material	DK	DK/L	DK/L	DK/L	DK/L	DK/L	DK/L	DK/L
Alberta XL	15	5.8	7.0	7.2	6.6	7.1	/6.3	5.1
Boston Es	28	10.8	13.3	13.5	12.3	13.3	17.2	9.5
Boston EQ	47	18.2	22.0	22.7	20.7	22.3	19.6	15.9
Boston ES2	50	19.4	23.5	24.2	22.0	23.7	20.9	16.9
Boston XO2	145	56.2	68.0	70.0	63.9	68.7	60.7	49.2
Paragon HDS	50	19.4	23.5	24.2	22.0	23.7	20.9	16.9
CM optimum extra	100	38.8	46.9	48.3	44.0	47.4	41.8	33.9
Largado onsi	56	21.7	26.3	27.0	24.7	26.5	23.4	19.0

Another important point is that the cornea changes its shape after each suture removal, thus making a new GP necessary [48]. Close cooperation with the surgeon is key to coordinating financial and organizational matters. In this way, the sutures can remain in place far longer in those patients who tolerate GP well.

Special attention is required in high-risk PK patients, that is, following caustic injury, with herpes simplex virus keratitis or existing epithelial defects. The healing process should not be interrupted or hindered and recurrences of the underlying disease should be avoided. Contraindications for fitting GPs are loose sutures, infiltrates, and infections [48].

7.4.5 Fitting Techniques

The modified contour fit is the best fitting technique that permits a distribution of pressure as uniform as possible over all of the irregularities (such as steps, edges, suture bulges, and small bumps) while maintaining adequate mobility. The pressure from the GP's back surface is distributed onto the center of the transplant and the host's cornea. The GP geometry necessary to achieve this goal depends on the condition and type of PK that was carried out. As opposed to the methods reported in most of the published articles on this subject [32, 33, 47, 49], 60–70% toric back surfaces was used, often with central radius differences of 0.8–2 mm for optimal pressure distribution and lens centering.

7.4.5.1 PK with One or Two Sutures

Miniscleral CL can be a good option in the patient whose cornea's midperiphery cannot be used as a CL fitting zone because of the presence of sutures. Pressure is distributed in the transplant center and sclera. If it can be centered, all kinds of corneal lens can be fitted, usually with large diameters.

7.4.5.2 CL Fitting Following Suture Removal

There are three types of PK relevant to GP in fitting terms:

Type 1: The transplant is steeper than the host's cornea (flat periphery);

Type 2: The transplant is flatter than the host's cornea (steeper periphery);

Type 3: A combination of types 1 and 2 with each meridian behaving differently.

Type 1. This is one of the easiest ways to treat; but they are found less often; more in conjunction with Fuchs' endothelial dystrophy than in KC. The GP geometries used to treat KC patients are also used for type 1 patients following PK. They become much flatter in the periphery and usually center very well around the highest point in the cornea where the transplant is located. The transplant's diameter (and thus that of the GP) plays a subsidiary role; a smaller diameter could be a good option in this type but not with the PK types described later.

Type 2. The transplant is flatter than the host's cornea. The cornea is oblong in shape, which makes it much more

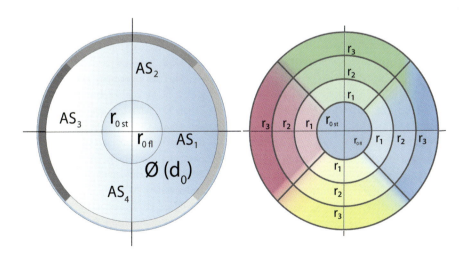

Fig. 7.3 Current production parameters of the Quadro-AS and Quadro-KA quadrant-differentiated lenses offer a plethora of fitting options. The back surface of this lenses can be rotation-symmetric or toric, the peripheral zones aspherical and/or multicurved, and the quadrants can differ in having reverse and/or oblong regions. Thus, it is possible to produce lenses possessing all of the abovementioned lens designs distributed over four quadrants. Should a lens with a rotation-symmetric central zone be required, a prism ballast is generally needed so that it inclines in the correct direction. An additional prism ballast is only necessary with toric back surfaces when the differences in the radii do not permit independent inclination

difficult to center the GP. A flatter periphery, which would otherwise facilitate natural centering around the cornea's highest point, is absent. It is often impossible to predict in which direction a normal rotation-symmetric GP will become decentered [50]. Reverse GP geometries [49], rotation symmetric, and toric combined with large GP diameters are used to achieve the best possible centering. They are often enhanced with extras such as ventilation holes to allow air bubbles to escape, and with oval GP shapes or ballast to reduce the upper lid's influence.

Type 3. This combination constitutes a variety of high central astigmatisms that change direction and size in the periphery. These corneal shapes cannot be satisfactorily accommodated by rotation-symmetric or toric back surfaces. Quadrant-differentiated lenses (Fig. 7.3), however, are an effective alternative. They are the only lenses that can accommodate the various toricities in the center and periphery, as well as the different eccentricities in individual quadrants that the PK patient often presents.

Large diameters are generally fitted in combination with many extras such as ventilation holes and prism ballast. Toric back surfaces are required in 60–70% of the GPs prescribed. The fitter's aim should be to obtain good edge lift for patient comfort and as broad a distribution of the lens' pressure over the corneal surface as possible.

Abbreviations

ABR	Aberration coefficient
CL	Contact lens
CT	corneal topographer
DALK	Deep Anterior Lamellar Keratoplasty
DK	Oxygen permeability
DK/L	Contact lens transmissibility
DSAEK	Descemet Stripping Automated Endothelial Keratoplasty
GP	Gas-permeable contact lens
KC	Keratoconus
PK	Penetrating keratoplasty
VA	Visual acuity
VCT	Video corneal topographer

Summary for the Clinician

- About 30% of PK patients require GP for visual rehabilitation (especially with high spherical and toric anisometropias and irregular astigmatism).
- The earliest fitting session should be 6 weeks after surgery, but 3 months later is even better, as the patient's visual status has stabilized by then.
- A new fitting session becomes necessary after each suture removal, since both the refraction and corneal contour change.
- The fitter must take special care, as the patient's central cornea has become hyposensitive; frequent follow-ups are required to monitor long-term tolerance.
- Be aware of patients with a history of allergies. Tolerance problems and lens deposits are more common than in other patients.
- GP fitting in patients with PK is safe, as they do not seem to present increased immune reactions.
- There is no standard, predictable back surface geometry associated with PK patients that would facilitate GP fitting. Toric-GP as well as quadrant-differentiated back surfaces are advisable in about 60–70% of GP back surfaces.
- Compared to patients with regularly contoured corneas, the PK patient following refractive surgery requires a wide knowledge about CL geometry and more diagnostic lenses [51].

References

1. Bürki E (2001) Neue Möglichkeiten der Hornhautdiagnostik mit Hilfe der Videokeratometrie. NOJ 10:52–55; 11:52–55; 12:52–57
2. Herrmann C, Ludwig U, Duncker G (2008) Korneale topographie. Ophthalmologe 105:193–206
3. Berentsen DA (2008) Imaging and instrumentation in contact lens practice. Contact Lens Spectrum 5:26–31
4. Jani BR, Szczotka LB (2000) Efficiency and accuracy of two computerizes topography software systems for fitting rigid gas permeable contact lenses. CLAO J 26(2):91–96
5. Lebow K (2007) Topographical maps can give you clues about how to best fit challenging contact lens cases. A map to contact lens wear success. Optom Manag 42(4):55–59
6. Neumann S, Seiwert A (1998) Die Verwendbarkeit des Oculus-Keratograph für die praktische Kontaktlinsenanpassung. NOJ 40(6):52–58
7. Szczotka L (2000) Enhancing your RGP fitting efficiency. Contact Lens Spectrum 5:54
8. Rosenthal P et al (2007) Use of fluid-ventilated GP scleral lens for management of severe keratoconjunctivitis sicca secondary to chronic graft-versus-host disease. Biol Blood Marrow Transplant 13(9):1016–1021
9. Muckenhirn D (1980) Ascon – mehr als nur eine neue Kontaktlinse. DOZ 35:240–249

10. Muckenhirn D (1981) Fitting individual contact lenses with the use of computer topometrie. Contacto Int Cont Lens J 25(6):28–34
11. Barr JT et al (2006) Estimation of the incidence and factors predictive of corneal scarring in the CLEK study. Cornea 25(1):16–25
12. Li X, Yang H, Rabinowitz Y (2007) Longitudinal study of keratoconus progression. Exp Eye Res 85:502–507
13. Edrington T et al (2004) Variables affecting rigid contact lens comfort in the CLEK study. Optom Vis Sci 81(3): 182–188
14. Lee JL, Kim MK (2004) Clinical performance and fitting characteristics with a multicurve lens for keratoconus. ECL 30(1):20–24
15. McMonnies Ch (2005) The biomechanics of keratoconus and rigid contact lenses. ECL 31(2):80–92
16. McMonnies Ch (2007) Abnormal rubbing and keratectasia. ECL 33(6):265–271
17. McMonnies Ch (2008) Management of chronic habits of abnormal eye rubbing. Cont Lens Anterior Eye 31(2): 95–102
18. Wagner H et al (2007) Collaborative longitudinal evaluation of keratoconus (CLEK) study. Methods and findings to date. Contact Lens Anterior Eye 30:223–232
19. Lema I et al (2008) Inflammatory response to contact lenses in patients with keratoconus compared with myopic subjects. Cornea 27(7):758–763
20. Griffiths M et al (1998) Masking of irregular corneal topography with contact lenses. CLAO J 24(2):76–81
21. Sonsino J (2006) Advanced concepts in fitting contact lenses. Contact Lens Spectrum 21(12):20–24
22. Zadnik K et al (2005) Comparison of flat and steep rigid contact lens fitting methods in keratoconus. Optom Vis Sci 82(12):1014–1021
23. Edwards M et al (2001) The genetics of keratoconus. Clin Exp Ophthalmol 29:345–351
24. Gundel RE et al (1996) Feasibility of fitting contact lenses with apical clearance in keratoconus. Optom Vis Sci 73(12): 729–732
25. Hu CY, Tung HC (2008) Managing keratoconus with reverse-geometry and dual-geometry contact lenses: a case report. ECL 34(1):71–75
26. Kusy PA, Barr JT (2006) Fitting reverse geometry lenses for keratoconus. Contact Lens Spectrum 10:24–27
27. Darlington JK et al (2006) Trends of PK in the US form 1980–2004. Ophthalmology 113(12):2171–2175
28. Geerling G et al (2005) Lamelläre keratoplastik. Ophthalmologe 102:1140–1151
29. Brahma A et al (2000) Visual function after PK for KC: a prospective longitudinal evaluation. BJO 84:60–66
30. Lim L, Resudovs K, Coster DJ (2000) Penetrating keratoplasty for keratoconus: visual outcome and success. Ophthalmology 107(6):1125–1131
31. Silbiger JS, Cohen E, Laibson PR (1996) CLAO J 22(4): 266–269
32. Szczotka L, Lindsay R (2003) Contact lens fitting following corneal graft surgery. Clin Exp Optom 86(4):244–249
33. Wietharn BE, Driebe WT (2004) Fitting contact lenses for visual rehabilitation after penetrating keratoplasty. ECL 30(1):31–33
34. Brierly SC et al (2000) PK for KC. Cornea 19(3):329–332
35. Ardjomand N et al (2007) Quality of vision and graft thickness in Deep anterior lamellar and Penetrating corneal allografts. Am J Ophthalmol 143(2):228–235
36. Bahar I et al (2008) Comparison of three different techniques of corneal transplantation for KC. Am J Ophthalmol 146(6):905–912
37. Bahar I et al (2008) Comparison of posterior lamellar keratoplasty techniques to penetrating keratoplasty. Ophthalmology 115(9):1525–1533
38. Ham L et al (2009) Visualr rehabilitation rate after isolated descemet membrane endothelial keratoplasty. Arch Ophthalmol 127(3):252–255
39. Macalister GO, Woodward EG, Buckley RJ (1993) The return of corneal sensitivity following transplantation. J Br cont lens Assoc 16(3):99–104
40. Ruben M, Colebrook E (1979) Keratoplasty sensitivity. BJO 63:265–267
41. Cornea donor study investigator group (2008) Donor age and corneal endothelial cell loss 5 years after successful corneal transplantation. Specular microscopy ancillary study results. Ophthalmology 115(4):627–632
42. Ing JJ et al (1998) Ten-year postoperative results of penetrating keratoplasty. Ophthalmology 105(10): 1855–1865
43. Reinhard T et al (2002) Endothelzellverlust nach PK. Klin Monatsbl Augenheilkunde 219:410–416
44. Zadok D et al (2005) Penetrating keratoplasty for keratoconus long term results. Cornea 24(8):959–961
45. Böhringer D et al (2003) Systematic EDP-supported acquisition of follow-up data of keratoplasty patients – report on ten years experience. Klin Monatsbl Augenheilkd 220: 253–256
46. Bourne WM, Shearer DR (1995) Effects of long-term rigid contact lens wear on the endothelium of corneal transplants for KC 10 years after PK. CLAO J 21(4): 265–267
47. Geerards A, Vreugdenhil W, Khazen A (2006) Incidence of RGP contact lens wear after KP for KC. ECL 32(4): 207–210
48. Yeung KK, Olson MD, Weissmann BA (2002) Am J Ophthalmol 133(5):607–612
49. Lim L et al (2000) Reverse geometry contact lens wear after photorefractive keratectomy, radial keratotomy, or penetrating KP. Cornea 19(3):320–324

50. Collins RS, Jarecke AJ, Traver R (2002) Contact lens stability after penetrating keratoplasty. Contact Lens Spectrum 17(12):26–32
51. Szczotka-Flynn L et al (2008) Disease severity and family history in keratoconus. BJO 92:1108–1111
52. Birnbaum F et al (2008) Perforierende Keratoplastik mit intrastromalem Hornhautring. Ophthalmologe 105: 452–456
53. Edrington T, Barr JT (2002) Post-PK contact lens care. Contact Lens Spectrum 17(8):50

Chapter 8

Allergic Disease of the Conjunctiva and Cornea

Andrea Leonardi

Core Messages

- Allergic conjunctivitis is not a single disease.
- Allergic conjunctivitis is characterized by one or more of the following symptoms: itching, tearing (commonly with anterior rhinorrhea), or lid swelling.
- The severity of allergic conjunctivitis ranges from mild and intermittent to seriously debilitating.
- Seasonal and perennial allergic conjunctivitis (PAC) are the most common entities and do not involve the cornea.
- The cornea may be involved in vernal keratoconjunctivitis (VKC), atopic keratoconjunctivitis (AKC), or contact blepharoconjunctivitis, but never in seasonal conjunctivitis or PAC.
- An accurate clinical history and evaluation of signs and symptoms allow the diagnosis of ocular allergy and the definition of possible sensitizing antigens.
- IgE-mediated hypersensitivity and mast cell degranulation are the initial pathophysiological mechanisms.
- Th2-type of cytokines, chemokines, and other multiple mediators are overexpressed in ocular allergy.
- Epitheliotoxic proteins, cytokines, and chemokines liberated from eosinophils and Th2 cells may act concomitantly in the pathogenesis of shield ulcer.
- Keratoconus (KC) is frequently associated with atopy.
- Infections can rarely complicate corneal inflammation in VKC and AKC.
- Allergic conjunctivitis is important in the context of corneal transplantation.
- Nonpharmacological measures and avoidance are extremely important for disease management.
- Therapy should not include vasoconstrictors and, if possible, corticosteroids.
- Mast cell stabilization and histamine antagonism are the main pharmacological interventions.
- Dual action drugs are the first choice in the treatment of ocular allergy.
- The cost of treating allergic conjunctivitis and indirect costs related to loss of workplace productivity from the disease are substantial.
- Severe cases need intense treatment.

8.1 Introduction and Classification

Ocular allergy can involve all the components of the ocular surface, including the lid and lid margin, the conjunctiva, and the lacrimal system. Corneal involvement is typically restricted to the two most severe forms of ocular allergy, vernal keratoconjunctivitis (VKC), and atopic keratoconjunctivitis (AKC). In fact, anatomical, physiological, and immunological properties of the cornea render it relatively protected from allergic inflammation. The cornea is more frequently involved in autoimmune diseases, at times as the initial presenting sign of a new autoimmune disease or as a new sign in patients with a long-standing history of autoimmune systemic disease.

Approximately one-third of the world population is affected by some form of allergic disease and ocular involvement is estimated to be present in 40–60% of this population. Allergic conjunctivitis is a localized allergic condition frequently associated with rhinitis but often observed as the only or prevalent allergic sensitization. This disease ranges in severity from mild forms, which can still interfere significantly with quality of life, to severe cases characterized by potential impairment of visual function.

The term allergic conjunctivitis refers to a collection of hypersensitivity disorders that affects the lid and the conjunctiva. Various clinical forms are included in the classification of ocular allergy (Table 8.1): seasonal (SAC) and perennial allergic conjunctivitis (PAC), VKC, AKC, giant papillary conjunctivitis (GPC), and contact or drug-induced dermatoconjunctivitis [1].

In 2001, the European Academy of Allergy and Clinical Immunology suggested a classification for allergic conjunctivitis, dividing the disorder into IgE-mediated and non-IgE-mediated conjunctivitis, thus trying to provide a more schematic immunopathological approach to classification [2]. IgE-mediated conjunctivitis can be divided into intermittent and persistent conjunctivitis, the latter of which is classified into vernal and AKC. However, this classification has limitations and may create more confusion [3]. For example, contact blepharitis or dermatoconjunctivitis (CDC) is a non-IgE-mediated form of localized contact dermatitis that is immunologically different from VKC or AKC. Contact lens-related GPC should be considered a non-IgE-mediated disease, mechanically related to lens microtrauma, which shares some immunopathological aspects with VKC. In this chapter, allergic conjunctivitis, allergic keratoconjunctivitis, and corneal problems related to allergy will be considered.

8.2 Clinical Forms

8.2.1 Seasonal and Perennial Allergic Conjunctivitis

Seasonal allergic conjunctivitis (SAC) is the most common form of ocular allergy. It is associated with sensitization and exposure to environmental allergens, particularly pollen. The perennial form, PAC, usually involves sensitization to mites or to multiple antigens. More than 95% of patients with seasonal conjunctivitis or PAC have allergic rhinitis, justifying the use of "allergic rhinoconjunctivitis" as a synonym for this disease. Allergic rhinoconjunctivitis may be associated with other airway disorders and is considered a predisposing factor for the development and exacerbation of asthma, sinusitis, otitis media with effusion, and nasal polyposis.

SAC and PAC are characterized by onset in childhood or early adulthood. They are typical IgE-mediated diseases, characterized by spikes of histamine and other mediators released from the conjunctival-activated mast cells that clinically correspond to episodes of ocular itching, redness, and lid swelling frequently associated with rhinitis. Other ocular signs of allergic conjunctivitis include mild serous or serous–mucous secretions, and/or slight papillary or follicular hypertrophy of the conjunctiva. Symptoms may be occasional, seasonal, or persistent. Apart from the presence of itching, no sign or symptom related to SAC or PAC is specific or pathognomic [1]. The most important diagnostic tool for SAC and PAC is a thorough medical history. Although these conditions are not serious, they are very disturbing to patients and can significantly affect their quality of life. Correlations between allergic symptoms and psychological disturbances have been reported. Allergic rhinoconjunctivitis significantly reduces the patient's overall energy and negatively affects behavior, leading to increased school absenteeism and decreased work productivity [4].

Acute or hyperacute episodes of ocular allergy, also called anaphylactoid reactions, are characterized by acute itching and eyelid swelling either as urticaria (hives and wheals) in the superficial layers of the skin, or angioedema in the deeper, subcutaneous tissues, or both. These reactions can be unilateral or bilateral and the conjunctiva may or may not be affected. Insect bites, food allergy, or contact hypersensitivity can be involved in the etiology of these reactions.

8.2.2 Vernal Keratoconjunctivitis

VKC is a severe ocular allergic disease that occurs predominately in children [1, 3, 5]. Most VKC patients complain of symptoms from early spring to fall, with differences among climate zones. Exacerbations of the disease and acute episodes arise, triggered by allergen exposure or, more frequently, by nonspecific stimuli such as wind, light, and dust. VKC is an IgE- and Th2-mediated disease; however, only 50% of patients present a clearly defined allergic sensitization [5, 6].

Intense itching, tearing, and photophobia are the classic symptoms of these patients. The presence of pain associated with photophobia is indicative of corneal involvement. Foreign body sensation may be caused by mucous hypersecretion, papillae hypertrophy, and superficial keratopathy. Various grades of conjunctival hyperemia and chemosis are always present in both forms of the disease. The tarsal form is characterized by irregularly sized hypertrophic papillae, leading to a cobblestone appearance on the upper tarsal plate and abundant mucus that may be incarcerated between them. A variation of the tarsal form of VKC may appear as diffuse upper tarsal conjunctival thickening with fine and diffuse subepithelial fibrosis without papillae formation. The limbal form

Table 8.1 Ocular allergic diseases

Condition	Prevalence	Severity	Causes	Sign/symptoms
SAC/PAC	Most frequent ocular allergic disease 10–15% of population	Mild/moderate	Genetic predisposition Associated with rhinitis Seasonal allergens (pollens, molds, chemicals) Perennial allergens (dust, animal dander, foods, chemicals)	Itching, redness, tearing, watery discharge, chemosis, lid swelling
VKC	Rare Ages 3–20 Under 14 M>F In adults M > F	Severe	Genetic predisposition? Associated with atopic disorders (50%) Th2 upregulation nonspecific eosinophil activation	Extreme itching, mucous discharge, giant papillae, trantas' dots, SPK/ulcer, conjunctival eosinophilia
AKC	Rare Second to fifth decade of life M>F	Severe/sight threatening	Genetic predisposition Associated with atopic dermatis Environmental allergens: food, dust, pollens, animal dander, chemicals	Itching, burning, tearing, photophobia, chronic redness, blepharitis, periocular eczema, mucous discharge, SPK/ulcer, conjunctival, and corneal scarring Cataract
GPC	Iatrogenic Second to fifth decade	Mild	Trauma induced by contact lens edge, ocular prosthesis, exposed sutures, aggravated by concomitant allergy	Lens intolerance, blurred vision, foreign body sensation, giant papillae
Contact Dermatitis of the eyelid	Not known	Moderate	Contact delayed type hypersensitivity Exogenous haptens (cosmetics, metals, chemicals) Topical preparation (drugs, preservatives)	Eyelid eczema, eyelid itching, redness, follicles, SPK
Drug induced conjunctivitis	Any age/adults	Moderate	Epithelial toxicity Hyperosmolarity Indirect toxicity	Redness, lid eczema, follicles, SPK
Urban allergy	Adults	Mild	Poor air Quality Pollution Oxidative stress	Itching, burning, redness

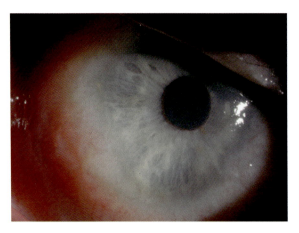

Fig. 8.1 Severe limbal vernal keratoconjunctivitis (VKC) with partial stem cell deficiency

of the disease is characterized by multiple gelatinous, yellow-gray limbal infiltrates and papillae, whose size and location may change over time. The limbus may appear thickened and opacified for 360°, accompanied by a peripheral, superficial neovascularization (Fig. 8.1). The apices of infiltrates may appear as punctiform calcified concretions called Trantas dots. In the mixed form of the disease, both tarsal and limbal signs are observed to varying degrees. Blepharospasm, tearing, and mucus hypersecretion may be present in all VKC forms, while pseudoptosis is usually secondary to the presence of heavy tarsal giant papillae.

Corneal involvement is common in VKC, and is more frequent in tarsal than limbal patients, taking the form of a superficial punctate keratitis, epithelial macroerosion or ulcers, plaque, neovascularization, subepithelial scarring, or pseudogerontoxon (Fig. 8.2). Ulcer formation is preceded by a progressive deterioration of the corneal epithelium, which appears irregularly stained and covered with fine filaments. The ocular complications that lead to visual loss include steroid-induced cataract, steroid-induced glaucoma, central corneal scars, irregular astigmatism, keratoconus (KC), limbal tissue hyperplasia, and dry eye syndrome.

8.2.3 Atopic Keratoconjunctivitis

AKC is a rare disease that comprises less than 1% of all ocular allergies. Generally, it emerges in children with active atopic dermatitis or in young adults and continues through the fifth decade of life, reaching its peak incidence between the ages of 30 and 50 [1, 7, 8]. A family history of allergic conditions is common, while 95% of patients have a history of eczema and 87% have a history of asthma. AKC presents as a chronic bilateral conjunctivitis with seasonal exacerbations corresponding to the offending allergen/s or food exposure. The common presenting symptoms are bilateral ocular itching, burning, tearing, and mucous discharge. The hallmark sign of AKC is erythematous, exudative lesions of the lids [1, 7, 8]. Eyelids tend to be thickened, indurated, erythematous, and fissurated, due to eczema, and is often associated with chronic blepharitis, meibomian gland dysfunction, and staphylococcal infection. The lids of about 90% of atopic patients are colonized with *Staphylococcus aureus* rather than the usual staphylococcal flora, however, their presence does not correlate with the incidence or severity of keratopathy [9]. The limbus may present Tranta's dots and the tarsal conjunctiva may present giant papillae, similar to those observed in VKC patients. Cicatrizing conjunctivitis, subepithelial fibrosis, and symblepharon have also been reported, with the lower fornix possibly shrinking subsequent to scarring. Reduced tear function and tear volume may also be observed. Punctate keratitis, persistent epithelial defects and ulcer with plaque formation are possible complications (Fig. 8.3). KC is also often associated with AKC (see later). Herpes keratitis and microbial infections may complicate the disease, particularly if chronic topical steroid therapy is required. Severe keratopathy with corneal neovascularization, pannus formation, and stromal keratitis may develop as a consequence of repeated corneal inflammation. This can result in marked astigmatic changes and permanent visual impairment. Anterior "atopic" or posterior subcapsular cataract contributes to the visual deterioration associated with AKC.

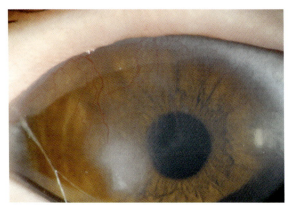

Fig. 8.2 Corneal ulcer in a VKC patient complicated by superficial and stromal neovascularization

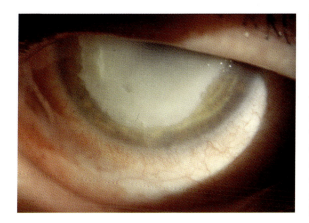

Fig. 8.3 Extensive, elevated corneal plaque complicated by initial corneal neovascularization in a severe AKC patient

8.2.4 Giant Papillary Conjunctivitis

GPC is a non-IgE-mediated inflammation induced most frequently by the use of all types of contact lenses, ocular prostheses, or the presence of corneoconjunctival sutures or protruding scleral buckling [10]. The upper tarsal conjunctiva is subjected to repetitive or constant microtrauma generated by a conjunctival "foreign body"; this phenomenon is then complicated by an immune reaction against a protein or residue deposited on the lens. Suspension of contact lens wear initiates the immediate regression of the disease. Previously considered an allergic condition, GPC has similarities with VKC for the morphology of giant papillae, and some immunopathological findings such as increased mast cell number, eosinophil and T cell infiltration, expression of Th2-type cytokines, such as IL-4 and chemokines [11]. GPC is mostly seen in young patients, is not related to gender but a history of atopy may be a predisposing factor. The early stages of GPC may be asymptomatic. In contact lens GPC, mild lens intolerance progresses to foreign body sensation, itching, blurred vision, and increased mucus production. Intolerance progresses until patients are no longer able to wear their lenses. In other forms of GPC, mild to severe irritation, discomfort, itching, and burning continue until removal of the external device or suture. The defining characteristic of GPC is the presence of giant papillae greater than 0.3 mm in diameter. There can be a single papilla or the entire tarsal plate may be covered. Conjunctival hyperaemia, limbal infiltrates, Tranta's dots, and conjunctival thickening are common findings. Mucous discharge and lens deposits are typical.

8.2.5 Contact Blepharoconjunctivitis

Contact blepharitis or dermatoconjunctivitis involves the skin of the eyelid and/or conjunctiva [12]. It is related to contact T cell-mediated delayed hypersensitivity reaction to haptens (incomplete antigens), which become immunogenic only after they bind to tissue protein. Various haptens and antigens that might come in contact with the eyelid and/or the conjunctiva have been implicated, including drugs, topical eye drops, preservatives, metals, nail polish, and cosmetics. An "allergic" reaction may occur following instillation of topical antiglaucoma agents, such as beta-blockers, prostaglandins and prostanoids, or mydriatics used for diagnostic purposes, usually phenylephrine. Other alpha-agonists are commonly used as decongestants in over-the-counter antiallergy eyedrops. Topical antibiotics such as neomycin, as well as ocular solutions based on herbal extracts can also provoke contact allergic reactions. Among preservatives, benzalkonium chloride, thimerosal, parabens, and ethylendiaminetetraacetic acid (EDTA) may cause either a toxic reaction or a cell-mediated (delayed) hypersensitivity (DH) response. The most prominent symptoms are itching and burning of the eyelid and eczematoid dermatitis. Other signs and symptoms are redness, eyelid swelling, tearing, and mucous discharge. The ocular surface may also be involved as conjunctival hyperemia, punctate staining of the cornea, and conjunctiva, especially on the inferonasal bulbar conjunctiva and a follicular reaction. Similar signs and symptoms and conjunctival staining patterns occur with drug or preservative toxicity. Marginal corneal infiltrates may rarely occur in reactions to neomycin, phenylephrine, dorzolamide, gentamicine, and atropine; however, the exact nature of these hypersensitivity reactions is not clear. Eczema on the eyelid skin in the absence of conjunctival hyperemia indicates that the cause of the reaction is due to something that has come in contact only with the eyelid. Diagnosis is based on accurate clinical history of agents/drug exposure and the results of patch tests on the dorsal skin.

8.2.6 Drug-Induced Conjunctivitis or Keratoconjunctivitis

Drug-induced ocular surface toxicity is more frequent than ocular allergy and is only second in frequency to keratoconjunctivitis sicca. Ocular discomfort may be the only manifestation after drug instillation. However, severe ocular surface reactions may develop. Often, these reactions develop slowly and exhibit subacute or chronic symptoms. Clinical manifestations of a drug's toxic effects may be mild with exacerbation occurring only several years later.

Moreover, during the chronic use of topical medications, burning, itching, and other signs of intolerance may be attributed to the initial disease manifestations and the potential side effects of the drug remain underestimated.

Conjunctival irritations may result from a direct cytotoxicity of drugs, a low or high pH of the formulation and/or a hyper- or hypo-osmolarity of the solution. Some substances can be allergenic at low concentrations and irritating at higher doses. Toxic compounds may cause corneal and conjunctival cell necrosis or induce cell death by apoptosis. Thus, initial impairment of ocular surface integrity stimulates a cycle of inflammatory reactions, with persistent inflammation leading to subepithelial fibrosis, symblepharon, corneal neovascularization, and scarring.

Unlike immunological reactions, which require prior sensitization, toxic effects can be observed after the first contact and can be dose dependent. Toxic adverse events may also be observed several months or even years after initiation of treatment when a cumulated concentration of the drug has been reached.

The toxicity of various topical medications can also be indirect as with the extensive use of antibiotics, antiviral agents, or corticosteroids due to toxicity on goblet cells, decreased lacrimal gland secretion or the detergent effect of preservatives on the lipid layer of the tear film, increased meibomian gland secretions, and seborrheic blepharitis.

Occlusion of the nasolacrimal system caused by inflammatory and fibrogenic mechanisms can induce alterations of tear film and bacterial flora that lead to secondary toxic effects on the ocular surface. Some types of drug may cause delayed wound healing (corticosteroids), deposits on the ocular surface (adrenaline) or pigment changes and growth of cilia (prostanoids).

8.2.7 Urban Eye Allergy Syndrome

A significant number of patients present with a type of conjunctivitis that is not strictly speaking of allergic, infectious, or dry eye origin. Clinical studies and experience have shown a cause–effect relationship between allergic-like symptoms and environmental factors, including outdoor air pollutants and poor indoor air quality [13]. Continuously increasing traffic, the ever-growing number of cars and trucks and their resultant fossil fuel emissions and airborne particulates, together with global warming and changing worldwide rainfall patterns have drastically modified air quality. Allergen susceptibility might be increased in individuals who live in areas with greater air pollution since the respiratory tract and eye are very sensitive to irritants during an ongoing allergic inflammation. Both allergens and pollutants can directly initiate mucosal inflammation through several mechanisms including oxidative stress, proinflammatory cytokine production, and cyclooxygenase, lipoxygenase, and/or protease activation. There has been speculation that a condition in the conjunctiva exists in which symptoms similar to allergic conjunctivitis can occur in the absence of an allergic response. The common signs and symptoms such as redness, itching, and burning could result from allergy, dry eye, toxicity, or none of these. Patients with these itchy and red eyes without an underlying apparent allergic mechanism and medical history of allergy, who report symptoms predominantly in periods when airborne allergens are not prevalent but when temperatures are high, wind speed is low and pollution levels are high, may be experiencing a pollution-related condition, which can be referred to as "urban eye allergy" [13]. These individuals certainly appear not to be *allergic* to pollutants, but rather pollutants stimulate the mucosal immune system to produce an allergic type response. Conjunctival redness associated with mild or occasional symptoms of itching, burning, and photophobia in response to nonspecific stimuli has been given many monikers such as pollution keratoconjunctivitis, occasional or perennial nonallergic conjunctivitis, perennial chronic conjunctivitis, vasomotor conjunctivitis, and discomfort eye syndrome. To be diagnosed with the "urban eye allergy" syndrome, dry eye, allergy, and toxic conjunctivitis need to be excluded. However, tear deficiency and allergy exacerbate the problems caused by pollution since these disease states allow longer contact of the conjunctiva with particulate matter and/or allergens, a prolonged mast cell activation and waves of inflammatory cascades. Urban eye syndrome may be considered as a transversal, crossover condition that has some common features of allergy, dry eye, and toxic conjunctivitis, related to poor air conditions and an urban environment. It also reflects changes in society's attitudes to relatively minor health problems and their impact on quality of life and productivity.

> **Summary for the Clinician**
> - Accurate history is essential.
> - If it does not itch, it is not allergy.
> - Diagnosis of SAC is usually clinical.
> - VKC and AKC have unique clinical features and typical signs.
> - Chronic forms of allergy require laboratory tests.
> - If lids are involved, suspect contact allergy.
> - Think of drug-induced conjunctivitis.
> - Air pollution may cause urban eye allergy.

8.3 Differential Diagnosis

Each of these clinical entities requires a differential diagnosis that is usually clinical, yet can be substantiated by objective laboratory parameters. Clinical characteristics allow a relatively convincing diagnosis of SAC, PAC, VKC, AKC, GPC, and contact blepharoconjunctivitis in the milder or initial stages of these diseases, but there can be some confusion as to which form of allergy is present. At times, pseudoallergic forms, with clinical manifestations similar to allergy but with a nonallergic equivocal pathogenesis, are difficult to distinguish from allergic forms that, in contrast, have precisely defined pathogenic mechanisms. Several clinical forms may mimic the clinical pictures of ocular allergy, including tear film dysfunction, subacute and chronic infections, and toxic and mechanical conjunctivitis (Table 8.2).

Bacterial, viral, or chylamydial infections should always be considered in the differential diagnosis of both acute and chronic conditions. In bacterial conjunctivitis, the discharge is usually purulent with morning crusting around the eyelids. It may be a unilateral condition, whereas allergy is usually bilateral. Viral conjunctivitis is often seen in conjunction with a recent upper respiratory infection. Conjunctival hyperemia, chemosis, serous discharge, and corneal subepithelial opacities indicate a viral infection. A chylamydial infection is caused by transfer of the organism from the genital tract to the eye. It is characterized by a follicular persistent or chronic conjunctivitis.

In most cases, allergy is confused with the different forms of dry eye that result from decreased tear production or disruption of tear stability. Even though dry eye is most common in adults or older people, and allergy in younger subjects, tear film dysfunction can occur at any age. Signs and symptoms include irritation, grittiness, burning, and foreign body sensation, but also itching. Dry eye may be worsened by certain medications including oral antihistamines, yet it can occur concomitantly to allergy.

Blepharitis is another common condition that can cause significant ocular irritation, itching and discomfort. It is caused by an inflammation of the eyelid margin caused by staphylococcal infection with or without seborrhea. It is frequently associated with dry eye, skin diseases such as seborrhea, psoriasis, atopic dermatitis, and acne rosacea.

Toxic and mechanical conjunctivitis are frequently confused with allergy. In these cases, careful medical history and examination can exclude an allergic pathogenesis. An intense and persistent follicular reaction is the typical feature, associated with mild to intense hyperaemia. Toxicity to single or repeated exposure to a particular chemical substance, eyedrop, or preservative does not produce a change in normal lysozyme or IgE levels but may result in low goblet cell levels, destruction of junctures between epithelial cells, and epithelial cell toxicity. The lacrimal puncta may be swollen or occluded by a cellular infiltrate with a consequent epiphora. The cornea is often involved as a diffuse punctate keratitis typically on

Table 8.2 Differential diagnosis of allergic from nonallergic conjunctivitis

	Allergy	Dry eye	Blepharitis	Toxic	Mechanical	Infections
History	Typical	Significant	–	±	–	–
Symptoms	Itching	Burning	Burning	Discomfort	Discomfort	Burning
	Tearing	Foreign body sensation	Itching	Burning	Pain	Discomfort
		Discomfort	Discomfort			Stickiness
		Pain				
Signs	Redness	SPK	Abnormal lid margin	Redness	Redness	Intense redness
	Lid swelling			Follicles	SPK	Secretion
	Papillae					Tearing
	Eczema					Swelling
Discharge	Serous/mucus	Mucus	Serous/mucus	Serous	Mucus	Mucopurulent/purulent
Cytology	Eosinophils/neutrophils/lymphocytes	Altered epithelial cells/lymphocytes	Neutrophils	Neutrophils/altered epithelial cells/lymphocytes	Neutrophils	Neutrophils

the entire corneal surface. Dermal involvement of the eyelids includes injection, swelling, and excoriation. Medicamentosa is essentially a toxic response with no underlying immune dysfunction; however, contact sensitivity to drugs, preservatives, or cosmetics may be present.

Molluscum contagiousum is a very similar, unilateral condition often included in the discussion of toxic keratoconjunctivitis and allergy. Typical lesions on the lid margin or the lid skin need to be carefully evaluated.

> **Summary for the Clinician**
> - Tear film dysfunction may simulate or overlap allergic conjunctivitis.
> - Blepharitis is usually not allergic.
> - Follicular conjunctivitis is more frequently toxic.
> - Consider chlamydial infection with persistent follicular conjunctivitis.

8.4 Diagnostic Tests in Ocular Allergy

The first step in diagnosing allergy is to determine definitively that the inflammation is not nonspecific but is allergic in origin, caused by an IgE-mediated sensitization to antigen. The second phase of the diagnosis consists in identifying the various forms of ocular allergy that are present based on the clinical characteristics observed. Diagnostic tests are shown in Table 8.3.

> **Summary for the Clinician**
>
> If allergy is suspected:
> - Complete an accurate clinical history and ocular examination.
> - Consult an allergist and results of skin prick tests.
> - Identify specific serum IgE levels.
> - Analyze blood cell count with the eosinophil count.
> - If all of these systemic tests are negative, consider local tests.
> - Defining the conjunctival allergic response to sensitizing allergens can be extremely helpful in understanding a patient's disease.
> - Cytological tests are useful in the active phase of the disease.
> - Low tear volume limits its potential usefulness in analytical diagnosis.

8.5 Ocular Immunity and the Allergic Reaction

8.5.1 Innate Immunity and Ocular Allergy

Innate immunity is the primary defense line for the ocular surface. It is essentially mechanical due to the anatomical characteristics and the position of the eye. These mechanical barriers are supported by nonspecific phagocytic and humoral responses produced by monocytes and macrophages and by ocular surface structural cells.

Induced immunity is the second specific defense line, involving the processing and recognition of antigen by antigen-presenting cells (APC) and lymphocytes and the development of a specific immune response through humoral or cell-mediated mechanisms.

How innate immunity of the ocular surface might interact with the mechanisms that drive toward an allergic reaction remains unclear. Some of the players of innate immunity are modified in ocular allergy. Toll-like receptors (TLRs) play a crucial role in the activation of several immune cells, as well as possibly modulating the Th1/Th2 lymphocyte equilibrium. Recently, TLRs studied in normal subjects, VKC [14] and AKC patients [15] showed different patterns when expressed in chronic allergic conjunctivitis. In VKC, TLR-4 was upregulated, TLR-9 was downregulated, and TLR-2 was slightly decreased relative to normal tissues. Whether this is a predisposing phenotype or a consequence of chronic inflammation remains a challenge for further studies. Activation of TLR-2 and TLR-4 induces mast cell degranulation and release of Th2 cytokines [16], suggesting a possible link between mechanisms that activate the adaptive immune response after microbial ocular infections and allergic inflammation.

There is also strong evidence supporting a role for a *S. aureus* infection in the pathogenesis of AKC. In fact, in one study, most affected individuals had this pathogen identifiable on lid swabs [9, 17]. It is believed that staphylococcal-derived superantigen is a potent adjuvant for allergen-specific Th2 responses and it may generically apply to other hypersensitivities, particularly when microorganisms have been implicated. In the ocular setting, these concepts are still unclear.

Recently, it was proposed that NK cells play a crucial role in the pathogenesis of allergic diseases by altering the balance between Th1/Th2 lymphocytes. NK cells might be triggered to secrete cytokines (IL-4, IL-5, and IL-13) that promote Th2 rather than Th1 responses. The recent finding of decreased circulating NK in VKC patients and significantly increased NK cells infiltrating the conjunctiva in inflamed VKC tissues [18] indicates that NK cells may be involved in the pathophysiology of chronic ocular allergy. By modulating allergic inflammation through the release of cytokines that influence the balance between

Table 8.3 Diagnostic tests for ocular allergy

Test	Indication	Advantages	Disadvantages
Skin prick test	Suspected sensitization to environmental (pollens, molds, mites, animal dander) and food allergens	Simple, rapid inexpensive	Not always correlated with eye symptoms
Patch test	Eczematous blepharitis Contact sensitivity Drug-induced conjunctivitis		Time consuming Eyelid skin is quite different from that of the back Increasing number of haptens
Serum specific IgE	In eczema, skin hyper-reactivity, prolonged use of drugs	Quantify sensitization-Diverse allergens simultaneously	Expensive Not always correlated with eye symptoms
Conjunctival provocation with allergens	Positive clinical history of allergic and prick test /IgE negative-Define the most important allergen in patients with several positive skin tests	Confirm conjunctival responsiveness	Few allergens available Expensive Time consuming Rare systemic side effects
Cytology	To evaluate the quality and quantity of inflammation	Presence of eosinophils indicative of allergy	Absence of eosinophils does not exclude allergy
Tear IgE	Suspected sensitization and negative allergy tests	Local IgE production	Low volume samples Not practical Not standardized

Th1 and Th2 responses, and the resulting conjunctival eosinophil infiltration, these cells may provide a link between innate and specific immunity in allergic diseases.

8.5.2 The Allergic Process

The conjunctiva is normally exposed to picogram quantities of environmental allergens such as pollens, dust mite fecal particles, animal dander, and other proteins. When deposited on the mucosa, these antigens are processed by Langerhans cells (LCs) or other APC in the mucosal epithelium, bind to the antigen recognition site of major histocompatibility complex (MHC) class II molecules, and present to naive CD4+ lymphocytes at some unknown location that could be the local draining lymph nodes. Complex and multiple simultaneous contacts and cytokine exchanges between APC and T cells expressing antigen-specific T cell receptors are necessary to trigger the antigen specific T cells to differentiate into Th2 lymphocytes [19]. Recently, more attention has been given to the role of dendritic cells (DCs) in ocular allergic diseases. B7-1 and B7-2, costimulatory molecules on APC, interact with CD28 located on Th2 cells [20, 21], activating them during the induction and effector phases. In contrast, CTLA-4 is expressed on activated T cells and transmits a negative signal that downregulates the ongoing T cell responses upon engagement by B7-1 or B7-2 [22]. Other ligand interactions may also be crucial in the production of IgE; for example, conjunctival B cells expressing the ligands CD23, CD21, and CD40 are activated in individuals with VKC. These B cells may be responsible for the IgE production associated with VKC [21]. A direct activation of allergen-specific T cells by T cell peptides or direct activation of DCs bearing high-affinity receptors for IgE may be alternate pathways for initiating an allergic reaction in patients with or without evidence of specific IgE sensitization. In fact, specific IgE sensitization is identified in only 50% of patients [6, 23], suggesting that non-IgE-mediated pathways may be present in VKC. It is still unclear why disease incidence changes with age and in different geographical regions. The risk of disease may be influenced by genetic susceptibility factors, some of which affect the immune response, e.g., polymorphisms of the FcεR1 and IL-4R genes [24]. We have shown recently that the number of DCs expressing the FcεRIg chain is increased and predominant in the substantia propria of the conjunctiva of VKC patients [25]. This increased expression of the receptor is likely to increase the ability of DCs to capture and subsequently process antigens for presentation to CD4+ T cells, thereby initiating the immune cascade.

It is still unknown why one subject becomes allergic and one is tolerant to the same allergen. Nonatopic subjects usually develop a low-grade immunological response to aeroallergens with the production of allergen-specific IgG1 antibodies and in vitro, a modest T cell proliferative response to allergens with the production of IFNγ, typical of Th1 cells. Nonatopics also appear to have a normal T-regulatory cell response [26]. In contrast, allergic subjects mount an exaggerated allergen-specific IgE response with elevated serum levels of IgE antibodies and positive skin tests to extracts of common aeroallergens. In fact, T cells derived from allergic subjects and grown in vitro proliferate in the presence of specific allergens, responding with the production of typical Th2-type cytokines, IL-4, IL-5, and IL-13 [27]. This may be the result of an inappropriate balance between allergen activation of regulatory T cells and effector Th2 cells.

The major driving force that polarizes CD4+ T cells to the Th2 phenotype is IL-4, whereas IL-12 favors a Th1 response. However, many other cytokines, chemokines, and mediators with potential relevance to allergy and allergic conjunctivitis, including histamine and histamine receptors, have been described since this initial definition of the Th1/Th2 paradigm. This may explain the disappointing results of single cytokine-directed therapy that have been recently observed in cases of allergy.

It has become evident that regulatory T cells (Treg) play a suppressive role in the development of allergy and that modulation of Treg function may be a possible therapy for allergic patients. However, the role of Treg and regulatory cytokines such as IL-10 and TGFβ in ocular allergy is still unclear [28]. It has been shown that IL-10 and TGFβ do not have immunosuppressive roles in the development of experimentally induced allergic conjunctivitis [29]. Moreover, these two cytokines increase the infiltration of eosinophils into the conjunctiva during the effector phase of experimentally induced allergic conjunctivitis.

8.5.3 Allergic Inflammation

Inflammatory mediators and inhibitors in the tear fluid have been extensively used in ocular allergy to find either a "disease marker," to better understand the immune mechanisms involved in the ocular surface inflammation, or to identify potential targets for therapeutic interventions. The presence of Th2 cells and Th2-type cytokines has been proven and confirmed in several studies.

However, during the active inflammatory phase of the disease, multiple cytokines are overexpressed and produced [30] including the typical Th1-type cytokine, INFγ, which probably contributes to increasing the ocular inflammation, similar to what has been shown in animal models. The presence and distribution of multiple mediators, proteases, and angiogenic and growth factors in normal tears and in those of active VKC patients has been demonstrated by using a modified microwell plate antibody array [31].

Massive infiltration of inflammatory cells is typical of chronic ocular allergy such as VKC, and differentiates this disease from SAC and PAC. Chemokines such as IL-8, MCP-1, RANTES, and eotaxin are actively secreted in VKC and produced by mast cells, macrophages, epithelial cells, and fibroblasts [32].

Several enzymatic systems may be activated in chronic disease, contributing to cell migration, tissue damage, and remodeling. Metalloproteases are overexpressed and activated in VKC [33], and urokinase, an extravascular fibrinolytic system activator, is highly produced in active patients and is expressed by inflammatory cells and conjunctival cell cultures exposed to cytokines involved in allergic inflammation [34]. Moreover, the activity of alpha-1 antitrypsin (AAT), the archetype of the serine protease inhibitor, is locally reduced in VKC creating an imbalance between protease and inhibitors, and facilitating or prolonging conjunctival inflammation [35]. In fact, tear trypsin inhibitory capacity is reduced, whereas tear MMP-1 and -9 activity is increased.

Multiple mediators, cytokines, chemokines, receptors, proteases, growth factors, intracellular signals, regulatory and inhibitory pathways, and other unknown factors and pathways are differently expressed, ultimately resulting in the many clinical manifestations of ocular allergic disease. A better understanding of the mechanisms involved in ocular surface immunity is necessary for identifying new classification criteria and new therapeutic strategies.

Summary for the Clinician

- Genetic and environmental influences determine IgE-mediated hypersensitivity.
- IgE/mast cell-dependent reactions are the basic mechanism in ocular allergy.
- There is a central role of Th2 cells in the allergic response.
- Th2 cells and Th2-type cytokines are involved in the pathological changes associated with chronic allergic disease.

8.6 The Cornea in Allergic Diseases

8.6.1 Corneal Immunology

The normal cornea is devoid of both blood and lymphatic vessels and actively maintains this avascularity. This so-called corneal "angiogenic privilege" is important for corneal transparency and vision. The cornea does not respond to environmental allergens and does not undergo inflammation in normal conditions. The absence of mast cells and vessels is the anatomical condition that renders the cornea nonresponsive to IgE-mediated (type I) ocular reactions.

From an immunologic point of view, the normal avascularity of the cornea contributes to maintaining an immune-privileged site. Corneal APCs were thought to reside exclusively in the peripheral cornea; however, recent evidence demonstrates that the central cornea is endowed with a heterogeneous population of bone marrow-derived cells, including epithelial LCs and anterior stromal DCs, which under certain conditions can function as APCs [36]. While the corneal periphery contains mature and immature resident bone marrow-derived DCs, the central cornea is endowed exclusively with highly immature/precursor-type DCs. During inflammation, a majority of resident DCs undergo maturation by acquiring high expression of MHC class II antigens and B7 (CD80/CD86) and CD40 costimulatory molecules [37]. These data revise the tenet that the cornea is immune privileged due to a lack of resident lymphoreticular cells per se, but suggest that the cornea is capable of actively participating in the immune response to foreign antigens and autoantigens, rather than being a passive bystander.

After allergic sensitization in an animal model, the cornea appears normal in terms of its APC and lymphatic content. The etiology of the keratopathy of chronic allergic eye disease is not known but may result from the release of toxic mediators from mast cells, eosinophils, and neutrophils in the inflamed conjunctiva. A histopathological study showed that patients with chronic allergic conjunctivitis with keratopathy have higher cell numbers in their conjunctiva than patients with no keratopathy, especially those staining for eosinophil cationic protein in the tarsal epithelium [38]. The role of APC in the development of allergic keratopathy is not known. It is also not clear why the cornea is not involved in IgE-mediated SAC and PAC but only in VKC and AKC.

8.6.2 Allergic Inflammation and Corneal Damage

During the ocular inflammatory process, allergic mediators are released onto the ocular surface and into the tear film, causing a wide range of corneal clinical manifestations.

Inflammatory cells, cytokines, and chemokines liberated from eosinophils, T helper type 2 (Th2) cells, and tear film instability may act concomitantly in the pathogenesis of shield ulcer. Eosinophils and eosinophil-derived major basic (MBP) and cationic protein (ECP), neurotoxins, and collagenases, in particular MMP-9, have been shown to damage the corneal epithelium and basement membrane [33, 39, 40].

In separate studies, tear levels of ECP, IL-5, and eotaxin-1, which contribute to eosinophil recruitment and activation, have been shown to correlate with the corneal clinical involvement in VKC [41].

The fact that human corneal keratocytes and conjunctival fibroblasts, but not epithelial cells, are capable of producing eotaxin by stimulation with IL-4 and TNFα suggests that eotaxin production in keratocytes may play an important role in eosinophil recruitment to corneal ulcers in allergic ocular disease [32, 41]. Thus eotaxin production by keratocytes, the increased production of cytokines on the ocular surface in the course of severe ocular allergies, and the increased expression of adhesion molecules by corneal epithelial cells stimulated by IL-4 and TNFα are all responsible for the corneal involvement observed in the most severe allergic ocular diseases.

8.6.3 Tear Instability and Corneal Involvement

Chronic ocular allergies may be associated with tear film instability, goblet cell loss and conjunctival squamous metaplasia. Goblet cell-derived mucine (MUC5AC) downregulation with upregulation of MUCs 1, 2, 4, and 16 mRNA expression has been shown in atopic eyes with allergic shield corneal ulcers compared with eyes without ulcers and eyes of control subjects [42–44]. These findings suggest that the presence of ocular surface inflammation, tear instability, decreased corneal sensitivity, and changes in conjunctival MUCs mRNA expression are important in the pathogenesis of atopic ocular surface disease. In particular, MUC16 upregulation, which is involved in the protection of the ocular surface epithelia, could be a manifestation of an ocular surface defense response that compensates for the ailing ocular surface health resulting from the decrease in MUC5AC [44]. Persistence of inflammation and further decline of expression of the major ocular surface mucin, MUC5AC, may stimulate upregulation of other epithelial mucins such as MUC16 to protect the ocular surface [44].

8.6.4 Corneal Clinical Manifestations in Ocular Allergy

Manifestations of corneal involvement among patients with VKC and AKC vary from Tranta's dots, superficial punctuate keratitis, shield ulcer, corneal plaque, corneal neovascularization, lipid infiltration, bacterial or fungal keratitis, KC, hydrops, pseudogerontoxon, and corneal opacification (Figs. 8.2 and 8.3). Punctate epithelial keratitis may coalesce to form an obvious corneal epithelial defect, known as shield ulcer, leaving the Bowman's layer intact. If left untreated, a plaque containing fibrin and mucus is deposited over the epithelial defect. Shield ulcers without plaque formation usually undergo rapid reepithelization, resulting in excellent visual outcome, however, patients with shield ulcers and visible plaque formation have delayed reepithelization. Tear film instability seen in the later stages of VKC adversely affects the reepithelization of shield ulcer.

Cameron classified shield ulcers on the basis of their clinical characteristics, response to treatment and complications [45]: Grade 1, shield ulcer with a clear base; these have a favorable outcome and reepithelization with mild scarring. Grade 2, ulcers with visible inflammatory debris at the base; such ulcers are prone to complications and exhibit delayed reepithelization and a poor response to medical therapy (Fig. 8.4). Grade 3, shield ulcers with elevated plaques (Fig. 8.5); these respond best to surgical therapy.

In addition to possible permanent vision loss, the longer the shield ulcer persists, the greater the likelihood of sterile ulceration, corneal scars, bacterial keratitis, amblyopia, and globe perforation [46].

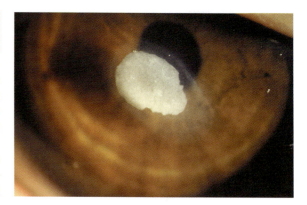

Fig. 8.5 Grade 3 corneal plaque in a VKC patient, according to Camerun classification

8.6.5 Confocal Microscopy and Allergic Keratoconjunctivitis

Confocal microscopy may be useful for elucidating the alterations of corneal morphology in allergic keratoconjunctivitis. Corneal disease in AKC has been associated with significant alterations of the basal epithelium, and subbasal and stromal corneal nerves, which relate to changes in tear function and corneal sensitivity [47]. The significantly lower number and density of subbasal long nerve fibers (LNF) and the total number of long nerves and their nerve branches (NB) may explain the lower corneal sensation observed in eyes with AKC [47]. In the stoma, thicker stromal nerves (probably due to edema and increased metabolic activity) with deflection and bifurcation abnormalities may be observed, indicating that the cornea attempts to regenerate and reconstitute a diseased stromal milieu when there is persistent ocular inflammation (Figs. 8.6 and 8.7). Corneal nerves have been shown to harbor neuropeptides and neurotransmitters such as calcitonin gene-related peptide and substance P with neurotrophic properties on corneal epithelium [48]. Altered expression of neurotransmitters, neuropeptides, and neuroreceptors has been demonstrated in VKC [49]. These abnormalities support the concept that corneal nerves exert a trophic effect on the corneal epithelium and that the loss of the trophic effect may lead to epithelial alterations that are frequently seen on the ocular surface by vital staining in the course of allergic keratoconjunctivitis.

Confocal microscopic observations also show that inflammatory cells are sometimes attached to the stromal nerves and that there are also numerous keratocytes close to the nerves (Figs. 8.6 and 8.7). Inflammatory cells have in fact been found in the superficial layer of the corneal stroma in AKC and VKC ulcers [39]. Keratocytes are known to be activated in states of corneal inflammation

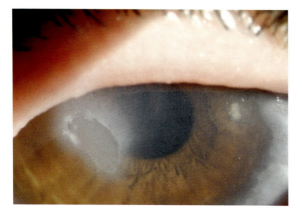

Fig. 8.4 Grade 2 corneal ulcer in VKC according to Camerun classification. Note the absence of epithelium, the presence of debris at the base of the ulcer, and the opacification of the Bowman layer

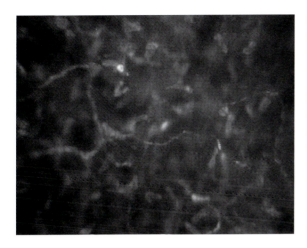

Fig. 8.6 Activated keratocytes, abnormal particles, and nerves in the anterior stroma of a VKC patient previously affected by corneal ulcer (Confoscan4, Nidek)

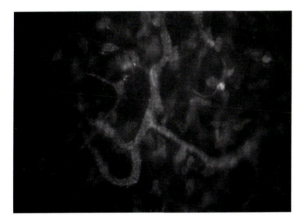

Fig. 8.7 Thick corneal stromal nerve with deflection and bifurcation abnormalities in the same patient of Fig. 8.6 (Confoscan4, Nidek)

and repair. Activated keratocytes can be seen in the corneal stroma of both AKC and VKC patients. They may overexpress nerve growth factors, which induce hypertrophy of the peripheral nervous system.

Loss of corneal epithelial trophism, decline in cellular functions, alteration of ocular surface mucin expressions, modification in the subbasal nerve plexus, modified corneal nerves, and increased expression and production of epitheliotoxic factors may explain some of the signs and symptoms and the hypersensitivity typical of patients affected by allergic keratoconjunctivitis.

8.6.6 Keratoconus and Allergic Conjunctivitis

The hypothesis that allergy, itch, and rubbing are relevant to the pathogenesis of KC is still unclear. The association between atopy and KC was first reported in 1937 [50] and this has been subsequently confirmed and contradicted [51, 52]. It was reported that there was no statistically significant difference between the group of KC patients and the control group with respect to the presence of atopy. Nevertheless, it has been reported that, in a healthy population, 3% of subjects had eczema, whereas in patients with KC, 32% of patients had eczema and itchy eyes [53]. In another study, the prevalence of asthma in the control group was 1%, whereas it was 17.9% in KC patients [54]. In a recent cohort study, asthma, eczema, and hay fever were associated to KC in 23, 14, and 30%, respectively [55], and 48% reported significant eye rubbing. It has also been reported that, in KC patients with atopy, the progression of KC takes place more rapidly, the need for keratoplasty surgery appears earlier, and that both refractive and immunologic complications are seen more frequently [56]. These findings have led to the concern of whether atopic KC patients should be evaluated as a separate entity in KC disease.

Children with VKC have a high incidence of KC if investigated by videokeratographic maps and have more abnormal topography patterns than expected compared with normal eyes [57]. A recent study showed that atopic KC eyes have steeper cones that appear to be thinner centrally, and both the thinnest point on the cornea and the cone are more peripherally located [58]. In a separate study, unlike in axial curvature maps, most apices in elevation maps were clustered in the inferotemporal quadrant [59]. Corneal topography characteristics in keratoconal eyes with atopy are different from those in keratoconal eyes without atopy; thus, atopic KC patients may indeed be a separate entity in this disease. The clinical approach to patients with KC and some form of allergy has not been standardized.

Central corneal thinning may result from corneal stromal cell apoptosis or be induced or perpetuated by the activation of matrix degrading enzymes, particularly members of the matrix metalloproteinase (MMP) family and decreased proteinase inhibitors [60–62]. Moreover, IL-6, TNF-α, and MMP-9 are overexpressed in the tears of patients with KC, indicating that the pathogenesis of KC may involve chronic inflammatory events [63]. Increased expression and activity of inflammatory cytokines and MMPs is typical of allergic conjunctivitis patients [33]; however, no comparison on the expression of these factors in allergic conjunctivitis patients with and without KC has been reported.

8.6.7 Keratoglobus

Keratoglobus is characterized by global corneal thinning and ectasia of the cornea and has been reported in patients with VKC [64]. Severe microbial keratitis in a patient with corneal hydrops in keratoglobus-associated VKC and atopic dermatitis has been described [65]. This rare comorbidity can impair corneal integrity and immunity and may allow for rapid penetration of infectious organisms. These patients are at high risk for developing a severe sight-threatening ocular infection that may respond poorly to intensive medical management.

8.6.8 Allergic Keratoconjunctivitis and Corneal Infection

Viral infections and allergy are linked in different ways. According to the "hygiene hypothesis," viral infections in the prenatal period or early childhood could prevent development of atopy by stimulating the Th-1 response and inhibiting the Th-2 immune response; however, acute viral infections are well known to exacerbate established allergic diseases, such as bronchial asthma, airway hyper-responsiveness, and atopic dermatitis. For example, respiratory syncytial virus (RSV) and chylamydial infection may be pathogenic factors in allergic diseases. However, a direct association between RSV or chylamydial infection and ongoing inflammation was not confirmed in VKC [66].

Although it is known that patients with atopic dermatitis are more susceptible to herpes simplex virus (HSV) infections that may involve the eye, the relationship between allergic eye disease and ocular herpetic disease is not well established. In a recent study, the age and gender adjusted relative risk of allergic vs. nonallergic patients to suffer a herpes event was higher in allergic patients. When stratified by age, the risk for HSV infections among allergic patients was significantly higher in all age groups [67]. This suggests that local allergic and inflammatory exacerbation could be the trigger for the herpetic attack. Allergic patients using topical steroids or cyclosporine need to be carefully followed since these drugs may trigger herpetic reactivation.

Bacterial colonization of the lid margins, particularly in AKC patients, may exacerbate chronic allergic conjunctivitis by delayed-type hypersensitivity. Long-term use of topical immunosuppressive drops may cause colonization of the lid margins by *S. aureus*, which can then induce superinfection of the cornea. Vernal corneal plaques are usually not complicated by infections; however, association with viral and bacterial keratoconjunctivitis has been reported [68, 69]. Though rare, fungal keratitis associated with shield ulcer may be observed in patients with VKC [70, 71]. Prompt diagnosis and treatment may prevent permanent complications and vision loss and should be considered in the differential diagnosis of infections associated with VKC.

> **Summary for the Clinician**
> - Corneal involvement is typical of VKC and AKC.
> - Ocular allergies may be associated with tear film instability.
> - Severe inflammationis more frequently associated with corneal complications.
> - KC is frequently associated with atopy.
> - KC and allergy may share some of multiple factors necessary for their expression.
> - Excessive eye rubbing and KC are associated.
> - Infections can rarely complicate corneal inflammation in VKC and AKC.

8.6.9 Allergy and Corneal Transplant

8.6.9.1 Immunology

Allergic conjunctivitis is important in the context of corneal transplantation for two reasons [72]. First, it is the most prevalent form of ocular inflammation, in general, and may actually be overrepresented in corneal transplant patients, given the association between allergic eye disease and KC. Second, atopy is associated with a skewing of the T helper cell immune responses toward Th2 [73]. Traditionally, allograft rejection has been thought to be a Th1-mediated process; however, Th2 and Th1 cells crossregulate each other. It has been hypothesized that by enhancing the Th2 response, the Th1 response would be attenuated and graft tolerance would be achieved [74]. However, the notion that Th2 immune responses might be deleterious rather than beneficial for corneal survival after transplant is supported by clinical observations, indicating that patients with severe ocular allergies are at a higher risk of corneal transplant rejection [75, 76].

Animal model studies on corneal graft mechanisms [72, 73, 77] demonstrate that: (1) atopic conjunctivitis promotes systemic Th2 immune responses to the alloantigens expressed on the corneal allograft; (2) corneal allografts transplanted to atopic hosts experience an increased incidence and a swifter time of rejection; (3) increased rejection is closely correlated with systemic Th2 cell-mediated responses to donor alloantigens and not local allergic inflammation; and (4) corneal allograft rejection in atopic hosts does not require the direct involvement of infiltrating eosinophils.

Graft infiltration by eosinophils has been described in rejected human allografts in patients with allergic conjunctivitis [76]. Although graft-infiltrating eosinophils were seen exclusively in allergic conjunctivitis, their absolute number is less than those of CD4 cells, CD8 cells, or macrophages. Eosinophils, as effector cells, may contribute to the accelerated rate of rejection seen after perioperative allergic conjunctivitis.

In addition, topical treatment with antihistamines did not prevent exacerbation of corneal allograft rejection associated with pollen conjunctivitis in an animal model [77]. The latter finding is consistent with the proposition that exacerbation of corneal allograft rejection in hosts expressing allergic conjunctivitis is due to a systemic Th2 immune response to donor histocompatibility antigens and not simply a nonspecific local effect produced by an inflamed eye. It is not clear if allergic inflammation in the perioperative period alone is sufficient to shorten graft survival. It is possible that allergen-induced conjunctival inflammation, immediately after transplantation, may influence the afferent and efferent limb of the allogeneic response. In avascular recipient corneas, the indirect route of alloantigen presentation is thought to be predominant, with APCs migrating to the graft from recipient conjunctiva and limbus. It may be that phenotypic or functional alterations in conjunctival APC in allergy alter the afferent component of the rejection response [72].

8.6.9.2 Clinical Outcomes

Several studies have shown that penetrating keratoplasty in eyes with KC and VKC has an excellent visual outcome and low complication rate. Graft rejection episodes occurred in 13.3% eyes, with irreversible graft failure occurring in 4.4% eyes. Bacterial keratitis occurred in 7.7% eyes, 2.2% of which developed irreversible graft failure [78]. In another report, the clinical outcome of PKP in eyes with KC and VKC was comparable to that in eyes with KC alone. However, because complications such as prematurely loosened sutures and steroid-induced cataract were more common in the coexistence of VKC, closer monitoring in these cases was recommended [79].

Recently, the 5-year graft survival was shown to be 97 and 95% in eyes with or without VKC, respectively, with no statistically significant differences in Kaplan-Meier graft survival and in postoperative complications between the 2 groups [80]. Postkeratoplasty atopic sclerokeratitis (PKAS) is a potentially severe complication in atopic patients undergoing keratoplasty [81, 82]. PKAS may develop within 1–4 weeks of keratoplasty, with acute onset characterized by discomfort, photophobia, hyperemia, and mucus production. Early loosening of sutures, wound leakage, microbial keratitis and graft rejection are early complications in these patients. Preoperative atopic blepharitis and corneal neovascularization were identified as risk factors for PKAS. Principal recommendations for these patients include the use of interrupted sutures and early immunosuppression with high-dose oral steroids at the onset of the inflammatory condition, together with control of risk factors for microbial keratitis. Systemic immunosuppression should be considered before PK in patients with active atopic blepharitis and corneal neovascularization [83, 84].

> **Summary for the Clinician**
>
> - Allergic conjunctivitis is a very important consideration in corneal transplantation.
> - Conjunctival inflammation is an important factor in accelerating rejection.
> - Sclerokeratitis is a potentially severe complication in atopic patients undergoing keratoplasty.

8.7 Treatment of Ocular Allergy

The most common diseases, SAC and PAC, are classic IgE-mediated disorders, in which the therapeutic focus is mostly confined to the local suppression of mast cells, their degranulation and the effects of histamine and other mast cell-derived mediators using topical drugs. Conversely, severe chronic disorders such as VKC and AKC are both IgE- and T cell-mediated, leading to a chronic inflammation in which eosinophil, lymphocyte, and structural cell activation characterizes the conjunctival allergic reaction. In these cases, stabilization of mast cells and histamine or other mediator receptor antagonists is frequently insufficient for control of conjunctival inflammation and the frequent corneal involvement.

Currently available topical drugs for allergic conjunctivitis belong to different pharmacological classes (Table 8.4): vasoconstrictors, antihistamines, mast cell stabilizers, "dual-acting" agents (with antihistaminic and mast cell stabilizing properties), and nonsteroidal antiinflammatory agents. Corticosteroids are usually not needed in SAC and PAC, and have potentially important side effects if used for periods longer than occasional short cycles to control severe recurrences, if any.

Table 8.4 Topical ocular allergy medications

Class	Drug	Indication	Comments
Vasoconstrictor/antihistamine combinations	Naphazoline/pheniramine	Rapid onset of action SAC, Episodic conjunctivitis	Short duration of action Tachyphylaxis Mydriasis Ocular irritation Hypersensitivity Hypertension Potential for inappropriate patient use
Antihistamines	Levocabastine Emedastine	Rapid onset of action Relief of itching Relief of signs/symptoms SAC, PAC, AKC, VKC, GPC	Short duration of action
Mast cell stabilizers	Cromolyn Nedocromil Lodoxamide NAAGA Pemirolast	Relief of signs and symptoms SAC, PAC, AKC, VKC, GPC	Long-term usage Slow onset of action Prophylactic dosing
Antihistamine/mast cell stabilizers (dual-acting)	Azelastine Epinastine Ketotifen Olopatadine	Treatment of signs and symptoms of SAC Rapid onset of action Long duration of action Excellent comfort SAC, PAC, AKC, VKC, GPC	Bitter taste (azelastine) No reported serious side effects Olopatadine once a day
Corticosteroids	Loteprednol Fluormetholone Desonide Rimexolone Dexamethasone	Treatment of allergic inflammation Use in severe forms of allergies (PAC) AKC, VKC	Risk for long-term side effects No mast cell stabilization Potential for inappropriate patient use Requires close monitoring

8.7.1 Nonpharmacological Management

The first treatment of ocular allergy should be avoidance of the offending allergens. This can be achieved usually for indoor, professional, or food allergens. Thus, the identification of allergens by skin or blood testing is necessary to allow for avoidance of precipitating factors. Nonpharmacologic treatments include tear substitutes and lid hygiene for the washing out of allergens and mediators from the ocular surface, and cold compresses for decongestion. Patients should be informed of the duration of the disease based on allergen diffusion and exposure.

8.7.2 Treatment of Allergic Conjunctivitis

Treatment of SAC and PAC includes topical ocular pharmacologic treatment, topical ocular nonpharmacologic treatments, topical nonocular pharmacologic treatment (see earlier), systemic pharmacologic treatments, and immunotherapy.

8.7.2.1 Topical Ocular Pharmacological Treatment

Topical treatment is the first line of pharmacological treatment of allergic conjunctivitis. Decongestant/vasoconstrictors are alpha-adrenergic agonists approved topically for relief of conjunctival redness. They have little place in the pharmacological treatment of SAC and PAC except for the immediate removal of injection for cosmetic reasons, but do have an adverse effect profile locally (glaucoma) and systemically (hypertension).

Topical antihistamines are H_1 receptor competitive antagonists of varying specificity, potency, and duration of action. The first generation antihistamines, pheniramine, and antazoline, are still available in over the counter products, particularly, in association with vasoconstrictors. The newer antihistamines have a longer duration of action (4–6 h) and are better tolerated than their predecessors [85]. These include levocabastine hydrochloride and emedastine difumarate. Both drugs are effective and well tolerated also in pediatric subjects with allergic conjunctivitis.

Mast cell stabilizers inhibit degranulation by interrupting the normal chain of intracellular signals resulting from the cross-linking and activation of the high-affinity IgE receptor (FceRI) by allergen [86]. These drugs inhibit the release of histamine and other preformed mediators and the arachidonic acid cascade of mediator synthesis. Several mast cell stabilizers are available for use in the eye: cromolyn sodium 4%, nedocromil sodium 2%, lodoxamide tromethamine ophthalmic solution 0.1%, spaglumic acid 4%, and pemirolast potassium ophthalmic solution 0.1%. These drugs are approved for the treatment of allergic conjunctivitis, VKC and GPC with four times daily dosing regimen. Both mast cell stabilizers and antihistamines have a good safety profile and may be used in treating seasonal and PAC.

The antihistamines, azelastine, epinastine, ketotifen, and olopatadine, which have mast cell stabilizing and additional antiinflammatory properties (called "double or multiple action"), are presently available and show evident benefits in treating all forms of ocular allergy. The advantage offered by these molecules is the rapidity of symptomatic relief given by immediate histamine receptor antagonism, which alleviates itching and redness, coupled with the long-term disease-modifying benefit of mast cell stabilization [87]. All these medications are well tolerated and none are associated with significant acute ocular drying effects [88]. The use of nonsteroidal anti inflammatory drugs (NSAIDS) can be considered, in some cases, for a short period of time, but have limited efficacy on ocular pruritus.

Corticosteroid formulations (including the so called "soft steroids") should be reserved for and carefully used only in the most severe cases that are refractory to other types of medications. Corticosteroids do not directly stabilize immune cell membranes and do not inhibit histamine release; however, they may modulate the mast cell response by inhibiting cytokine production and inflammatory cell recruitment and activation. Thus, they are not the ideal therapy choice for inhibiting the acute allergic reaction, however, clinically, are the most effective antiinflammatory agents in active ocular allergy. Fluorometholone, medrysone, lotepredno, rimexolone, and desonide, called "soft" steroids, are considered to be those of choice when a mild, weakly penetrating drug is needed.

8.7.2.2 Topical Nonocular Pharmacological Treatment

The efficacy of intranasal corticosteroids in treating allergic nasal symptoms is well established. Recent data show a promising effect of intranasal corticosteroids on ocular symptoms of allergic rhinoconjunctivitis [89]. In SAC and PAC associated with allergic rhinitis, topical nasal steroids (and particularly new molecules with low systemic bioavailability, such as mometasone furoate and fluticasone furoate) have been shown to control the nasal-ocular reflex component of eye symptoms without increasing the risk of cataracts or of an increased ocular pressure. In fact, intranasal corticosteroids are considered safe due to their low systemic bioavailability. Analysis of an intranasal corticosteroid on individual ocular symptoms supported the positive impact of mometasone furoate on ocular symptoms [90]. Mometasone improved individual symptoms (eye itching, tearing, and redness) and subject-reported total ocular symptom scores compared with placebo, in addition to its established efficacy in reducing nasal symptoms of seasonal allergic rhinitis [90].

8.7.2.3 Systemic Pharmacological Treatment

Systemic antihistamines should be used in patients with concomitant major nonocular allergic manifestations. In fact, allergic rhinoconjunctivitis is an equally frequent condition generally treated with systemic antihistamines that have been proven effective in relieving nasal and conjunctival signs and symptoms [85]. When allergic symptoms are isolated, focused therapy with topical (ophthalmic) antihistamines is often efficacious and clearly superior to systemic antihistamines, either as monotherapy or in conjunction with an oral or intranasal agent. First-generation H1 receptor antagonists may provide some relief of ocular itching, but are sedating and have anticholinergic effects such as dry mouth, dry eye, blurred vision, and urinary retention. Second-generation antihistamines offer the same efficacy as their predecessors, but with a low-sedating profile and lack of anticholinergic activity. These drugs include acrivastine, cetirizine, ebastine, fexofenadine, loratadine, and mizolastine. However, even their use has been associated with drying effects, particularly of the ocular surface [85]. Desloratadine and levocetirizine are considered a subsequent evolution of these second generation agents.

8.7.2.4 Specific Immunotherapy

Allergen-specific immunotherapy (SIT) is indicated only when a clearly defined systemic hypersensitivity to identified allergens exists. The choice of the allergen to be employed for SIT should be made in accordance with the combination of clinical history and results of skin prick test. SIT is one of the cornerstones of allergic rhinoconjunctivitis treatment. Since the development of noninvasive formulations with better safety profiles, there is an increasing tendency to prescribe immunotherapy in youngsters. In these cases, sublingual immunotherapy (SLIT), which is better tolerated in children [91], can be considered since it is equally effective as traditional subcutaneous injections. Since the approval of SLIT by the World Health Organization in 1988, the efficacy and safety of SLIT have been confirmed in several new double-blind, placebo-controlled studies for mono-sensitized patients who are allergic to house dust mites, grass pollens, ragweed, and birch pollen. Documented immunologic responses to SLIT have included decreased serum eosinophilic cationic protein and interleukin 13 (IL-13) levels, an elevation in IL-12 levels, a reduction in late-phase responses, and increases in IgG4/IgE ratios [91]. However, successful treatment requires at least 2 years of therapy and adjustment of tolerated doses during the pollen season.

SLIT and treatment with anti-IgE antibody may be complementary approaches to treating allergic rhinoconjunctivitis, which may be used for single or combined treatment [92].

8.7.3 Treatment of GPC

Prevention is the most important management step in GPC. This involves prescription of the appropriate lens type and edge design, and education on strict lens hygiene. Enzymatic cleaning of the lens is essential in minimizing the accumulation of lens coatings and removing protein build-up. The most essential treatment of early stage GPC is removal of the device that is causing the condition. In fact, patients are asymptomatic several days after discontinuation or removal of the contact lens, device, or suture. Reinitiation of lens wear with a clean lens, or lens of a different type or design may be attempted within days of symptom resolution. Mild GPC symptoms may be alleviated by mast cell stabilizers or antihistamine agents. Tear substitutes can be used to minimize conjunctival trauma.

8.7.4 Treatment of Vernal Keratoconjunctivitis

Treatment of VKC requires a multiple approach that includes conservative measures and the use of drugs. Patients and parents should be made aware of the long duration of disease, its chronic evolution, and possible complications. The potential benefits of frequent hand and face washing along with avoiding eye rubbing have to be emphasized. Exposure to nonspecific triggering factors such as sun, wind, and salt water should be avoided. The use of sunglasses, hats with visors, and swimming goggles are recommended.

The use of drugs should be well planned in patients with a history of the disease. Mast cell stabilizers, including disodium cromoglycate, nedocromil, spaglumic acid and lodoxamide, and topical antihistamines are initially used and continued at a decreasing frequency if effective. Newer topical formulations with combined mast cell stabilizing properties and histamine receptor antagonist, such as olopatadine and ketotifen, may be more effective. Nonsteroidal antiinflammatory drugs such as ketorolac, diclofenac, and pranoprofen may be considered as steroid-sparing options. However, these drugs should be used for a limited period of time only. Oral aspirin at doses of 0.5–1 g/day may be beneficial. In VKC patients with extraocular allergies, systemic treatment with oral antihistamines or antileukotrienes can reduce the severity of ocular flare-ups.

8.7.4.1 Corticosteroids

Moderate to severe VKC may require repeated topical steroid treatment to downregulate conjunctival inflammation. "Soft corticosteroids" such as clobetasone, desonide, fluorometholone, loteprednol, and rimexolone may be considered preferentially as the first corticosteroid preparations to be used carefully. A "pulsed" corticosteroid treatment is recommended, in addition to the continuous use of mast cell stabilizers and or topical antihistamines. Doses are chosen based on the inflammatory state. Instillation frequency of 4 times/day for 5–10 days is recommended. The "harder" corticosteroids formulations of prednisolone, dexamethasone, or betamethasone have to be used as a second line and as a last resort for the management of the most severe cases [5]. If a systemic hypersensitivity to identified allergens exists, SIT may be considered.

8.7.4.2 Cyclosporine and Other Immunosuppressive Treatments

Cyclosporine A (CsA) is effective in controlling VKC-associated ocular inflammation by blocking Th2 lymphocyte proliferation and interleukin-2 production. It inhibits histamine release from mast cells and basophils through a reduction in interleukin-5 production, and may reduce eosinophil recruitment and effects on the conjunctiva and cornea. Cyclosporine is lipophilic and thus must be dissolved in an alcohol–oil base. Unavailability of a commercial preparation of topical cyclosporine, technical difficulties in dispensing cyclosporine eye drops, and legal restrictions in many countries on its topical use preclude its widespread use in the treatment of VKC.

CsA 1 or 2% emulsion in castor or olive oil can be considered for treatment of severe VKC and can serve as a good alternative to steroids [93–97]. Cyclosporine 1% was reported to be the minimum effective concentration in the treatment of vernal shield ulcer, with recurrence observed at lower concentrations [98]. In a randomized, controlled trial, the effects of 0.05% topical cyclosporine were similar to placebo in the treatment of VKC [83]. Conversely, in another study, topical CsA 0.05% decreased the severity of symptoms and clinical signs significantly after 6 months, and the need for steroids was reduced, suggesting that CsA at low doses is an effective steroid-sparing agent in severe allergic conjunctivitis [99]. Frequent instillation may be inconvenient but no significant side effects of topical cyclosporine, except for a burning sensation during administration, have been reported. Thus, topical cyclosporine can control the symptoms of VKC but further trials are required to establish the optimal concentration needed to treat the disease.

Short-term, low-dose, topical mitomycin-C 0.01% has been considered for acute exacerbation periods of patients with severe VKC refractory to conventional treatment. A significant decrease in signs and symptoms compared with the placebo group was shown at the end of the 2 week treatment period [100]. Nevertheless, mitomycin-C is not approved for treatment of VKC.

Tacrolimus is a potent drug similar to cyclosporine in its mode of action, but chemically distinct. A skin ointment of tacrolimus has recently been licensed for the treatment of moderate to severe atopic eyelid diseases [101]. Treated patients may be at increased risk of folliculitis, acne, and HSV. A recent study reported great efficacy of tacrolimus 0.1% ointment in the treatment of severe VKC patients [102].

Severe cases that do not respond to any of these topical therapies may require treatment with systemic corticosteroids (prednisone 1 mg/kg a day) for a short period of time.

8.7.5 Treatment of AKC

The overall management of AKC involves a multidisciplinary approach. Identification of allergens by skin or blood testing is important for preventive measures. Cold compresses and regular lubrication may provide symptomatic relief. Tear substitutes help remove and reduce the effects of allergens and the release of mediators, thus reducing the potential for corneal involvement. Lid hygiene is essential: it prevents infectious blepharitis, improving meibomian gland function and tear-film quality.

Prolonged use of topical antiallergic drugs and mast cell stabilizers may be required. Topical antihistamines may be useful for the relief of itching, redness, and mucous discharge. Topical corticosteroids are effective, but should be used only when other topical treatments are not providing sufficient benefits. Brief periods of intensive topical corticosteroid therapy are often necessary to control the local inflammation in severe cases. Topical cyclosporine may improve the signs and symptoms in steroid-dependent patients, thus reducing the need for corticosteroids to control the ocular surface inflammation. Systemic antihistamines are often used to reduce itching and control widespread inflammation in patients with active skin involvement. Systemic corticosteroids may be necessary in severe cases.

8.7.5.1 Cyclosporine and Other Immunosuppressive Treatments

Topical CsA 2% is an effective and safe steroid-sparing agent in AKC and, despite difficulties in patient tolerance, improves symptoms and signs [103]. The lower dose of topical CsaA 0.05% seems to be safe and have some effect in alleviating signs and symptoms of severe AKC refractory to topical steroid treatment [7]. In a multicentered randomized controlled trial, 0.05% cyclosporine 6 times per day followed by 4 times per day was found to be effective in alleviating the signs and symptoms of AKC [7]. Although cyclosporine in a higher (1%) concentration has been shown to be more effective, frequent instillations may compensate for the low concentration of cyclosporine in the currently available commercial preparations in the US and South America.

Topical immunomodulators such as tacrolimus have revolutionized the treatment of atopic dermatitis.

Application of topical tacrolimus on eyelid skin may be effective for treatment of severe atopic dermatitis of the eyelids, and may have secondary benefits for AKC [101, 104, 105]. Topical tacrolimus can be used for at least 1 year without apparent adverse reaction in some patients, although possible adverse reaction should be carefully monitored.

Systemic cyclosporine may be an alternative to systemic corticosteroids for treatment of AKC. Atopic dermatitis patients with and without KC deteriorates graft prognosis statistically significantly. Systemic cyclosporin A improves graft prognosis in atopic dermatitis with KC and the dermatitis as long as the drug is used [84].

In severe cases, systemic treatment with T lymphocyte signal transduction inhibitors such as cyclosporine or tacrolimus may ameliorate both the dermatologic and ocular manifestations in severe patients who are refractory to conventional treatment [106, 107].

8.7.6 Surgical Treatment of Keratoconjunctivitis

Corneal complications have to be carefully monitored and antiinflammatory therapy adjusted accordingly. Secondary microbial infection can be prevented by prescription of antibiotics for a period of 1 week.

Surgical removal of corneal plaques is recommended to alleviate severe symptoms and to allow for corneal reepithelization. Giant papillae excision with or without combined cryotherapy may be indicated in cases of mechanical pseudoptosis or the presence of coarse giant papillae and continuous active disease. A combined treatment regime consisting of surgical removal of giant papillae and supratarsal corticosteroid injection followed by cyclosporine (0.05%) and cromolyn sodium eye drops applied 5 times daily has been proposed for the treatment of severe treatment-resistant shield ulcers [108, 109].

Amniotic membrane grafts following keratectomy have been described as a successful treatment in deep ulcers, in cases with slight stromal thinning [110, 111]. The amniotic membrane patch may be enough to achieve epithelization. This procedure prevents the presence of membrane remains under the epithelium, which can affect postoperative corneal transparency.

Excimer laser phototherapeutic keratectomy and CO_2-assisted removal of giant papillae have been attempted in the treatment of shield ulcer with or without plaque [112].

More invasive procedures such as oral mucosal grafting or supratarsal corticosteroid injections should be avoided.

Summary for the Clinician

- Make the proper diagnosis.
- Educate on avoidance of the offending allergens.
- Stress the importance of nonpharmacologic treatments (lubricants, lid hygiene, and cold compresses).
- Warn against use and abuse of decongestant/vasoconstrictors, which have little place in the pharmacological treatment of ocular allergic disease.
- Recommend systemic antihistamines only in patients with concomitant major nonocular allergic manifestations.
- Specific immune therapy is especially indicated if extra-allergic manifestations are also present.
- Use topical corticosteroid formulations only in the most severe cases.
- In SAC/PAC associated with allergic rhinitis, topical nasal steroids should improve the nasal-ocular reflex.
- Dual acting components are first line in the treatment of ocular allergy.
- Avoid abuse of steroids.
- Severe diseases must be treated with two or more drugs.
- Removal of corneal plaques is the only surgical procedure recommended in cases of corneal complications.

References

1. Ono SJ, Abelson MB (2005) Allergic conjunctivitis: update on pathophysiology and prospects for future treatment. J Allergy Clin Immunol 115:118–122
2. Johansson SG, Hourihane JO, Bousquet J et al (2001) A revised nomenclature for allergy. An EAACI position statement from the EAACI nomenclature task force. Allergy 56:813–824
3. BenEzra D (2006) Classification of conjunctivitis and blepharitis. In: BenEzra D (ed) Blepharitis and conjunctivitis. Guidelines for diagnosis and treatment. Editorial Glosa, Barcelona, Spain
4. Blaiss MS (2007) Allergic rhinoconjunctivitis: burden of disease. Allergy Asthma Proc 28:393–397
5. Leonardi A (2002) Vernal keratoconjunctivitis: pathogenesis and treatment. Prog Ret Eye Res 21:319–339

6. Bonini S, Bonini S, Lambiase A et al (2000) Vernal keratoconjunctivitis revisited. A case series of 195 patients with long-term follow up. Ophthalmology 107:1157–1163
7. Akpek EK, Dart JK, Watson S et al (2004) A randomized trial of topical cyclosporin 0.05% in topical steroid-resistant atopic keratoconjunctivitis. Ophthalmology 111: 476–482
8. Foster CS, Calonge M (1990) Atopic keratoconjunctiuvitis. Ophthalmology 97:992–100
9. Nivenius E, Montan PG, Chryssanthou E et al (2004) No apparent association between periocular and ocular microcolonization and the degree of inflammation in patients with atopic keratoconjunctivitis. Clin Exp Allergy 34:725–730
10. Allansmith MR, Korb DR, Greiner JV (1978) Giant papillary conjunctivitis induced by hard or soft contact lens wear: quantitative histology. Ophthalmology 85:766–778
11. Irkec MT, Orhan M, Erdener U (1999) Role of tear inflammatory mediators in contact lens-associated giant papillary conjunctivitis in soft contact lens wearers. Ocul Immunol Inflamm 7:35–38
12. Wilson FM (2003) Allergy to topical medication. Int Ophthalm Clin 43:73–81
13. Leonardi A, Lanier B (2008) Urban eye allergy syndrome: a new clinical entity? Curr Med Res Opin 24:2295–2302
14. Bonini S, Micera A, Iovieno A et al (2005) Expression of Toll-like receptors in healthy and allergic conjunctiva. Ophthalmology 112:1548–1549
15. Cook EB, Stahl JL, Esnault S et al (2005) Toll-like receptor 2 expression on human conjunctival epithelial cells: a pathway for Staphylococcus aureus involvement in chronic ocular proinflammatory responses. Ann Allergy Asthma Immunol 94:486–497
16. Varadaradjalou S, Feger F, Thieblemont N et al (2003) Toll-like receptor 2 (TLR2) and TLR4 differentially activate human mast cells. Eur J Immunol 33:899–906
17. Tabuchi K, Inada N, Shoji J et al (2004) The relationship between Staphylococcus aureus and atopic keratoconjunctivitis. Nippon Ganka Gakkai Zasshi 108:397–400
18. Lambiase A, Normando EM, Vitiello L et al (2007) Natural killer cells in vernal keratoconjunctivitis. Mol Vis 13: 1562–1567
19. Manzouri B, Flynn T, Ohbayashi M et al (2008) The dendritic cell in allergic conjunctivitis. Ocul Surf 6:70–78
20. Abu El Asrar AM, Fatani RA, Missotten L et al (2001) Expression of CD23/CD21 and CD40/CD40 ligand in vernal keratoconjunctivitis. Eye 15:217–224
21. Abu El Asrar AM, Al-Kharashi SA, Al-Mansouri S et al (2001) Langerhans' cells in vernal keratoconjunctivitis express the costimulatory molecole B7-2 (CD86) but not B7-1 (CD80). Eye 15:648–654
22. Sumi T, Fukushima A, Fukuda K et al (2007) Differential contributions of B7-1 and B7-2 to the development of murine experimental allergic conjunctivitis. Immunol Lett 108:62–67
23. Leonardi A, Busca F, Motterle L et al (2006) Case series of 406 vernal keratoconjunctivitis patients: a demographic and epidemiological study. Acta Ophthalmol Scand 84:406–410
24. Toda M, Ono SJ (2002) Genomics and proteomics of allergic disease. Immunology 106:1–10
25. Manzouri B, Ohbayashi M, Leonardi A, et al (2008) Characterization of dendritic cell phenotype in allergic conjunctiva: increased expression of FcvarepsilonRI, the high-affinity receptor for immunoglobulin E. Eye [Epub ahead of print]
26. Maggi L, Santarlasci V, Liotta F et al (2007) Demonstration of circulating allergen-specific CD4+ CD25highFoxp3+ T-regulatory cells in both nonatopic and atopic individuals. J Allergy Clin Immunol 120:429–436
27. Woodfolk JA (2007) T-cell responses to allergens. J Allergy Clin Immunol 119:280–294
28. Fukushima A, Yamaguchi T, Sumi T et al (2007) Roles of CD4+ CD25+ T cells in the development of experimental murine allergic conjunctivitis. Graefes Arch Clin Exp Ophthalmol 245:705–714
29. Fukushima A, Sumi T, Fukuda K et al (2006) Interleukin 10 and transforming growth factor b contribute to the development of experimentally induced allergic conjunctivitis in mice during the effector phase. Br J Ophthalmol 90: 1535–1541
30. Leonardi A, Curnow SJ, Zhan H et al (2006) Multiple cytokines in human tear specimens in seasonal and chronic allergic eye disease and in conjunctival fibroblast cultures. Clin Exp Allergy 36:777–784
31. Sack RA, Conradi L, Beaton A et al (2007) Antibody array characterization of inflammatory mediators in allergic and normal tears in the open and closed eye environments. Exp Eye Res 85:528–538
32. Kumagai N, Fukuda K, Fujitsu Y et al (2006) Role of structural cells of the cornea and conjunctiva in the pathogenesis of vernal keratoconjunctivitis. Prog Retin Eye Res 25: 165–187
33. Leonardi A, Brun P, Abatangelo G et al (2003) Tear levels and activity of matrix metalloproteinase (MMP)-1 and MMP-9 in vernal keratoconjunctivitis. Invest Ophthalmol Vis Sci 44:3052–3058
34. Leonardi A, Brun P, Sartori MT et al (2005) Urokinase plasminogen activator, uPA receptor and its inhibitor in veronal keratoconjunctivitis. Invest Ophthalmol Vis Sci 46: 1364–1370

35. Ghavami S, Hashemi M, de Serres FJ et al (2007) Trypsin inhibitory capacity in vernal keratoconjunctivitis. Invest Ophthalmol Vis Sci 48:264–269
36. Hamrah P, Dana MR (2007) Corneal antigen-presenting cells. Chem Immunol Allergy 92:58–70
37. Hamrah P, Huq SO, Liu Y et al (2003) Corneal immunity is mediated by heterogeneous population of antigen-presenting cells. J Leukoc Biol 74:172–178
38. Bacon AS, Tuft SJ, Metz DM et al (1993) The origin of keratopathy in chronic allergic eye disease: a histopathological study. Eye 7(Suppl):21–25
39. Messmer EM, May CA, Stefani FH et al (2002) Toxic eosinophil granule protein deposition in corneal ulcerations and scars associated with atopic keratoconjunctivitis. Am J Ophthalmol 134:816–821
40. Trocme SD, Kephart GM, Allansmith MR et al (1989) Conjunctival deposition of eosinophil granule major basic protein in vernal keratoconjunctivitis and contact lens-associated giant papillary conjunctivitis. Am J Ophthalmol 108:57–63
41. Leonardi A, Jose P, Zhan H et al (2003) Tear and mucus eotaxin-1 and eotaxin-2 in allergic keratoconjunctivitis. Ophthalmology 110:487–492
42. Dogru M, Okada N, Asano-Kato N et al (2005) Ocular surface and MUC5AC alterations in atopic patients with corneal shield ulcers. Curr Eye Res 30:897–905
43. Dogru M, Okada N, Asano-Kato N et al (2006) Alterations of the ocular surface epithelial mucins 1, 2, 4 and the tear functions in patients with atopic keratoconjunctivitis. Clin Exp Allergy 36:1556–1565
44. Dogru M, Matsumoto Y, Okada N et al (2008) Alterations of the ocular surface epithelial MUC16 and goblet cell MUC5AC in patients with atopic keratoconjunctivitis. Allergy 63:1324–1334
45. Cameron JA (1995) Shield ulcers and plaques of cornea in vernal keratoconjunctivitis. Ophthalmology 102:985–993
46. Tabbara KF (1999) Ocular complications of vernal keratoconjunctivitis. Can J Ophthalmol 34:88–92
47. Hu Y, Matsumoto Y, Adan ES et al (2008) Corneal in vivo confocal scanning laser microscopy in patients with atopic keratoconjunctivitis. Ophthalmology 115:2004–2012
48. Lambiase A, Manni L, Bonini S et al (2000) Nerve growth factor promotes corneal healing: structural, biochemical, and molecular analyses of rat and human corneas. Invest Ophthalmol Vis Sci 41:1063–1069
49. Motterle L, Diebold Y, Enriquez de Salamanca A et al (2006) Altered expression of neurotransmitter receptors and neuromediators in vernal keratoconjunctivitis. Arch Ophthalmol 124:462–468
50. Hilgartner HL, Hilgartner HL Jr, Gilbert JT (1937) A preliminary report of a case of keratoconus successfully treated with organotherapy, radium and shortwave diathermy. Am J Ophthalmol 20:1032–1039
51. Galin MA, Berger R (1958) Atopy and keratoconus. Am J Ophthalmol 45:904–906
52. Spencer WH, Fisher JJ (1959) The association of keratoconus with atopic dermatitis. Am J Ophthalmol 47:332–334
53. Copeman PWM (1965) Eczema and keratoconus. BMJ 2:977–979
54. Gasset AR, Hinson WA, Frias JL (1978) Keratoconus and atopic disease. Ann Ophthalmol 10:991–994
55. Weed KH, MacEwen CJ, Giles T et al (2008) The Dundee University Scottish Keratoconus study: demographics, corneal signs, associated diseases, and eye rubbing. Eye 22:534–541
56. Lapid-Gortzak R, Rosen S, Weitzman S et al (2002) Videokeratography findings in children with vernal keratoconjunctivitis versus those of healthy children. Ophthalmology. 109:2018–2023
57. Totan Y, Hepşen IF, Cekiç O et al (2001) Incidence of keratoconus in subjects with vernal keratoconjunctivitis: a videokeratographic study. Ophthalmology 108:824–827
58. Kaya V, Karakaya M, Utine CA et al (2007) Evaluation of the corneal topographic characteristics of keratoconus with orbscan II in patients with and without atopy. Cornea 26:945–948
59. Demirbas NH, Pflugfelder SC (1998) Topographic pattern and apex location of keratoconus on elevation topography maps. Cornea 17:476–484
60. Smith VA, Hoh HB, Littleton M et al (1995) Over-expression of a gelatinase A activity in keratoconus. Eye 9:429–433
61. Smith VA, Easty DL (2000) Matrix metalloproteinase 2: involvement in keratoconus. Eur J Ophthalmol 10:215–226
62. Smith VA, Matthews FJ, Majid MA et al (2006) Keratoconus: matrix metalloproteinase-2 activation and TIMP modulation. Biochim Biophys Acta 1762:431–439
63. Mackiewicz Z, Määttä M, Stenman M et al (2006) Collagenolytic proteinases in keratoconus. Cornea 25:603–610
64. Cameron JA, Al-Rajhi AA, Badr IA (1989) Corneal ectasia in vernal keratoconjunctivitis. Ophthalmology 96:1615–1623
65. Nguyen DQ, Sidebottom R, Bates AK (2007) Microbial keratitis in keratoglobus-associated vernal keratoconjunctivitis and atopic dermatitis. Eye Contact Lens 33:109–110
66. Koulikovska M, van der Ploeg I, Herrmann B et al (2001) Respiratory syncytial virus and chlamydia are not detectable by PCR in ongoing vernal keratoconjunctivitis. Ocul Immunol Inflamm 9:253–257
67. Kaiserman I, Kaiserman N, Elhayany A et al (2006) Increased risk for herpetic eye disease in patients with allergic conjunctivitis. Curr Eye Res 31:721–725
68. Gedik S, Akova YA, Gür S (2006) Secondary bacterial keratitis associated with shield ulcer caused by vernal conjunctivitis. Cornea 25:974–976
69. Kerr N, Stern GA (1992) Bacterial keratitis associated with vernal keratoconjunctivitis. Cornea 11:355–359

70. Arora R, Gupta S, Raina UK et al (2002) Penicillium keratitis in vernal Keratoconjunctivitis. Indian J Ophthalmol 50:215–216
71. Sridhar MS, Gopinathan U, Rao GN (2003) Fungal keratitis associated with vernal keratoconjunctivitis. Cornea 22:80–81
72. Niederkorn JY (2007) Immune mechanisms of corneal allograft rejection. Curr Eye Res 32:1005–1016
73. Beauregard C, Stevens C, Mayhew E et al (2005) Cutting edge: atopy promotes Th2 responses to alloantigens and increases the incidence and tempo of corneal allograft rejection. J Immunol 174:6577–6581
74. Chen N, Field EH (1995) Enhanced type 2 and diminished type 1 cytokines in neonatal tolerance. Transplantation 59:933–941
75. Ghoraishi M, Akova YA, Tugal-Tutkun I et al (1995) Penetrating keratoplasty in atopic keratoconjunctivitis. Cornea 14:610–613
76. Hargrave S, Chu Y, Mendelblatt D et al (2003) Preliminary findings in corneal allograft rejection in patients with keratoconus. Am J Ophthalmol 135:452–460
77. Flynn TH, Ohbayashi M, Ikeda Y et al (2007) Effect of allergic conjunctival inflammation on the allogeneic response to donor cornea. Invest Ophthalmol Vis Sci 48:4044–4049
78. Mahmood MA, Wagoner MD (2000) Penetrating keratoplasty in eyes with keratoconus and vernal keratoconjunctivitis. Cornea 19:468–470
79. Egrilmez S, Sahin S, Yagci A (2004) The effect of vernal keratoconjunctivitis on clinical outcomes of penetrating keratoplasty for keratoconus. Can J Ophthalmol 39:772–777
80. Wagoner MD, Ba-Abbad R, King Khaled Eye Specialist Hospital Cornea Transplant Study Group (2009) Penetrating keratoplasty for keratoconus with or without vernal keratoconjunctivitis. Cornea 28:14–18
81. Lyons CJ, Dart JK, Aclimandos WA et al (1990) Sclerokeratitis after keratoplasty in atopy. Ophthalmology 97:729–733
82. Tomita M, Shimmura S, Tsubota K et al (2008) Postkeratoplasty atopic sclerokeratitis in keratoconus patients. Ophthalmology 115:851–856
83. Daniell M, Constantinou M, Vu HT et al (2006) Randomized controlled trial of cyclosporine A in steroid dependent allergic conjunctivitis. Br J Ophthalmol 90: 461–464
84. Reinhard T, Möller M, Sundmacher R (1999) Penetrating keratoplasty in patients with atopic dermatitis with and without systemic Cyclosporin A. Cornea 18:645–651
85. Bielory L, Lien KW, Bigelsen S (2005) Efficacy and tolerability of newer antihistamines in the treatment of allergic conjunctivitis. Drugs 65:215–228
86. Cook EB, Stahl JL, Barney NP et al (2002) Mechanisms of antihistamines and mast cell stabilizers in ocular allergic inflammation. Curr Drug Targets Inflamm Allergy 1:167–180
87. Abelson MB (2004) A review of olopatadine for the treatment of ocular allergy. Expert Opin Pharmacother 5:1979–1994
88. Torkildsen GL, Ousler GW 3rd et al (2008) Ocular comfort and drying effects of three topical antihistamine/mast cell stabilizers in adults with allergic conjunctivitis: a randomized, double-masked crossover study. Clin Ther 30:1264–1271
89. Origlieri C, Bielory L (2008) Intranasal corticosteroids and allergic rhinoconjunctivitis. Curr Opin Allergy Clin Immunol 8:450–456
90. Bielory L (2008) Ocular symptom reduction in patients with seasonal allergic rhinitis treated with the intranasal corticosteroid mometasone furoate. Ann Allergy Asthma Immunol 100:272–279
91. Röder E, Berger MY, de Groot H et al (2008) Immunotherapy in children and adolescents with allergic rhinoconjunctivitis: a systematic review. Pediatr Allergy Immunol 19:197–207
92. Rolinck-Werninghaus C, Hamelmann E, Keil T et al (2004) The co-seasonal application of anti-IgE after preseasonal specific immunotherapy decreases ocular and nasal symptom scores and rescue medication use in grass pollen allergic children. Allergy 59:973–979
93. BenEzra D, Pe'er J, Brodsky M, Cohen E (1986) Cyclosporine eyedrops for the treatment of severe vernal keratoconjunctivitis. Am J Ophthalmol 101:278–282
94. Kilic A, Gurler B (2006) Topical 2% cyclosporine A in preservative-free artificial tears for the treatment of vernal keratoconjunctivitis. Can J Ophthalmol 41:693–698
95. Pucci N, Novembre E, Cianferoni A et al (2002) Efficacy and safety of cyclosporine eyedrops in vernal keratoconjunctivitis. Ann Allergy Asthma Immunol 89:298–303
96. Secchi AG, Tognon MS, Leonardi A (1990) Topical use of Cyclosporine in the treatment of vernal keratoconjunctivitis. Am J Ophthalmol 110:137–142
97. Spadavecchia L, Fanelli P, Tesse R et al (2006) Efficacy of 1.25% and 1% topical cyclosporine in the treatment of severe vernal keratoconjunctivitis in childhood. Pediatr Allergy Immunol 17:527–532
98. Cetinkaya A, Akova YA, Dursun D et al (2004) Topical cyclosporine in the management of shield ulcers. Cornea 23:194–200
99. Ozcan AA, Ersoz TR, Dulger E (2007) Management of severe allergic conjunctivitis with topical cyclosporin a 0.05% eyedrops. Cornea 26:1035–1038
100. Akpek EK, Hasiripi H, Christen WG et al (2000) A randomized trial of low-dose, topical mitomycin-C in the treatment of severe vernal keratoconjunctivitis. Ophthalmology 107:263–269
101. Virtanen HM, Reitamo S, Kari M et al (2006) Effect of 0.03% tacrolimus ointment on conjunctival cytology in patients with severe atopic blepharoconjunctivitis: a retrospective study. Acta Ophthalmol Scand 84:693–695

102. Vichyanond P, Tantimongkolsuk C, Dumrongkigchaiporn P et al (2004) Vernal keratoconjunctivitis: Result of a novel therapy with 0.1% topical ophthalmic FK-506 ointment. J Allergy Clin Immunol 113:355–358
103. Hingorani M, Calder VL, Buckley RJ et al (1999) The immunomodulatory effect of topical cyclosporin A in atopic keratoconjunctivitis. Invest Ophthalmol Vis Sci 40:392–399
104. Miyazaki D, Tominaga T, Kakimaru-Hasegawa A et al (2008) Therapeutic effects of tacrolimus ointment for refractory ocular surface inflammatory diseases. Ophthalmology 115:988–999
105. Rikkers SM, Holland GN, Drayton GE et al (2003) Topical tacrolimus treatment of atopic eyelid disease. Am J Ophthalmol 135:297–302
106. Anzaar F, Gallagher MJ, Bhat P et al (2008) Use of systemic T-lymphocyte signal transduction inhibitors in the treatment of atopic keratoconjunctivitis. Cornea 27:884–888
107. Stumpf T, Luqmani N, Sumich P et al (2006) Systemic tacrolimus in the treatment of severe atopic keratoconjunctivitis. Cornea 25:1147–1149
108. Fujishima H, Fukagawa K, Satake Y, Saito I, Shimazaki J, Takano Y, Tsubota K (2000) Combined medical and surgical treatment of severe vernal ketatoconjunctivitis. Jpn J Ophthalmol 44:511–515
109. Tanaka M, Takano Y, Dogru M et al (2004) A comparative evaluation of the efficacy of intraoperative mitomycin C use after the excision of cobblestone-like papillae in severe atopic and vernal keratoconjunctivitis. Cornea 23:326–329
110. Pelegrin L, Gris O, Adán A et al (2008) Superficial keratectomy and amniotic membrane patch in the treatment of corneal plaque of vernal keratoconjunctivitis. Eur J Ophthalmol 18:131–133
111. Rouher N, Pilon F, Dalens H et al (2004) Implantation of preserved human amniotic membrane for the treatment of shield ulcers and persistent corneal epithelial defects in chronic allergic keratoconjunctivitis. J Fr Ophtalmol 7:1091–1097
112. Belfair N, Monos T, Levy J et al (2005) Removal of giant vernal papillae by CO2 laser. Can J Ophthalmol 40:472–476

Chapter 9

Trachoma

Matthew J. Burton

Core Messages

- Trachoma is the leading infectious cause of blindness worldwide.
- It is caused by the bacterium *Chlamydia trachomatis*.
- Repeated conjunctival infection produces scarring, trichiasis, and corneal opacification (CO).
- Over 40 million people have the active inflammatory stages of the disease, and eight million have trichiasis.
- Trachoma control is through the implementation of the SAFE Strategy.
- Trichiasis surgery reduces the risk of corneal blindness.
- Antibiotics (oral azithromycin or topical tetracycline) are used in mass treatment programs to control chlamydial infection.
- Face washing and environmental improvements help to suppress the transmission of the infection.

9.1 Introduction

9.1.1 Overview

Trachoma begins in early childhood with repeated infection of the conjunctiva by *Chlamydia trachomatis*, the causative agent. This triggers recurrent episodes of chronic conjunctival inflammation (active trachoma). Conjunctival scarring, which is believed to be immunopathologically mediated, develops progressively over many years. The scar may contract, pulling the eyelids in (entropion), resulting in contact between the eyelashes and the eye (trichiasis). This damages the cornea, and blinding opacification often follows.

Trachoma is the leading infectious cause of blindness worldwide. It is a considerable public health problem, afflicting some of the poorest regions of the globe, predominantly in sub-Saharan Africa and Asia. In 2003, the WHO estimated that there were 84 million people having active trachoma and 7.6 million with sight-threatening trichiasis requiring surgery [88]. Recent estimates for the number of blind vary between 1.3 and 3.8 million [33, 60]. The disease prospers in communities with crowded living conditions and limited hygiene, which favor transmission of *C. trachomatis*. The impact of blinding trachoma on the individual is devastating. The corneal blindness is effectively irreversible as keratoplasty is rarely an option in endemic countries. Trachoma has major social and economic consequences for effected families and communities. Previously healthy productive adults are rendered dependent on others and are unable to work or care for themselves, compounding poverty. It is estimated that trachoma costs up to US$ 8 billion in lost productivity worldwide every year [34].

The World Health Organization is leading a global effort to eliminate blinding trachoma through the implementation of the SAFE strategy. This involves surgery for trichiasis, antibiotics for infection, facial cleanliness (hygiene promotion), and environmental improvements to reduce transmission of the organism. This program has met with some success wherever it has been fully implemented. However, there are significant gaps in the evidence base, and optimal management remains uncertain.

9.1.2 History

Trachoma is a disease of antiquity [2]. It was endemic in ancient Egypt. The *Ebers Papyrus*, dating from the sixteenth century BC, describes the condition and its treatment; epilation forceps have been found in tombs from that time. Later, Hippocrates wrote about trachoma and trichiasis. The name *trachoma*, from the Greek *trachus*, meaning rough, was first recorded by Discordes in *Materia Medica* in around 60 AD. Arab ophthalmologists, working in the eighth to fourteenth century AD, wrote extensively about trachoma; they considered it to be an infectious disease with acute and chronic manifestations. Treatments included scalp incisions, cauterisation, and the application of ferrous sulfate. The limited records from Medieval Europe suggest that trachoma was widespread, and that epilation was practiced and exotic ointments prescribed. Trachoma was a major public health problem in Europe at the beginning of the nineteenth century. Many of the major ophthalmic hospitals of Europe (including Moorfields Eye Hospital, London) were originally established to care for patients with trachoma. The disease gradually declined in Western Europe during the nineteenth century. This change is attributed to improvements in living conditions and sanitation rather than to any specific medical intervention.

9.2 Clinical Features

9.2.1 Symptoms and Signs

Clinically, trachoma is subdivided into Active (early) and Cicatricial (late-stage) disease. Active disease is more commonly found in children. The individual may have minimal symptoms of ocular irritation and a slight watery discharge. In more severe cases, there may be photophobia and copious watering. However, it is not uncommon to find asymptomatic individuals with significant conjunctival inflammation. Active disease is characterized by a chronic, recurrent follicular conjunctivitis, most prominently involving the upper tarsal conjunctiva (Fig. 9.1a) [25]. Follicles are collections of lymphoid cells subjacent to the conjunctival epithelium. They range from 0.2 to 2 mm in diameter, but only those greater than 0.5 mm are considered significant in the WHO classification scheme. Intense cases are characterized by the presence of papillary hypertrophy. When mild, there is engorgement of the small vessels appearing as small red dots with surrounding oedema within the tarsal conjunctiva. In more severe

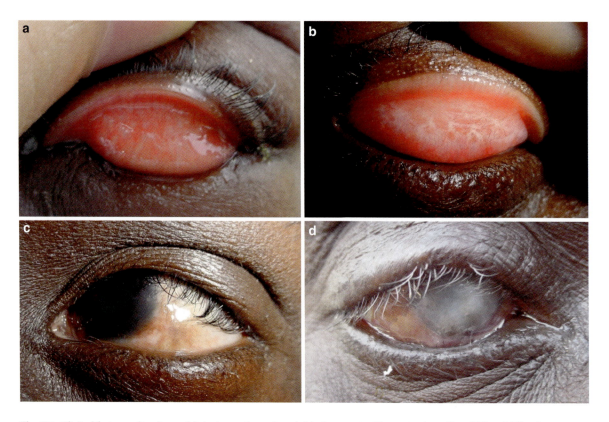

Fig. 9.1 *Clinical features of trachoma.* (**a**) Active trachoma in a child, characterized by a mixed papillary (TI) and follicular response (TF). (**b**) Tarsal conjunctival scarring (TS). (**c**) Entropion and trichiasis (TT). (**d**) Blinding corneal opacification (CO) with entropion and trichiasis (TT)

cases, there is a pronounced inflammatory thickening and oedema of the conjunctiva that obscures the normal deep tarsal blood vessels. During an episode of active disease, the cornea can be affected in a number of ways: superficial vascular pannus, punctate epithelial keratopathy, superficial infiltrates, swelling of the limbus, and development of limbal follicles. As the limbal follicles resolve, they leave characteristic small depressions called Herbert's pits.

The cicatricial sequelae of trachoma tend to become apparent from the third decade of life, although in hyperendemic settings trichiasis may be found in children [52]. Individuals with entropion and trichiasis frequently experience pain as the in-turned lashes rub on the cornea. Tarsal conjunctival scarring (TS) ranges from a few linear or stellate scars to thick distorting bands of fibrosis (Fig. 9.1b). Arlt's Line is a characteristic feature: a horizontal band of fibrosis running across the tarsal conjunctiva a few millimeters above the lid margin. The fornix can be shortened, and symblepheron sometimes develop. Contraction of the scar tissue causes in-turning of the eyelids (entropion). Trichiasis, the contact between the eyelashes and the globe, may be a direct result of the entropion (Fig. 9.1c). However, in many cases, the trichiasis may be the result of either misdirected (arising from the lash-line) or metaplastic lashes (arising from aberrant positions), in the absence of frank entropion. Trachomatous corneal opacification (CO) has varying phenotypes, ranging from a few small opacities in areas directly traumatized by an in-turned lash, through to total opacification of the cornea, and sometimes phthisis bulbi (Fig. 9.1d).

9.2.2 Trachoma Grading Systems

Over the last 80 years, several trachoma grading systems have been developed. For research purposes, the WHO published a detailed system, which independently grades five separate features, each on a four-point scale [25]. However, this system is too detailed for programmatic purposes; therefore, the essential clinical signs were distilled down to the Simplified WHO Trachoma Grading System (Table 9.1) [75]. This is reliable and easy to use, yielding useful information on the prevalence of active and cicatricial disease.

9.2.3 Differential Diagnosis

The differential diagnosis of a chronic follicular conjunctivitis includes a number of infections: various viruses

Table 9.1 The simplified WHO system for the assessment of trachoma [75]

Grade	Description
TF	Trachomatous inflammation – follicular: the presence of five or more follicles (>0.5 mm) in the upper tarsal conjunctiva
TI	Trachomatous inflammation – intense: pronounced inflammatory thickening of the tarsal conjunctiva that obscures more than half of the deep normal vessels
TS	Trachomatous scarring: the presence of scarring in the tarsal conjunctiva
TT	Trachomatous trichiasis: at least one lash rubs on the eyeball
CO	Corneal opacity: easily visible corneal opacity over the pupil

(adenovirus, *molluscum contagiosum*) and bacteria (*S. aureus* and *Moraxella*). The genital strains (D to K) of *C. trachomatis* cause adult inclusion conjunctivitis, characterized by large opalescent follicles. Occasionally, chronic follicular conjunctivitis is caused by topical medication.

In endemic regions, the vast majority of upper lid cicatricial entropion is caused by trachoma. However, a number of alternative conditions occasionally arise which have similar features: Stevens-Johnson syndrome (sulphonamides are in more frequent use), chemical injury, mucus membrane pemphigoid, and sarcoidosis. These are usually readily distinguished by the history.

> **Summary for the Clinician**
>
> - Trachoma has two distinct phases: (1) active disease and (2) cicatricial disease
> - Active disease is characterized by a chronic follicular conjunctivitis
> - Cicatricial disease is characterized by a progression: conjunctival scarring, entropion/trichiasis, CO

9.3 Chlamydia Trachomatis

Chlamydia trachomatis is an obligate intracellular bacterium, with 19 different serovars. These are sub-divided into two biovars; the trachoma biovar (serovars A to K) and the lymphogranuloma venereum biovar (serovars L1,

L2, L2a, and L3). Endemic trachoma is caused by serovars A, B, Ba, and C [77]. Genital chlamydial infection, which causes pelvic inflammatory disease and infertility, is associated with serovars D to K. This tissue tropism is poorly understood. Some differences between genital and ocular strains have been identified, with the genital strains maintaining the capacity to synthesize tryptophan [21]. Recent studies have demonstrated significant variation in the virulence of different strains of *C. trachomatis*, both in vitro and in animal studies [40].

During the course of its developmental cycle, *C. trachomatis* has two principle forms: reticulate bodies (RB) and elementary bodies (EB) [78]. EB are the small (0.3 μm), hardy, metabolically inactive extracellular form of the organism. Nuclear material is tightly packed with histone-like proteins. It is in this form that *Chlamydiae* are transferred between host cells and organisms. They have a protective cellular envelope similar to that of gram-negative bacteria, having both an inner and an outer membrane with a periplasmic layer in-between, ensuring osmotic stability in the extracellular environment. The Major Outer Membrane Protein (MOMP) accounts for 60% of the surface protein. Variations in MOMP epitopes define serovar specificity and may be an important target for the immune response to *C. trachomatis*. Other surface expressed molecules have been investigated more recently. The Polymorphic Membrane Proteins have been found to be quite variable and may turn out to be important in the immune response to the infection [22]. The chlamydial developmental cycle commences with the attachment of the EB to the surface of epithelial cells which triggers endocytosis of the bacteria. Inside the host cell, the EB transforms into the reticulate body form. The RB is larger (1 μm) than the EB, and they are contained within a peri-nuclear inclusion body. They are metabolically active, replicating by binary fission. After some hours, the newly produced RB transform into EB; nuclear material is condensed and there is an overall reduction in size. The newly formed EB are released either by lysis of the host cell or by the fusion of the inclusion body with the plasma membrane. In vitro, the chlamydial development cycle takes between 36 and 70 h to complete.

Summary for the Clinician

- Endemic trachoma is caused by the ocular serovars of *Chlamydia trachomatis*: A, B, Ba, and C.
- *C. trachomatis* is an obligate intracellular bacteria with a biphasic developmental cycle.

9.4 Laboratory Diagnosis

The detection of *C. trachomatis* infection is problematic. Trachoma control programs have to rely on the clinical signs of disease for diagnosis, as there is currently no point-of-care test available which is suitable for use in an operational setting (reliable, rapid, and cheap). For research studies, it is usually important to know the individual *C. trachomatis* infection status, and various different tests have been used over the years [69]. Unfortunately, there is no "Gold Standard" test.

The earliest studies used cytological analysis of conjunctival smears, usually stained with Giemsa, to demonstrate the chlamydial inclusion body. Whilst this is specific, it lacks sensitivity. It has the advantage of allowing the adequacy of the specimen to be assessed, and provides information about the presence of inflammatory cells and bacteria, but requires a skilled microscopist. The sensitivity of microscopy can be increased by direct immunofluorescence with monoclonal antibodies to *C. trachomatis* antigens. *C. trachomatis* can be grown in cell culture and then detected by microscopy. Several systems were developed, and for many years, this was the reference technique. It is the only method that can assess the viability of the organism. Although tissue culture is very specific, it too lacks sensitivity. In addition, samples have to be handled very carefully. It is expensive, requires sophisticated laboratory equipment, as well as a high degree of expertise. Enzyme-linked immunoassays, which detected chlamydial antigens were produced commercially. However, these had moderate sensitivity, and could cross-react with other bacteria, reducing specificity.

Over the last 15 years, nucleic acid amplification tests, such as the polymerase chain reaction (PCR), have become the preferred method for detection of *C. trachomatis*. These tests are both highly specific and sensitive, identifying many more individuals harboring *C. trachomatis* in endemic populations than previously recognized. However, PCR is not practical for routine use by control programs in endemic countries because of its cost and complexity. Considerable care needs to be taken in collecting and processing conjunctival swab specimens for PCR to avoid contamination, leading to false positive results. Recently, quantitative real-time PCR has been used to measure the load of *C. trachomatis* infection in members of trachoma-endemic communities to better define the major reservoirs of infection and monitor response to treatment [19, 67, 68].

> **Summary for the Clinician**
>
> - The detection of *C. trachomatis* infection is problematic, with no option that is practical for use in trachoma control programs.
> - Several alternatives have been used in research settings: Microscopy, Culture, ELISA, PCR.
> - Currently, nucleic acid amplification tests are generally preferred.

9.5 Clinical Signs and Infection

Trachomatous conjunctival inflammation is believed to be triggered by *Chlamydia trachomatis*. However, there is a complex relationship between disease and infection in trachoma. Many studies, using a range of tests, have demonstrated a mismatch between clinical signs and detection of *C. trachomatis*: active trachoma without detectable *C. trachomatis*, and conversely, *C. trachomatis* detected in clinically normal individuals [18, 63, 90]. This mismatch is a significant problem for trachoma control programs, which rely on signs to guide antibiotic treatment. It also indicates the importance of the host response in the disease process.

There are several potential contributory reasons for this mismatch. Firstly, there may be an "incubation period" during which infection is present but disease has not yet developed. Secondly, the resolution of signs of disease lags behind the resolution of infection, often by many weeks [35]. The duration of both disease and infection episodes are modified by age, lasting longer in children. Thirdly, it is possible that a sub-clinical persistent form of infection may develop under certain conditions in which the organism is not replicating, but lies dormant and may not provoke the disease phenotype. Fourthly, the signs of conjunctival inflammation are not exclusive to trachoma and could be initiated by other pathogens. Other bacterial infections have more recently been associated with conjunctival inflammation in individuals with established scarring and trichiasis, and may contribute to progressive disease [15, 20]. Finally, the presence of detectable chlamydial antigen or DNA does not necessarily equate to an established, replicating infection. Tests may be positive as a result of a transient inoculation of the conjunctiva with *C. trachomatis*, following close contact with a heavily infected individual or the activities of eye seeking flies, or through cross contamination in the field or the laboratory.

Recently, the relationship between disease and infection has been explored using quantitative PCR for *C. trachomatis*, to measure the relative load of infection in members of several trachoma endemic communities [18, 19, 67, 68]. The majority of infected individuals had relatively low infection loads, whilst a smaller number have high loads. The highest infection loads are usually found in preschool children, especially those with intense conjunctival inflammation. Clinically, normal individuals with detectable *C. trachomatis* tend to have lower infection loads.

> **Summary for the Clinician**
>
> - There is a mismatch between the clinical signs of active trachoma and the detection of *C. trachomatis* infection.
> - Clinically, occult infection and persistent disease without detectable *C. trachomatis* are frequent.
> - This has implications for which members of a trachoma endemic community should be offered antibiotic treatment.

9.6 Epidemiology

9.6.1 Prevalence and Distribution

Trachoma accounts for about 3–4% of global blindness [60]. This most recent estimate from the WHO suggests that there are about 1.3 million people blind from trachoma (visual acuity less than 3/60), with many more having moderate to severe visual impairment. Other recent estimates have been higher, at around four million blind people [33]. In 2008, it was estimated that about 40 million people had active trachoma concurrently, and 8.2 million had trichiasis [45]. The highest prevalence of trachoma is reported from Ethiopia and Sudan, where active trachoma is often found in more than 50% of children under 10 years, and trichiasis is found in up to 5% of adults [10, 51]. Despite the limitations and potential unreliability of the available data, there does appear to be an encouraging downward trend in the overall numbers compared to earlier estimates [76]. The global burden of disease from trachoma has been variably estimated to be within 1.3–3.6 million Disability-Adjusted Life Years (DALYs) lost annually [33, 87]. The economic cost has been estimated to be between US$ 5 billion and US$ 8 billion) [34].

Trachoma is currently endemic in more than 50 countries worldwide in Sub-Saharan Africa, the Middle East, South and South-East Asia [53]. In addition, there are some isolated pockets in South America and Australia. Countries in Sub-Saharan Africa carry the greatest burden of trachoma. Here, it is predominantly found in two broad belts: the first runs across the Sahal from West Africa to the Horn. The second runs down the Eastern side of the continent, from Egypt in the north to Tanzania further south. Ethiopia and Sudan currently report some of the highest prevalence figures, with active trachoma in children often greater than 50%, and trichiasis prevalent in 5% of adults. For many trachoma-endemic countries, the socio-economic developments that might promote the disappearance of the disease are likely to be very slow in arriving, which in the light demographic trends and in the absence of effective control programs was predicted to lead to an increase in the amount of trachoma blindness in the absence of an effective control program [62].

9.6.2 Age and Gender

The clinical manifestations of trachoma change with age. Active disease is most commonly found in young children, declining to relatively low levels in adulthood, leading one author to dub it "the disease of the crèche" [70]. However, if adults in endemic communities are examined frequently enough, they too are found to have episodes of active disease and infection, albeit brief [5, 35]. In studies using diagnostic tests, the detection of *C. trachomatis* infection has generally paralleled the clinical observations, with infection being most prevalent in children, and where the load of infection has been measured, the highest loads have generally been found in the preschool children [5, 19, 35, 63, 68]. The prevalence of trachomatous conjunctival scarring increases with age, reflecting the cumulative nature of the damage from the repeated episodes of infection and inflammation [27, 84].

Most epidemiological studies have found that signs of active trachoma tend to be equally prevalent between male and female children. In contrast, the scarring complications of the disease, including trichiasis and CO are usually more common in women [27, 84]. About 75% of trichiasis and corneal blindness cases are in women. This probably reflects differences in the lifetime exposure of women to *C. trachomatis* infection through greater contact with children in most endemic settings [23].

9.6.3 Risk Factors for Active Trachoma and *C. Trachomatis* Infection

Individual and community level risk factors for active trachoma and *C. trachomatis* infection have been investigated in numerous epidemiological studies [19, 36, 38, 64, 73, 74]. Understanding the epidemiology is crucial, as it has pointed the way forward in trachoma control by identifying potential intervention strategies against the disease (Fig. 9.2). A general conclusion arising from this work is that the major risk factors are things that favor the transmission of infection between individuals within endemic communities.

Central to transmission of *C. trachomatis* from one person to the next are dirty faces. A dirty face is a common finding in individuals with active trachoma (usually young children); they can produce copious amounts of conjunctival discharge [19, 38, 64, 73, 74]. It would seem logical that this discharge, which is known to contain *C. trachomatis*, is the starting point and vehicle for the journey of the organism from one person to the next. By regular removal of infected secretions by regular face washing, transmission may be suppressed. Various factors contribute to whether or not a child's face is dirty. The key determinants are: (1) presence of active trachoma, (2) availability of water for washing, and (3) how the available water is used. Today, trachoma is most prevalent in regions that typically have limited access to water [31]. However, studies have demonstrated that it is not only how much water enters the house, but also how it is used that matters [4, 54, 64].

Trachoma epidemiology studies have consistently demonstrated a high degree of clustering, particularly within families [6, 18, 41, 84]. Crowded living conditions, for example, multiple children sleeping in the same bed, has been also associated with active trachoma and infection [6, 54]. This suggests that probably most *C. trachomatis* transmission events occur during close contact between individuals. It is likely that several different routes of transmission from infected to uninfected individuals exist (Fig. 9.2): direct spread from eye to eye during close contact (e.g., sharing a bed, during play), spread on fingers, indirect spread on fomites (e.g., face cloths, bed sheets), and transmission by eye-seeking flies. There is probably a combination of these and other modes of transmission that functions in most environments. Therefore, a variety of interventions may be necessary to interrupt transmission. From the trachoma control perspective, clustering is a problem; it increases the sample size required to accurately estimate the prevalence within a region [41].

Eye-seeking flies are a common feature of life in many trachoma endemic communities. They constantly buzz around people, and are particularly attracted to eyes with peri-ocular secretions. The species accounting for the majority of contacts in many environments is *Musca sorbens* [29]. These flies, caught whilst leaving the faces of children, have been shown to carry *C. trachomatis* by PCR [47]. They also breed preferentially in the faeces of

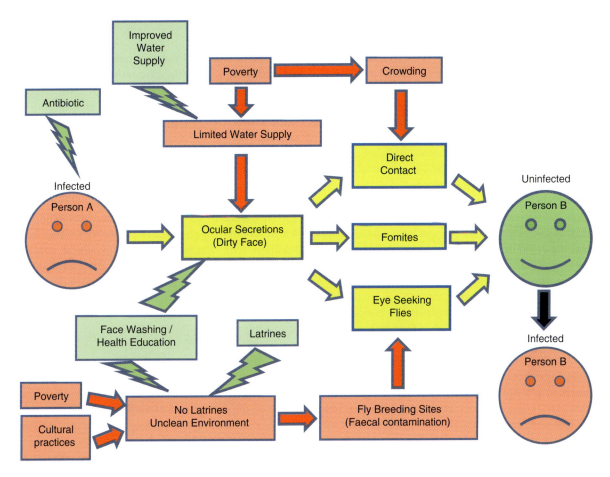

Fig. 9.2 *Routes and risk factors for transmission of C. trachomatis.* There are several potential routes of transmission of *C. trachomatis* between an infected person (Person A, *red face*) and a susceptible uninfected person (Person B, *green face*), which are indicated by *yellow arrows*. Infected individuals frequently have dirty faces associated with ocular secretions; these contain the transmissible form of *C. trachomatis*. Various factors probably promote the transmission of infection (contained in ocular secretions), these are identified in *red*. Potential interventions to limit transmission are indicated in *green* ("lightening" arrows)

children [30]. It has been observed for some time that communities, where latrine usage is low, appear to be at higher risk of trachoma. The "protective" effect of latrines is thought to work through suppressing the fly population by depriving them of their favored breeding material, in addition to reflecting a higher general standard of hygiene.

Summary for the Clinician

- Trachoma accounts for about 4% of global blindness
- Today, it is largely found in poor rural communities, in parts of Africa and Asia
- Major risk factors include limited access to water, poor sanitation, crowded living conditions

9.7 Pathophysiology of Trachoma

9.7.1 The Stimulus for Inflammation and Scarring in Trachoma

Chronic inflammation is a central event in the development of scar tissue in many human diseases. The ocular surface is no exception; inflammation leads to scarring in conditions such as mucus membrane pemphigoid and Stevens – Johnson syndrome. Clinically, active trachoma is characterized by episodes of chronic conjunctivitis. In children, the median duration has been estimated to be 36 weeks, and in adults, 7 weeks [35]. It seems likely that this chronic, recurrent inflammatory process results in the development of conjunctival scarring. Long-term epidemiological studies examining the development of scarring have identified a sub-group of people who have severe inflammatory trachoma (TI) on repeated examination. These individuals are at greatest risk of developing scarring and trichiasis in later life [26, 83, 86].

What is driving inflammation in trachoma? There is a consensus in the literature that, for the majority of people, serial reinfection of the conjunctiva by *C. trachomatis* is the major stimulant to the development of the cicatricial complications, although direct microbiological evidence for this from long-term epidemiological studies is very limited [86]. In primate models, conjunctival scarring only developed after many episodes of *C. trachomatis* reinfection [71]. An alternative view, which may be true for a minority, is that the infection becomes persistent, driving the inflammation [66]. In vitro studies suggest that the organism may transform into a persistent non-replicating form when stressed, although, evidence for this has not been found in vivo. From studies on monkeys, it has been found that conjunctival inflammation develops in response to chlamydial Heat Shock Protein 60 (HSP60), which is found within live whole organisms [72]. Heat shock proteins are found in both eukaryotic and prokaryotic cells, and have extensive sequence homology; they are induced when a cell is under stress. It has been suggested that the chronic inflammatory reaction in trachoma could be partly an autoimmune reaction to the human equivalent of HSP60; however, the evidence for this is limited.

The mismatch between the signs of disease and the detection of infection has been discussed above (Sect. 5). The signs of trachomatous inflammation can often be found in the absence of detectable *C. trachomatis*. One possible explanation for this is that other nonchlamydial bacterial pathogens could also be provoking an inflammatory response. Such pathogens are more commonly found in individuals with conjunctival scarring and inflammation compared to controls, particularly where trichiasis is also present [15, 20]. This has led to the suggestion that at least in the cicatricial stages of the disease, they could promote disease progression, and are highly likely to contribute to the corneal pathology.

9.7.2 Histopathology

Histopathology studies of active trachoma in children have demonstrated a widespread inflammatory cell infiltrate of T and B lymphocytes, macrophages, plasma cells, and neutrophils [14]. Sometimes B-cell follicles form which can be seen clinically as small pearl-like elevations in the conjunctiva. The conjunctival epithelium is hyperplastic, and chlamydial intracellular inclusion bodies can be seen within epithelial cells. Staining for collagen sub-types shows increased collagen type I, III, and IV (normally found in the stroma) and deposition of new type V [13].

In adults with trachomatous scarring, the conjunctival epithelium is atrophic, often only one cell thick and goblet cells are lost [1]. The loose sub-epithelial stroma (normally collagen types I and III) is replaced with a thick scar of collagen type V. Along the conjunctival basement membrane, collagen type IV is laid down [12]. These new fibers are orientated vertically, and are firmly attached to the posterior surface of the tarsal plate, causing distortion [1]. Biopsies from some scarred individuals have an inflammatory infiltrate dominated by T-cells, corresponding to clinical conjunctival inflammation, which is frequently observed in people with established trichiasis [58]. The tarsal plate is usually of normal thickness, but there is often atrophy of the meibomian glands and a chronic inflammatory infiltrate [1].

9.7.3 The Immune Response in Trachoma

C. trachomatis infection stimulates a poorly understood immune response. The resolution of infection probably depends on a cell-mediated response, which may also contribute to the pathogenesis of trachomatous scarring. The limited data from human challenge experiments indicate that some strain-specific immunity can develop. When previously uninfected volunteers were challenged with *C. trachomatis*, almost all developed infection. In contrast, only half of those challenged for a second time became infected [39]. When rechallenged with a different strain of *C. trachomatis*, infection developed. The finding that duration of *C. trachomatis* infection decreases with increasing age is also consistent with an acquired immune response [35].

There is probably an initial innate immune response to *C. trachomatis* infection at the epithelial surface. In vitro studies indicate that *C. trachomatis* infection triggers production of pro-inflammatory cytokines by epithelial cells (IL-1, IL-6, IL-8, and TNF-α) [56]. This triggers the rapid recruitment of neutrophils and macrophages into the conjunctiva, which may help to limit the initial infection through phagocytosis. Conjunctival biopsies from children with active trachoma reveal increased numbers of macrophages, which produce IL-1β and TNF-α [14]. Ongoing activation of macrophages even after infection has resolved probably plays an important part in the development of scarring, perhaps through the release of factors such as macrophage metalloelastase (MMP-12), which would continue to break down the extracellular matrix (ECM) and promote the influx of additional inflammatory cells.

An adaptive response to *C. trachomatis* develops with both antibody-meditated (humoral) and cell-mediated components. Current evidence suggests that a predominately T_H1 response is associated with a more favorable outcome in chlamydial infections. Antichlamydial antibodies can be found in the tears and serum of patients with active trachoma: antichlamydial IgG has been associated with increased risk of active disease subsequently developing, possibly through facilitating the entry of *C. trachomatis* into conjunctival epithelial cells, and this may reflect a predominantly T_H2 type response [9]. Antichlamydial IgA appears to reduce the risk of subsequent active disease, possibly by interfering with chlamydial attachment to host cells.

In animal models of chlamydial infection, a cell-mediated immune (CMI) response has been shown to be necessary for the resolution of infection [55]. Athymic mice are unable to clear genital infection with *C. trachomatis*, but this ability can be restored by the adoptive transfer of chlamydia-specific T-cells. Individuals who resolve clinically active trachoma have stronger lymphocyte proliferation responses to chlamydial antigens compared to people with persistent clinical disease [8]. In contrast, individuals with established trachomatous conjunctival scarring had weaker lymphocyte proliferation responses to chlamydial antigens compared with normal controls [37]. Interferon-γ (IFN-γ) appears to be the critical cytokine. It is primarily released by T_H1 lymphocytes. Individuals with *C. trachomatis* infection have increased conjunctival expression of IFN-γ, IL-2, and IL-12, consistent with a T_H1 response [16]. IFN-γ has several antichlamydial actions [61]. Firstly, indoleamine 2,3-dioxygenase (IDO) is induced by IFN-γ. IDO metabolizes L-tryptophan to N-formylkynurenine, depriving *C.trachomatis* of an essential amino acid. Secondly, IFN-γ increases inducible nitric oxide synthase (iNOS), generating nitric oxide, which is toxic to chlamydia. Thirdly, IFN-γ depletes intracellular iron, reducing the infectivity of EB. It is primarily released by T_H1 lymphocytes. Individuals with *C. trachomatis* conjunctival infection have increased conjunctival expression of IFN-γ, IL-2, and IL-12, consistent with a T_H1 response [16].

CD8+ Cytotoxic Lymphocytes (CTL) are present in the conjunctiva in active trachoma, however, their importance is uncertain [12]. They may have their effect through triggering the apoptosis of infected cells or through IFN-γ mediated pathways. The expression of Perforin, which is mainly produced by CTL, was found to be elevated in the conjunctiva of individuals with *C. trachomatis* infection from a trachoma-endemic community [16].

9.7.4 Immunopathogenesis of Conjunctival Scarring

Clinically, active trachoma often persists long after the infection becomes undetectable. Active disease, irrespective of the presence of *C. trachomatis* infection, is associated with increased expression of the pro-inflammatory cytokines IL-1β and TNF-α, particularly by macrophages [12, 16]. TNF-α has been found more frequently in the tears of individuals with trachomatous scarring compared with controls, especially when chlamydial infection was present [24, 65]. A single nucleotide polymorphism (SNP) in the *TNF-α* promoter region, TNFA-308A, which leads to increased levels of TNF-α, has been associated with increased risk of trachomatous scarring and trichiasis [49]. The antiinflammatory cytokine IL-10 also appears to influence the outcome of trachoma. It is produced by various cells, including Regulatory T-cells and Type 2 T-Helper cells. It counteracts pro-inflammatory responses. However, IL-10 also opposes the action of the T_H1 response mediated through IFN-γ, and so may impede the resolution of infection. IL-10 is expressed at increased levels in the conjunctiva of individuals with active trachoma, and certain genetic polymorphisms have been associated with increased scarring, although their functional significance is uncertain [16, 50, 65].

The fibrogenic process leading to trachomatous scarring remains to be elucidated. As with other fibrotic diseases, it is likely that TGF-β is important. Other fibrogenic cytokines associated with a T_H2 response, such as IL-13, may also contribute to promoting fibrosis. Matrix metalloproteinases (MMP) are a family of proteolytic enzymes which are central to the regulation of the ECM, and have been implicated in many scarring disorders. They degrade the ECM and facilitate scar contraction. The expression of MMP-9 is increased in conjunctival macrophages in active trachoma, becoming more marked with increasing severity of inflammatory disease [16, 28]. A SNP in the catalytic domain of *MMP-9*, possibly resulting in reduced function, is associated with a reduced risk of scarring complications in trachoma [48]. MMP-9 has many ECM substrates, but also activates pro-IL-1β and TGF-β, possibly helping to perpetuate the disease process.

Summary for the Clinician

- Blinding trachoma is the end-stage of a chronic inflammatory process in the conjunctiva, which produces scarring
- The main stimulus for this inflammation is *C. trachomatis*; however, it is the immune response to the infection that damages the tissue and leads to scarring

9.8 Trachoma Control

9.8.1 The SAFE Strategy

Trachoma is a major public health problem in many endemic countries, and controlling it requires a "public health" approach that goes beyond the ophthalmology clinic. Many countries have had organized control programs for decades. These have taken different approaches to prevent the blinding disease, which have met with variable success. To meet this challenge, in 1998 the World Health Assembly resolved to eliminate blinding trachoma by the year 2020 [89]. The Global Alliance for the Elimination of Blinding Trachoma (GET2020) was formed, which includes representatives from the WHO, national blindness control programs from endemic countries, NGOs working in the field, industry, and academics. The GET2020 alliance recognized the importance of a multifaceted approach to controlling trachoma by adopting and promoting the SAFE Strategy. The four components of SAFE are Surgery for trichiasis, Antibiotics for infection, Facial cleanliness, and Environmental improvements to reduce transmission. In the following sections, supporting evidence and important issues around the implementation of the SAFE Strategy will be reviewed.

9.8.2 Surgery for Trichiasis

There are about eight million people with trachomatous trichiasis (TT) worldwide [45]. TT is probably the main risk factor for developing blinding CO, although other factors may also contribute to the process [20]. It is believed that surgical correction of TT probably reduces the risk of developing blinding CO. Several surgical procedures are in use by trachoma control programs: bilamellar tarsal rotation and several variations on the posterior tarsal rotation (PLTR) [59]. Some of these have been compared in formal trials: of the procedures that were compared, the bilamellar tarsal rotation had the lowest TT recurrence rate, and was therefore endorsed by the WHO [57]. The indication for TT surgery varies between control programs. Some advocate surgery when one or more lashes touch the eye, whilst others recommend epilation until more severe TT develops. Both approaches have their advocates: the "immediate surgery" camp point out that since many patients with mild TT live in areas where access to ophthalmic services is limited, the progression to more severe disease can be swift, and so blinding complications can arise before surgery if this is delayed until more severe TT develops. The "epilate until more severe" camp point out that a significant proportion of eyes with mild TT do not have frank entropion; moreover, many people with one or two peripheral misdirected or metaplastic lashes are being operated on; given that a proportion of operated cases (perhaps 10%) will have surgical failure (discussed below), there is potentially a risk of doing more harm than good. As perhaps around half of the cases of TT fall into this mild group, this question has operational significance, and is being addressed currently in a clinical trial.

A major issue limiting the effectiveness of surgery in preventing blindness is the relatively high trichiasis recurrence rate following surgery in operational settings: this can be as high as 30–60% [17, 20, 42, 79]. Various factors may contribute, and can be broadly sub-divided into early recurrence due to "surgical failure" and late recurrence, which relate to the primary disease process: the type of operation, suture type, inter-surgeon variability, infection, preoperative disease severity, and ongoing cicatrizing conjunctivitis. Significant inter-surgeon variation has been found, particularly in operational studies [20, 79]. Trials examining whether peri-operative antibiotic (azithromycin) reduces the risk of recurrence found that for hyperendemic regions, this adjunctive therapy was associated with less recurrent trichiasis, but this was not the case in meso-endemic settings [20, 85]. Despite these disappointing results, there can be a small improvement in vision following surgery of about a line of Snellen visual acuity [20, 57].

In many trachoma-endemic countries, trichiasis surgery is performed by trained nurses and other paramedical staff, as there are insufficient ophthalmologists to perform the volume of surgery needed to deal with the backlog. The outcomes of surgery performed by ophthalmologists and para-medical staff have been compared and were similar [3]. The uptake of surgery is low in many endemic countries for a variety of reasons. A leading barrier to surgery is access; to make this easier many programs offer the services at community level, with comparable outcomes and much improved patient uptake [11].

9.8.3 Antibiotics

The rationale for using antibiotics to control trachoma is that by reducing the burden of ocular *C. trachomatis* infection at the individual and community level, the driving force for progressive trachomatous scarring is removed. Trachoma was first treated with antibiotics in the 1940s. Initially, oral sulphonamides were used.

Subsequently, several other antibiotics were evaluated, with topical tetracycline becoming the treatment of choice until the late 1990s. However, there are few placebo-controlled trial data, which demonstrates the limited efficacy of these antibiotics in treating active trachoma [44]. These studies were conducted at a time when the standard practice was to only treat individuals with active disease; excluding people without signs of inflammation. This approach would have probably left a large pool of untreated but infected individuals within a community to subsequently reinfect treated individuals, undermining the effectiveness of the intervention.

More recently, azithromycin, an azalide antibiotic, was shown to be as effective as topical tetracycline in trachoma control [7]. In a large study conducted in three endemic countries, mass community-wide azithromycin treatment produced a marked reduction in the prevalence of chlamydial infection, which was sustained for the 12 months of the study [63]. Similar responses have been observed in subsequent cohort studies [19, 67]. Currently, the WHO recommends that trachoma control programs use either tetracycline eye ointment applied twice a day for 6 weeks or a single oral dose of azithromycin (20 mg/kg up to a maximum dose of 1 g). Azithromycin has several advantages: treatment can be directly observed, compliance is high, and extra-ocular sites of infection are treated. Fifteen trachoma-endemic countries currently receive azithromycin as part of a philanthropic donation from the manufacturer (Pfizer Inc.).

Uncertainty remains over how these antibiotics should be used to the greatest effect to control trachoma. A key problem, discussed above, is the mismatch between the signs of active trachoma and the detection of chlamydial infection. How should control programs decide who should be offered antibiotic treatment? If only those with signs of trachoma are given antibiotics, many infected individuals with significant loads of infection would be left untreated [18]. There is a consensus that treatment needs to include people living alongside those with signs of active disease, in the form of mass community treatment or more targeted family based treatment. The WHO has developed guidelines for determining how treatment should be distributed to endemic populations, depending on the prevalence of the disease (Fig. 9.3) [88].

Whilst studies have reported significant reductions in the prevalence of disease and infection following a single dose of azithromycin, the impact is variable, and in some studies, there has been rapid reemergence of infection [19, 82]. This is probably due to a combination of inadequate treatment coverage, introduction of new chlamydial infections, and primary treatment failures. A mathematical model of antibiotic treatment for trachoma control suggested that for hyperendemic regions (>50%), mass antibiotic treatment would probably be

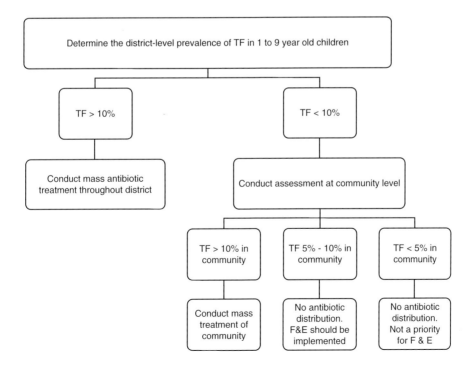

Fig. 9.3 WHO recommendations for initiating antibiotic treatment for trachoma [88]

needed twice a year, and for regions with moderate prevalence (<35%), annual treatment is probably sufficient; this projection has now been confirmed in clinical trials [43, 46]. There are only limited long-term data to guide programs as to how long mass antibiotic treatment should be given, and this remains a difficult area which requires further research. The current recommendation from the WHO is that three annual rounds of mass treatment should initially be given [88]. After this, the community should then be reassessed to see whether the prevalence of active disease has dropped sufficiently to discontinue treatment.

9.8.4 Face Washing

The importance of dirty faces in the transmission of *C. trachomatis* infection among people within endemic communities has been discussed earlier. It was suggested that by washing away potentially infected ocular secretions, the transmission of *C. trachomatis* might be interrupted. This hypothesis was tested in a community randomized trial of an intensive participatory face-washing strategy conducted in Tanzania; a moderate reduction in severe TI was achieved in the intervention villages [80]. The promotion of facial cleanliness, particularly of children, is a key message in trachoma health education.

9.8.5 Environmental Improvements

Environmental risk factors that promote the transmission of *C. trachomatis* have been discussed earlier. As part of the full implementation of the SAFE Strategy, these risk factors need to be addressed in a locally appropriate manner. The evidence base for the effectiveness of environmental interventions in trachoma control is limited. The most extensive work relates to fly control. A community randomized trial in The Gambia tested the hypothesis that controlling the fly population could suppress the transmission of *C. trachomatis* and reduce the prevalence of active trachoma [32]. Communities were randomized to one of three arms: (1) insecticide spray, (2) latrine provision, and (3) control. Latrine provision removes faecal material from the environment, the breeding sites for flies. Both intervention arms (spray and latrines) had a significant reduction in the fly population. However, only in the spray villages was this sufficient to significantly suppress the prevalence of active trachoma. A community randomized controlled trial conducted in Tanzania did not find that the addition of insecticide spraying to azithromycin distribution improved trachoma control [81].

Trachoma control programs advocate for environmental improvements such as improved water supply (face washing) and sanitation (fly control), although in reality they are not usually in a position to provide these improvements themselves. Rather, they often collaborate with other agencies to identify areas of greatest need. Several changes that would tend to promote improved control of trachoma are things that are of benefit to the general health of a population. The United Nations' seventh Millennium Development Goal aims to halve the number of people without safe water and basic sanitation by 2015. This is a timely coincidence for trachoma control, as many more resources are being made available than would ever be possible for a single ophthalmic disease.

> **Summary for the Clinician**
>
> - The SAFE Strategy is being implemented by prevention of blindness programs to control trachoma
> - Surgery for trichiasis reduces the risk of corneal blindness, but the recurrence rates are high
> - Antibiotics can be effective in controlling the endemic infection if community wide treatment with high coverage rates is given
> - Face washing and environmental improvements help to limit the transmission of infection

9.10 Conclusion

Trachoma remains the commonest infectious cause of blindness worldwide, and in many endemic regions, it is second only to cataract. During the last few decades, real progress has been made in controlling the disease. Trachoma was endemic in Europe 100 years ago, where it declined in the face of general improvements in living standards: less crowding, improved sanitation and water supply. Similar improvements have happened or are happening in parts of currently endemic countries. However, for many communities, it may take many decades for these general improvements to arrive and have an impact on trachoma. Therefore, it is necessary to actively implement the SAFE Strategy as the best validated approach to the prevention of blindness from trachoma.

References

1. al-Rajhi AA, Hidayat A, Nasr A et al (1993) The histopathology and the mechanism of entropion in patients with trachoma. Ophthalmology 100:1293–1296
2. al-Rifai KM (1988) Trachoma through history. Int Ophthalmol 12:9–14
3. Alemayehu W, Melese M, Bejiga A et al (2004) Surgery for trichiasis by ophthalmologists versus integrated eye care workers: a randomized trial. Ophthalmology 111:578–584
4. Bailey R, Downes B, Downes R et al (1991) Trachoma and water use, a case control study in a Gambian village. Trans R Soc Trop Med Hyg 85:824–828
5. Bailey R, Duong T, Carpenter R et al (1999) The duration of human ocular Chlamydia trachomatis infection is age dependent. Epidemiol Infect 123:479–486
6. Bailey R, Osmond C, Mabey DC et al (1989) Analysis of the household distribution of trachoma in a Gambian village using a Monte Carlo simulation procedure. Int J Epidemiol 18:944–951
7. Bailey RL, Arullendran P, Whittle HC et al (1993) Randomised controlled trial of single-dose azithromycin in treatment of trachoma. Lancet 342:453–456
8. Bailey RL, Holland MJ, Whittle HC et al (1995) Subjects recovering from human ocular chlamydial infection have enhanced lymphoproliferative responses to chlamydial antigens compared with those of persistently diseased controls. Infect Immun 63:389–392
9. Bailey RL, Kajbaf M, Whittle HC et al (1993) The influence of local antichlamydial antibody on the acquisition and persistence of human ocular chlamydial infection: IgG antibodies are not protective. Epidemiol Infect 111:315–324
10. Berhane Y, Worku A, Bejiga A (2006) National survey on blindness, low vision and trachoma in ethiopia. Federal Ministry of Health of Ethiopia
11. Bowman RJ, Soma OS, Alexander N et al (2000) Should trichiasis surgery be offered in the village? A community randomised trial of village vs. health centre-based surgery. Trop Med Int Health 5:528–533
12. bu El-Asrar AM, Geboes K, Al-Kharashi SA et al (1998) An immunohistochemical study of collagens in trachoma and vernal keratoconjunctivitis. Eye 12:1001–1006
13. bu El-Asrar AM, Geboes K, Al-Kharashi SA et al (1998) Collagen content and types in trachomatous conjunctivitis. Eye 12:735–739
14. bu El-Asrar AM, Geboes K, Tabbara KF et al (1998) Immunopathogenesis of conjunctival scarring in trachoma. Eye 12:453–460
15. Burton MJ, Adegbola RA, Kinteh F et al (2007) Bacterial infection and trachoma in the gambia: a case control study. Invest Ophthalmol Vis Sci 48:4440–4444
16. Burton MJ, Bailey RL, Jeffries D et al (2004) Cytokine and fibrogenic gene expression in the conjunctivas of subjects from a Gambian community where trachoma is endemic. Infect Immun 72:7352–7356
17. Burton MJ, Bowman RJ, Faal H et al (2005) Long term outcome of trichiasis surgery in the Gambia. Br J Ophthalmol 89:575–579
18. Burton MJ, Holland MJ, Faal N et al (2003) Which members of a community need antibiotics to control trachoma? Conjunctival Chlamydia trachomatis infection load in Gambian villages. Invest Ophthalmol Vis Sci 44:4215–4222
19. Burton MJ, Holland MJ, Makalo P et al (2005) Re-emergence of Chlamydia trachomatis infection after mass antibiotic treatment of a trachoma-endemic Gambian community: a longitudinal study. Lancet 365:1321–1328
20. Burton MJ, Kinteh F, Jallow O et al (2005) A randomised controlled trial of azithromycin following surgery for trachomatous trichiasis in the Gambia. Br J Ophthalmol 89:1282–1288
21. Caldwell HD, Wood H, Crane D et al (2003) Polymorphisms in Chlamydia trachomatis tryptophan synthase genes differentiate between genital and ocular isolates. J Clin Invest 111:1757–1769
22. Carlson JH, Porcella SF, McClarty G et al (2005) Comparative genomic analysis of Chlamydia trachomatis oculotropic and genitotropic strains. Infect Immun 73:6407–6418
23. Congdon N, West S, Vitale S et al (1993) Exposure to children and risk of active trachoma in Tanzanian women. Am J Epidemiol 137:366–372
24. Conway DJ, Holland MJ, Bailey RL et al (1997) Scarring trachoma is associated with polymorphism in the tumor necrosis factor alpha (TNF-alpha) gene promoter and with elevated TNF-alpha levels in tear fluid. Infect Immun 65:1003–1006
25. Dawson CR, Jones BR, Tarizzo ML (1981) Guide to Trachoma Control. World Health Organization, Geneva
26. Dawson CR, Marx R, Daghfous T et al (1990) What clinical signs are critical in evaluating the intervention in trachoma? In: Bowie WR (ed) Chlamydial Infections. Cambridge University, Cambridge
27. Dolin PJ, Faal H, Johnson GJ et al (1998) Trachoma in The Gambia. Br J Ophthalmol 82:930–933
28. El-Asrar AM, Geboes K, Al-Kharashi SA et al (2000) Expression of gelatinase B in trachomatous conjunctivitis. Br J Ophthalmol 84:85–91
29. Emerson PM, Bailey RL, Mahdi OS et al (2000) Transmission ecology of the fly Musca sorbens, a putative vector of trachoma. Trans R Soc Trop Med Hyg 94:28–32
30. Emerson PM, Bailey RL, Walraven GE et al (2001) Human and other faeces as breeding media of the trachoma vector Musca sorbens. Med Vet Entomol 15:314–320

31. Emerson PM, Cairncross S, Bailey RL et al (2000) Review of the evidence base for the 'F' and 'E' components of the SAFE strategy for trachoma control. Trop Med Int Health 5:515–527
32. Emerson PM, Lindsay SW, Alexander N et al (2004) Role of flies and provision of latrines in trachoma control: cluster-randomised controlled trial. Lancet 363:1093–1098
33. Frick KD, Basilion EV, Hanson CL et al (2003) Estimating the burden and economic impact of trachomatous visual loss. Ophthalmic Epidemiol 10:121–132
34. Frick KD, Hanson CL, Jacobson GA (2003) Global burden of trachoma and economics of the disease. Am J Trop Med Hyg 69:1–10
35. Grassly NC, Ward ME, Ferris S et al (2008) The natural history of trachoma infection and disease in a gambian cohort with frequent follow-up. PLoS Negl Trop Dis 2: e341
36. Harding-Esch EM, Edwards T, Sillah A et al (2008) Risk factors for active trachoma in The Gambia. Trans R Soc Trop Med Hyg 102(12):1255–1262
37. Holland MJ, Bailey RL, Hayes LJ et al (1993) Conjunctival scarring in trachoma is associated with depressed cell-mediated immune responses to chlamydial antigens. J Infect Dis 168:1528–1531
38. Hsieh YH, Bobo LD, Quinn TC et al (2000) Risk factors for trachoma: 6-year follow-up of children aged 1 and 2 years. Am J Epidemiol 152:204–211
39. Jawetz E, Rose L, Hanna L et al (1965) Experimental inclusion conjunctivitis in man: measurements of infectivity and resistance. JAMA 194:620–632
40. Kari L, Whitmire WM, Carlson JH et al (2008) Pathogenic diversity among Chlamydia trachomatis ocular strains in nonhuman primates is affected by subtle genomic variations. J Infect Dis 197:449–456
41. Katz J, Zeger SL, Tielsch JM (1988) Village and household clustering of xerophthalmia and trachoma. Int J Epidemiol 17:865–869
42. Khandekar R, Mohammed AJ, Courtright P (2001) Recurrence of trichiasis: a long-term follow-up study in the Sultanate of Oman. Ophthalmic Epidemiol 8: 155–161
43. Lietman T, Porco T, Dawson C et al (1999) Global elimination of trachoma: how frequently should we administer mass chemotherapy? Nat Med 5:572–576
44. Mabey D, Fraser-Hurt N, Powell C (2005) Antibiotics for trachoma. Cochrane Database Syst RevCD001860
45. Mariotti SP, Pascolini D, Rose-Nussbaumer J (2009) Trachoma: global magnitude of a preventable cause of blindness. Br J Ophthalmol 93:563–568
46. Melese M, Alemayehu W, Lakew T et al (2008) Comparison of annual and biannual mass antibiotic administration for elimination of infectious trachoma. JAMA 299:778–784
47. Miller K, Pakpour N, Yi E et al (2004) Pesky trachoma suspect finally caught. Br J Ophthalmol 88:750–751
48. Natividad A, Cooke G, Holland MJ et al (2006) A coding polymorphism in matrix metalloproteinase 9 reduces risk of scarring sequelae of ocular Chlamydia trachomatis infection. BMC Med Genet 7:40
49. Natividad A, Hanchard N, Holland MJ et al (2007) Genetic variation at the TNF locus and the risk of severe sequelae of ocular Chlamydia trachomatis infection in Gambians. Genes Immun 8:288–295
50. Natividad A, Wilson J, Koch O et al (2005) Risk of trachomatous scarring and trichiasis in Gambians varies with SNP haplotypes at the interferon-gamma and interleukin-10 loci. Genes Immun 6:332–340
51. Ngondi J, Ole-Sempele F, Onsarigo A et al (2006) Blinding trachoma in postconflict southern Sudan. PLoS Med 3:e478
52. Ngondi J, Reacher MH, Matthews FE et al (2008) Risk factors for trachomatous trichiasis in children: cross-sectional household surveys in Southern Sudan. Trans R Soc Trop Med Hyg 102:432–438
53. Polack S, Brooker S, Kuper H et al (2005) Mapping the global distribution of trachoma. Bull World Health Organ 83:913–919
54. Polack S, Kuper H, Solomon AW et al (2006) The relationship between prevalence of active trachoma, water availability and its use in a Tanzanian village. Trans R Soc Trop Med Hyg 100:1075–1083
55. Ramsey KH, Rank RG (1991) Resolution of chlamydial genital infection with antigen-specific T-lymphocyte lines. Infect Immun 59:925–931
56. Rasmussen SJ, Eckmann L, Quayle AJ et al (1997) Secretion of proinflammatory cytokines by epithelial cells in response to Chlamydia infection suggests a central role for epithelial cells in chlamydial pathogenesis. J Clin Invest 99:77–87
57. Reacher MH, Munoz B, Alghassany A et al (1992) A controlled trial of surgery for trachomatous trichiasis of the upper lid. Arch Ophthalmol 110:667–674
58. Reacher MH, Pe'er J, Rapoza PA et al (1991) T cells and trachoma. Their role in cicatricial disease. Ophthalmology 98:334–341
59. Reacher MH, Taylor HR (1990) The management of trachomatous trichiasis. Rev Int Trach Pathol Ocul Trop Subtrop Sante Publique 67:233–262
60. Resnikoff S, Pascolini D, Etya'ale D et al (2004) Global data on visual impairment in the year 2002. Bull World Health Organ 82:844–851
61. Rottenberg ME, Gigliotti-Rothfuchs A, Wigzell H (2002) The role of IFN-gamma in the outcome of chlamydial infection. Curr Opin Immunol 14:444–451
62. Schachter J, Dawson CR (1990) The epidemiology of trachoma predicts more blindness in the future. Scand J Infect Dis Suppl 69:55–62

63. Schachter J, West SK, Mabey D et al (1999) Azithromycin in control of trachoma. Lancet 354:630–635
64. Schemann JF, Sacko D, Malvy D et al (2002) Risk factors for trachoma in Mali. Int J Epidemiol 31:194–201
65. Skwor TA, Atik B, Kandel RP et al (2008) Role of secreted conjunctival mucosal cytokine and chemokine proteins in different stages of trachomatous disease. PLoS Negl Trop Dis 2:e264
66. Smith A, Munoz B, Hsieh YH et al (2001) OmpA genotypic evidence for persistent ocular Chlamydia trachomatis infection in Tanzanian village women. Ophthalmic Epidemiol 8:127–135
67. Solomon AW, Holland MJ, Alexander ND et al (2004) Mass treatment with single-dose azithromycin for trachoma. N Engl J Med 351:1962–1971
68. Solomon AW, Holland MJ, Burton MJ et al (2003) Strategies for control of trachoma: observational study with quantitative PCR. Lancet 362:198–204
69. Solomon AW, Peeling RW, Foster A et al (2004) Diagnosis and assessment of trachoma. Clin Microbiol Rev 17:982–1011
70. Taylor HR (2008) Trachoma: a blinding scourge from the Bronze age to the twenty-first century. Centre for Eye Research Australia, Melbourne
71. Taylor HR, Johnson SL, Prendergast RA et al (1982) An animal model of trachoma II. The importance of repeated reinfection. Invest Ophthalmol Vis Sci 23:507–515
72. Taylor HR, Johnson SL, Schachter J et al (1987) Pathogenesis of trachoma: the stimulus for inflammation. J Immunol 138:3023–3027
73. Taylor HR, Velasco FM, Sommer A (1985) The ecology of trachoma: an epidemiological study in southern Mexico. Bull World Health Organ 63:559–567
74. Taylor HR, West SK, Mmbaga BB et al (1989) Hygiene factors and increased risk of trachoma in central Tanzania. Arch Ophthalmol 107:1821–1825
75. Thylefors B, Dawson CR, Jones BR et al (1987) A simple system for the assessment of trachoma and its complications. Bull World Health Organ 65:477–483
76. Thylefors B, Negrel AD, Pararajasegaram R et al (1995) Global data on blindness. Bull World Health Organ 73: 115–121
77. Treharne JD (1988) The microbial epidemiology of trachoma. Int Ophthalmol 12:25–29
78. Ward ME (1995) The immunobiology and immunopathology of chlamydial infections. APMIS 103:769–796
79. West ES, Mkocha H, Munoz B et al (2005) Risk factors for postsurgical trichiasis recurrence in a trachoma-endemic area. Invest Ophthalmol Vis Sci 46:447–453
80. West S, Munoz B, Lynch M et al (1995) Impact of face-washing on trachoma in Kongwa, Tanzania. Lancet 345: 155–158
81. West SK, Emerson PM, Mkocha H et al (2006) Intensive insecticide spraying for fly control after mass antibiotic treatment for trachoma in a hyperendemic setting: a randomised trial. Lancet 368:596–600
82. West SK, Munoz B, Mkocha H et al (2005) Infection with Chlamydia trachomatis after mass treatment of a trachoma hyperendemic community in Tanzania: a longitudinal study. Lancet 366:1296–1300
83. West SK, Munoz B, Mkocha H et al (2001) Progression of active trachoma to scarring in a cohort of Tanzanian children. Ophthalmic Epidemiol 8:137–144
84. West SK, Munoz B, Turner VM et al (1991) The epidemiology of trachoma in central Tanzania. Int J Epidemiol 20: 1088–1092
85. West SK, West ES, Alemayehu W et al (2006) Single-dose azithromycin prevents trichiasis recurrence following surgery: randomized trial in Ethiopia. Arch Ophthalmol 124:309–314
86. Wolle MA, Munoz BE, Mkocha H et al (2008) Constant Ocular Infection with Chlamydia trachomatis Predicts Risk of Scarring in Children in Tanzania. Ophthalmology 116(2):243–247
87. World Health Organization (2008) The global burden of disease: 2004 update. World Health Organization, Geneva
88. World Health Organization (2003) Report of the 2nd global scientific meeting on trachoma. World Health Organization, Geneva
89. World Health Organization (1998) Global elimination of blinding trachoma. Resolution WHA 51.11. Adopted by the World Health Assembly 16 May 1998
90. Wright HR, Taylor HR (2005) Clinical examination and laboratory tests for estimation of trachoma prevalence in a remote setting: what are they really telling us? Lancet Infect Dis 5:313–320

Chapter 10

Keratoprosthesis

Jason J. Jun, Donna E. Siracuse-Lee, Mary K. Daly, Claes H. Dohlman

Core Messages

- Despite the widespread use of standard keratoplasty, there continues to be a worldwide need for alternative therapies due to:
  (a) Substantial rates of graft failure on long-term follow-up
  (b) Poor prognosis in patients with underlying inflammation or chemical burns
  (c) Limited access to resources including donor tissue
- Experience with keratoprosthesis (Kpro) has grown rapidly over the past two decades, and has resulted in improved outcomes and decreased complications for a large number of patients.
- A key lesson learned is that long-term prognosis is linked to underlying diagnosis.
- Kpro patients should be divided into two categories and examined separately:
  (a) In patients who have experienced failed grafts for corneal dystrophies, trauma, and infection, but lack underlying severe ocular inflammation, Kpro has yielded promising results in terms of device retention and improved visual acuity.
  (b) In patients with cicatrizing autoimmune diseases and chemical burns, the prognosis for Kpro has been more guarded.
- A variety of Kpro designs are currently in use, and may have specific applications based on underlying patient subtype.
- Assessment of current and future Kpro technology should account for this prognostic hierarchy.
- Experimental "biologic" designs that aim to better integrate Kpro material with corneal tissue wcomplications, but are yet to be proven.

10.1 Introduction

An estimated eight million people worldwide are blind due to corneal disease [53], making it the third leading cause of blindness after cataract and glaucoma [55]. Since the early twentieth century, keratoplasty has offered hope to many people suffering from corneal blindness due to a variety of conditions. In fact, keratoplasty has become the most frequently performed organ transplant worldwide [17]. However, keratoplasty is not without its limitations. Graft failure remains a persistent problem [58]. In a large retrospective study, grafts for all causes remained clear in only 70% of cases after 5 years [6, 58]. Examined separately, regrafts fare even worse. Bersudsky et al. found that only 20% of first regrafts were clear after 5 years, while all repeat regrafts had failed over that same period [5]. In addition, the prognosis for standard keratoplasty is significantly worse in certain "high-risk" diagnostic categories including autoimmune conditions and chemical burns [6, 36, 55, 56]. Finally, in large parts of the world, keratoplasty is unfeasible due to lack of health resources or cultural impediments, resulting in an inadequate supply of donor corneas [10]. Given these limitations, the need for a safe and effective keratoprosthesis (Kpro) as an alternative to keratoplasty remains strong.

The concept of Kpro has captured the attention of scientists and physicians for more than 200 years [43]. For a detailed history of Kpro, the reader is referred to previous review articles on this subject [12, 33]. Development of an effective Kpro was initially slow due to significant early and late-stage complications, often resulting in loss of the eye. However, over the past several decades, renewed interest and improved technology have allowed great strides to be made. In 1992, there were only 15 Kpro operations attempted in the United States [13]. In 2008, the corresponding number was over 800. While this number is small compared to the approximately 100,000 standard keratoplasties performed worldwide per year [13], this rapid expansion in experience has brought forth key lessons for the present and future use of Kpro as a viable therapy for severe corneal opacities.

10.2 Prognostic Hierarchy

One key principle that has emerged from recent experience with Kpro is that prognosis is clearly linked to diagnosis. A retrospective study by Yaghouti et al. [56] demonstrated the existence of a prognostic hierarchy among diagnostic categories for patients undergoing Boston Kpro surgery. Eyes with prior graft failure from nonautoimmune conditions (dystrophies, degenerations, or viral/bacterial infections) fared best, with 83% of those achieving better than 20/200 vision and maintaining it after 2 years, followed by ocular cicatrizing pemphigoid (OCP) (72%), chemical burns (64%), and Stevens-Johnson syndrome (SJS) (33%) [52]. Subsequent studies of Boston Kpro have confirmed consistently better outcomes among patients with nonautoimmune graft failure [7, 8, 59]. In contrast, patients with underlying autoimmune conditions and chemical burns have been shown to have worse outcomes and increased complications [8, 41, 59]. In a review of 227 patients receiving either osteo-odonto keratoprosthesis (OOKP) or tibial keratoprosthesis (TKpro), Michael et al. found that primary diagnosis was the only significant factor associated with anatomical retention, with OCP having the worst prognosis [37]. Despite continued advances in Kpro materials and technique, options for these high-risk patients remain limited. It has become clear that Kpro patients should be separated into two broad subtypes, and that experience with Kpro falls along these two lines.

10.3 Defining Patient Subtypes

10.3.1 Patient Subtype A: The Noninflamed Eye

The first subtype consists of patients undergoing Kpro who lack significant history of ocular inflammation, and have normal blink mechanism and tear secretion. These patients have experienced graft failure with underlying diagnoses such as dystrophy, infection, trauma, aphakic/pseudophakic bullous keratopathy [7, 13, 56, 59].

10.3.2 Patient Subtype B: The Inflamed Eye

The second subtype consists of patients with acute and/or chronic inflammation due to underlying cicatrizing autoimmune disorders. Conditions such as SJS, OCP, graft-vs.-host disease (GVHD), and severe uveitis often lead to severe ocular surface damage due to destruction of limbal stem cells, corneal neovascularization, stromal scarring, and conjunctival fibrosis [41, 46, 49]. Patients with chemical burns were initially considered high risk due to increased rates of endophthalmitis, corneal melt, retinal detachment, and glaucoma [56]. Although recent studies have suggested that outcomes in patients with chemical burns may be improving [7, 21, 59], these patients should still be approached with caution.

10.4 Experience with Kpro in Patient Subtype A

There is a growing body of data showing that patients who lack a significant history of ocular inflammation experience good outcomes after Kpro. Given that 15% of all keratoplasties in the U.S. are performed for graft failure, and that subsequent regrafts get progressively worse [5], Kpro should be considered as a viable alternative to further keratoplasty in these patients [15, 35].

10.4.1 Boston Type 1 Kpro

The most commonly implanted device in the U.S. and worldwide is the Boston Type 1 Kpro. The Boston Kpro was approved by the FDA for patient use in 1992. This device is based on a "collar-button" design in which a central optical stem is stabilized by a front and back plate, all of which are made of poly (methyl methacrylate) (PMMA, Fig. 10.1). Donor corneal tissue is sandwiched between the front and back plates and then used as a carrier (Fig. 10.2). Technical details regarding its implantation have been reported elsewhere [11, 14, 15]. In a multicenter prospective study examining outcomes from 141 Boston Type 1 KPro surgeries, patients with preoperative diagnosis of noncicatrizing graft failure demonstrated BCVA ≥20/200 in 90% and anatomic retention in 97% at a median follow-up of 8.5 months [59]. Ciolino et al. have subsequently reported a retention rate of 91.6% after extending the average follow-up to 13 months [8]. Eighty-three percent of patients had preoperative diagnoses of graft rejection, chemical injury, or aphakic/pseudophakic bullous keratopathy. In a longer-term study of 30 eyes with average follow-up of 19 months, Bradley et al. found postoperative BCVA ≥20/200 in 77% of eyes and 83.3% device retention [7]. In their single-surgeon series of 57 Boston Type 1 Kpro implantations, the largest to date, Aldave et al. report an 84% retention rate at an average follow-up of 17 months [1]. Of the patients for whom VA was checked postoperatively, BCVA was ≥20/100 in 67% (30/45) at 6 months, 75% (21/28) at 1 year, and 69% (9/13) at 2 years. Although Kpro is typically reserved for patients with repeat graft failure, eight eyes in this cohort had no

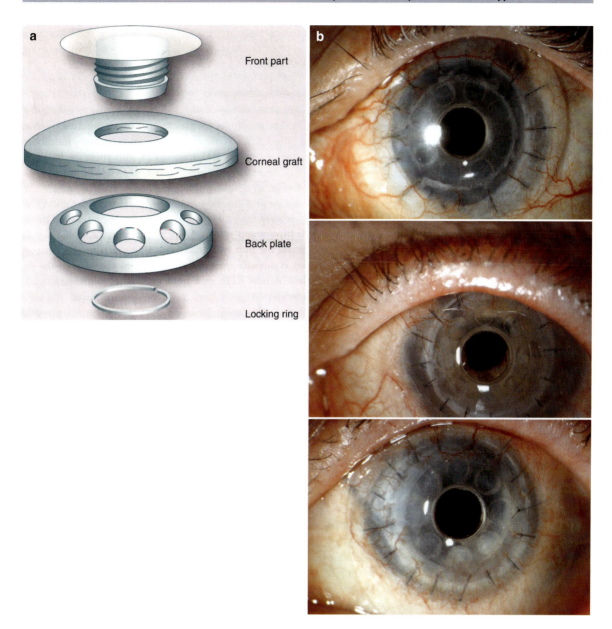

Figs. 10.1 (**a**) Schematic diagram of Boston type 1 keratoprosthesis. (**b**) Clinical photo of Boston type 1 keratoprosthesis. Courtesy of Claes Dohlman, MD, PhD

history of prior corneal surgery. With a 100% retention rate in these eight eyes and postoperative BCVA ≥20/80 in seven of eight eyes at an average follow-up of 22 months, the authors suggest that Kpro should be considered as the initial procedure in certain cases of visually significant corneal limbal stem cell deficiency. Prior dreaded complications of Boston Kpro surgery such as endophthalmitis have been reduced or eliminated due to improved technique and postoperative management including the use of life-long prophylactic antibiotic drops [13, 27]. Currently, the primary limitations to meaningful recovery of vision are: end-stage glaucoma, retinal detachment, and age-related macular degeneration [14, 59, 40].

10.4.1.1 Pediatric Application of Boston Type 1 Kpro

Another major advance has been the application of the Boston Type 1 Kpro in the pediatric population. The treatment of pediatric corneal opacity by standard keratoplasty renders patients at high risk for deprivation and refractive amblyopia due to the duration of postoperative corneal opacity, graft rejection, or irregular astigmatism [3]. Kpro not only provides a clear visual axis and stable refraction within days after surgery but also eliminates concerns over graft rejection and its sequellae, factors which are critical for amblyopia prevention in this population [3]. In a retrospective review of 21 cases of Boston Type 1 Kpro implanted into patients 1.5–136 months of age, Aquavella et al. report 100% retention at a mean follow-up of 9.7 months [3]. The visual axis remained clear in 100% of cases. In seven patients aged 4 or older, VA ranged from counting fingers to 20/30. In the remaining cases, all infants were able to follow light, fingers, and objects. There were no cases of surface infection or endophthalmitis. These results suggest that Boston Type 1 Kpro offers a viable alternative to standard keratoplasty in the pediatric population, where rapid restoration of a clear optical pathway is critical.

10.4.2 AlphaCor Kpro

Another design, the Alphacor Kpro (previously known as the Chirila Kpro) has been studied in patients without evidence of inflammation. The Alphacor is a one-piece device consisting of a transparent core and an opaque porous skirt made from poly(2-hydroxyethyl methacrylate) (PHEMA). PHEMA is a so-called "hydrogel" consisting of cross-linked hydrophilic polymers, which in theory has improved biocompatibility due to permeability to oxygen and other water-soluble metabolites [22]. Technical details regarding its use and clinical outcome have been reported elsewhere [21]. The AlphaCor Kpro is approved by the FDA for implantation into adults who lack current inflammation, have a satisfactory tear film, and have no history of ocular herpes simplex virus (HSV). Patients with severe ocular surface disease were excluded from early clinical trials. A review of the 322 AlphaCor implantations [21] showed retention rates of 92, 80, and 62% at 6 months, 1 year, and 2 years, respectively. Preoperative diagnoses were similar to those in the multicenter Boston Type 1 Kpro trial. Patients (44.4%) had corneal dystrophies and trauma (both mechanical and chemical), while 38.2% had bullous keratopathy. Despite the AlphaCor's approved indications, this study found that HSV was not a significant risk factor for corneal melt. Despite the exclusion of high-risk patients, postoperative stromal melting occurred in 26.4% of cases and led to device explantation in 64.5% of cases in which the device was removed [21]. The authors report that the incidence of stromal melting decreased over the course of the study.

10.5 Experience with Kpro in Patient Subtype B

The application of Kpro in Patient Subtype B has proven more problematic. These patients suffer from autoimmune conditions that lead to chronic inflammation and severe ocular surface damage. Experience with Boston Type 1 Kpro in this patient subtype clearly demonstrates worse outcomes and increased complications such as endophthalmitis, retinal detachment, uncontrolled glaucoma, necrosis, and device extrusion [8, 41, 46, 59]. Among these patients, SJS represents the highest risk category [13, 16, 46, 59]. These issues are not unique to Kpro surgery, as these patients tend to do poorly after standard keratoplasty as well [6, 32, 51, 52]. Sadly, patients in this category are often young, suffer bilateral disease, and are in desperate need of good long-term results with Kpro [13, 46, 39]. Other Kpro designs have shown more promise in this challenging cohort, but may place additional demands on both patients and caregivers alike.

10.5.1 Osteo-Odonto Keratoprosthesis (OOKP)

The OOKP procedure was first introduced by Strampelli in the 1960s, and has since been modified by Falcinelli, Liu, and others [18, 23, 30, 47, 49]. It is a complex, two-stage procedure in which the destroyed ocular surface is replaced with a full-thickness buccal mucosal graft. A PMMA optic is implanted into an autologous tooth, which is then inserted onto the cornea. A related procedure, tibial bone keratoprosthesis (TKPro) uses autologous tibial bone as the optical carrier [9, 37, 50]. Falcinelli et al. reported on the long-term results of 181 patients receiving modified OOKP between 1973 and 1999 [18]. They estimated an 85% retention rate 18 years after surgery. In addition, mean BCVA ranged from 20/30 to 20/20. Twenty-four percent of these patients had diagnoses of OCP, SJS, or GVHD. More recently, Tan et al. examined the use of OOKP in 15 patients with severe end-stage corneal disease [49]. Seven out of fifteen patients had underlying SJS. At a mean follow-up of 19.1 months, device retention was 100%, and 73.3% of patients had achieved a BCVA of 20/40 or better. While other studies have reported similarly high retention rates [24, 34], Michael et al. found slightly more tempered results, with an overall 10-year mean anatomic survival of 62% in their retrospective review of 227 patients who underwent either TKPro or OOKP [37]. Interestingly, primary diagnosis was the only significant factor associated with anatomical survival in this cohort, with OCP having the worst prognosis. Overall, the use of OOKP in patients with end-stage corneal disease secondary to autoimmune conditions

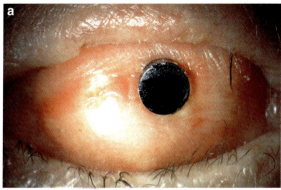
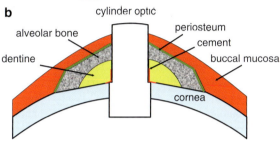

Fig. 10.2 (**a**) Clinical photo of osteo-odonto keratoprosthesis (OOKP). (**b**) Schematic of osteo-odonto keratoprosthesis (OOKP). Courtesy of Lippincott Williams & Wilkins (K Hille, et al. Cornea 2005 Nov; 24 (8): 895-908.)

remains promising. Limitations to OOKP include the complexity of the procedure involving multiple surgical specialties, and the need for the patient to donate a healthy, rooted tooth. Hille et al. found that one-third of patients referred to them for Kpro did not have a suitable tooth [24].

10.5.2 Boston Type 2 Kpro

A slightly modified version of the Boston Type 1 Kpro was developed to improve outcomes in patients with severe ocular surface disease secondary to underlying inflammation. The Boston Type 2 Kpro is similar in design to the Type 1 except for the addition of a 2-mm anterior nub to the optical stem, which is meant to penetrate through the lid skin after concurrent, permanent tarsorraphy. In theory, protecting the ocular surface from drying by tarsorraphy reduces the rate of tissue melt [13]. Sayegh et al. conducted a retrospective study of 16 eyes with SJS undergoing Boston Kpro surgery [46]. Ten eyes (63%) underwent Type 2 surgery, and the rest Type I. Fifty percent of eyes had VA of 20/200 or better after 5 years. There were no spontaneous extrusions of the implant in this cohort. However, aqueous leakage necessitated the replacement of the device in two Type 2 eyes.

While these results show improvement over previous experience with the Type I only, no specific comment was made regarding differences in outcomes between Type 1 and Type 2. A complication of Boston Type 2 Kpro surgery is the retraction of lid skin around the device requiring surgical revision. Another limitation, shared by the OOKP, is the inability to exactly measure the intraocular pressure and control it other than with oral medications [46].

10.6 Other Kpro Designs

10.6.1 Pintucci Kpro

The Pintucci Kpro consists of an optical cylinder made of PMMA fixed to a woven Dacron membrane skirt, which allows for tissue in-growth. Pintucci et al. initially reported their results in 20 patients, 60% of whom suffered from mucous membrane pemphigoid [45]. At a mean follow-up of 58.9 months, there were two cases of device extrusion and one case of endophthalmitis. Thirty-five percent of patients had BCVA >20/40. A more recent study of 31 Indian patients found no device extrusions at a mean follow-up of 3.2 years. However, only 6.5% of these patients achieved BCVA >20/40 [35].

10.6.2 Seoul-Type Kpro

The Seoul-type Kpro (S-Kpro) utilizes an optic and skirt, but has additional haptics to increase postimplantation biomechanical stability. The device is anchored to the patient's eye both by suturing the skirt to the cornea and by attachment of the additional haptics onto the sclera. Lee et al. reported their results in nine patients, six of whom had a diagnosis of SJS and one with OCP [28]. While they report a 66.7% anatomic retention rate at 68 months, all devices developed corneal melt leading to full exposure of the skirt, and four devices needed to be exchanged. All four eyes requiring Kpro exchange subsequently developed retinal detachments. Visual acuity of finger counting or higher was maintained for a mean 31.6 months [28].

10.6.3 Worst-Singh Kpro

Also known as the "champagne cork" Kpro, this device consists of a hood, anticonical PMMA shaft, and stainless-steel loops which secure the hood to the sclera. The Worst-

Singh Kpro is implanted either in the center of the cornea or as a paralimbal scleral window [2]. While this device is currently utilized in India, primarily by Singh and colleagues, long-term outcomes data are not available.

10.6.4 Russian/Ukrainian Experience

It has been estimated that over 2,000 Kpro procedures have been done at the Fyodorov Institute in Moscow, the Filatov Institute in Odessa, and other centers across the former Soviet Union [26]. Yakimenko reported on 502 cases using their design of a central PMMA optical core and tantalum-titanium alloy haptics [57]. Eyes (51.5%) had a primary diagnosis of chemical burn. Long-term results demonstrated an extrusion rate of 12.1%, and approximately 48% of eyes achieved 20/200 vision or better. Yakimenko reported that improved surgical techniques and implants have lowered the extrusion rate to approximately 3.5%. However, subsequent data regarding the design, implementation, and outcomes of Kpro from this and other centers has been very limited.

10.7 New Directions in Kpro Research

New research is focusing on ways to "biointegrate" Kpro with one or more layers of the cornea. According to Ciolino, integration with the corneal epithelium could theoretically stabilize the tear film and offer a barrier to infection, while stromal integration could offer improved structural stability and greater retention [9]. Several research groups are developing materials and methods for enhancing the biologic compatibility of Kpro.

10.7.1 Hydroxyapatite Biologic Haptics

Success with autologous bone in OOKP and TKP has led to interest in other materials with similar properties to be used as Kpro haptics. Made of phosphate and calcium, hydroxyapatite has a similar mineral composition to both bone and teeth, and is frequently used as a bone substitute within the orbit [4]. In other studies, hydroxyapatite has been found to have superior keratocyte proliferation and adhesion over other materials currently used as Kpro haptics [36]. Leon et al. have developed a Kpro which utilizes a Coralline hydroxyapatite skirt to stabilize a central optic [29]. Their HAKpro has demonstrated fibrovascular tissue in-growth when implanted into rabbits. Although hydroxyapatite has promising biocompatibility profile, it is inherently brittle and rigid. Another group has combined porous nano-hydroxyapatite with hydrogel to create a Kpro haptic [19]. Preliminary results in rabbits show in-growth of host tissue, deposition of collagen, and vascularization in the skirt material without intrastromal inflammation.

10.7.2 Biologic Coatings

Other researchers have focused on improving in-growth and biocompatibility of corneal epithelial cells with Kpro materials. While most current Kpro haptic materials are inert and noncell-adhesive, coating these synthetic materials with bio-active extracellular matrix proteins may stimulate epithelial proliferation and adhesion. Several groups have found success with fibronectin, laminin, and collagen in encouraging epithelial cell growth on synthetic materials [42, 44, 48]. Sweeney et al. found collagen I, collagen IV, and laminin to support consistent multilayered epithelialization of synthetic material implanted into rabbit eyes. In collagen I-coated implants, they observed formation of a basement-membranes and adhesion complexes [48].

10.7.3 Biologic Scaffolds and Enhanced Hydrogels

Other groups have furthered the development of hydrogel technology first seen in clinical use with the AlphaCor Kpro. Fabrications have varied from collagen-based copolymers [20, 25] to interpenetrating polymer networks (IPN) [38]. These enhanced hydrogels are intended to support not only peripheral tissue integration but also corneal epithelialization and diffusion of bioactive substances such as glucose [38]. Results in vitro have so far been promising. Myung et al. demonstrated good retention, optical clarity, and multilayering of corneal epithelium of a poly(ethylene glycol)/poly(acrylic acid) (PEG/PAA) IPN implanted intrastromally in rabbit corneas [39]. This group has also fabricated a single-piece keratoprosthesis (the "Stanford Kpro"), composed entirely of a PEG/PAA IPN, and further testing is ongoing [38].

10.8 Conclusion

Keratoplasty has been the dominant therapy for rehabilitation of severely opaque corneas over the past century. However, limitations such as graft failure, poor prognosis in severe ocular surface disease, and high resource demands have fueled continued interest in

Kpro as a viable alternative to standard keratoplasty. Practical experience with Kpro has grown rapidly over the past few decades, and has brought forth key lessons in this evolving field. It is clear that diagnosis is a key determinant of prognosis, and that patients should be separated into two different categories based on the presence or absence of underlying inflammation. Recognition of these principles allows the promise of Kpro to emerge in the treatment of a large number of patients suffering from repeat graft failures. Patients with severe ocular surface disease from autoimmune conditions and chemical burns continue to challenge Kpro practitioners and researchers alike. The use of autologous biologic haptics as in OOKP and TKP shows promise for long-term device retention in cases of severe ocular surface disease, but may place greater demands on patients and practitioners. New directions in Kpro research will likely introduce biologically active materials into the clinical arena.

References

1. Aldave AJ, Kamal KM, Vo RC et al (2009) The Boston type 1 keratoprosthesis: improving outcomes and expanding indications. Ophthalmology 116:640–651
2. Andel P, Worst J, Singh I (1993) Results of champagne cork keratoprosthesis in 127 corneal blind eyes. Refract Corneal Surg 9:189–190
3. Aquavella JV, Gearinger MD, Akpek EK et al (2007) Pediatric keratoprosthesis. Ophthalmology 114:989–994
4. Asworth JL, Rhatigan M, Sampath R et al (1996) The hydroxyapatite orbital implant: a prospective study. Eye 10(Pt 1):29–37
5. Bersudsky V, Blum-Hareuveni T, Rehani U et al (2001) The profile of repeated corneal transplantation. Ophthalmology 108:461–469
6. Bishop VL, Robinson LP, Wechsler AW et al (1986) Corneal graft survival: a retrospective Australian study. Aust N Z J Ophthalmol 14:133–138
7. Bradley JC, Hernandez EG, Schwab IR et al (2009) Boston type 1 keratoprosthesis: the University of California Davis experience. Cornea 28:321–327
8. Ciolino JB, Ament JW, Zerbe BL et al (2008) Etiology of keratoprosthesis loss: results from the Boston keratoprosthesis multicenter study. Invest Ophthalmol Vis Sci 49:E-Abstract 5712
9. Ciolino JB, Dohlman CH (2009) Biologic keratoprosthesis materials. Int Ophthalmol Clin 49:1–9
10. Dandona L, Naduvilath TJ, Janarthanan M et al (1997) Survival analysis and visual outcome in a large series of corneal transplants in India. Br J Ophthalmol 81:726–731
11. Doane MG, Dohlman CH, Bearse G (1996) Fabrication of keratoprosthesis. Cornea 15:179–184
12. Dohlman CH (1994) Keratoprostheses. In: Albert D, Jakobiec FJ (eds) Principles and practice of ophthalmology. WB Saunders, Philadelphia, PA, pp 338–342
13. Dohlman CH, Harissi-Dagher M, Khan BF et al (2006) Introduction to the use of the Boston Keratoprosthesis. Expert Rev Ophthalmol 1:41–48
14. Dohlman CH, Barnes S, Ma J (2007) Keratoprosthesis. In: Krachmer JH, Mannis MJ, Holland EJ (eds) Cornea. CV Mosby, St. Louis, MO, pp 1719–1728
15. Dohlman CH, Schneider HA, Doane MG (1974) Prosthokeratoplasty. Am J Ophthalmol 77:694–700
16. Dohlman CH, Terada H (1998) Keratoprosthesis in pemphigoid and Stevens-Johnson syndrome. Av Exp Med Biol 438:1021–1025
17. Eye Bank Association of America. Eye banking statistical report. Eye Bank Association of America 2007, Washington DC, USA
18. Falcinelli G, Falsini B, Taloni M et al (2005) Modified osteoodonto-keratoprosthesis for treatment of corneal blindness: long-term anatomical and functional outcomes in 181 cases. Arch Ophthalmol 123:1319–1329
19. Fenglan X, Yubao L, Xiaoming Y et al (2007) Preparation and in vivo investigation of artificial cornea made of nano-hydroxyapatite/poly (vinyl alcohol) hydrogel composite. J Mater Sci Mater Med 18:635–640
20. Griffith M, Hakim M, Shimmura S et al (2002) Artificial human corneas: scaffolds for transplantation and host regeneration. Cornea 21:S54–S61
21. Hicks CR, Crawford GJ, Dart JK et al (2006) AlphaCor: clinical outcomes. Cornea 25:1034–1042
22. Hicks CR, Crawford GJ, Lou X et al (2003) Corneal replacement using a synthetic hydrogel cornea, AlphaCor: device, preliminary outcomes and complications. Eye 17: 385–392
23. Hille K, Grabner G, Liu C et al (2005) Standards for modified osteoodontokeratoprosthesis (OOKP) surgery according to Strampelli and Falcinelli: the Rome-Viena Protocol. Cornea 24:895–908
24. Hille K, Hille A, Ruprecht KW (2006) Medium term results in keratoprostheses with biocompatible and biological haptic. Graefes Arch Clin Exp Ophthalmol 244:696–704
25. Huang YX, Li QH (2007) An active artificial cornea with the function of inducing new corneal tissue generation in vivo – a new approach to corneal tissue engineering. Biomed Mater 2:S121–S125
26. Khan BF, Harissi-Dagher M, Dohlman CH (2008) Keratoprosthesis. In: Albert DM, Miller JW (eds) Albert and Jakobiec's Principles and Practice of Ophthalmology, 3rd edn. WB Saunders, Philadelphia, PA, pp 895–903
27. Khan BF, Harissi-Dagher M, Khan DM et al (2007) Advances in keratoprosthesis: enhancing retention and

prevention of infection and inflammation. Int Ophthalmol Clin 47:61–71
28. Lee MK, Lee SM, Lee JL et al (2007) Long-term outcome in ocular intractable surface disease with Seoul-type keratoprosthesis. Cornea 26:546–551
29. Leon CR, Barraquer JI Jr, Barraquer JI Sr (1997) Corraline hydroxyapatite keratoprosthesis in rabbits. J Refract Surg 13:74–78
30. Liu C, Paul B, Tandon R et al (2005) The osteo-odonto-keratoprosthesis (OOKP). Semin Ophthalmol 20:113–128
31. Ma J, Dohlman CH (2005) Repeat Penetrating keratoplasty versus the Boston keratoprosthesis in graft failure. Int Ophthalmol Clin N Am 45:49–59
32. Maguire MG, Stark W, Gottsch J (1994) Risk factors for corneal graft failure and rejection in the collaborative corneal transplantation studies (CTTS). Ophthalmology 101:1536–1547
33. Mannis MJ (1999) Dohlman CH (2005) The artificial cornea: a brief history. In: Mannis MJ, Mannis AA (eds) Corneal Transplantation: A History of Profiles (Hirschberg History of Ophthalmology). JP Wayenborgh, Oostende, Belgium, pp 321–335
34. Marchi V, Ricci R, Pecorella I et al (1994) Osteo-odonto-keratoprosthesis. description of surgical technique with results in 85 patients. Cornea 13:125–130
35. Maskati QB, Maskati BT (2006) Asian experience with Pintucci keratoprosthesis. Indian J Ophthalmol 54(2): 89–94
36. Mehta JS, Futter CE, Sandeman SR et al (1997) Hydroxyapatite promotes superior keratocyte adhesion and proliferation in comparison with current keratoprosthesis in rabbits. J Refract Surg 13:74–78
37. Michael R, Charoenrook V, Fideliz de la Paz M et al (2008) Long-term functional and anatomical results of osteo- and osteoodonto-keratoprosthesis. Graefes Arch Clin Exp Ophthalmol 246:1133–1137
38. Myung D, Duhamel PE, Cochran JR et al (2008) Development of hydrogel-based keratoprostheses: a materials perspective. Biotechnol Prog 24:735–741
39. Myung D, Farooqui N, Waters D et al (2008) Glucose-permeable interpenetrating polymer network hydrogels for corneal implant applications, a pilot study. Curr Eye Res 33:29–43
40. Netland PA, Terada H, Dohlman CH (1998) Glaucoma associated with keratoprosthesis. Ophthalmology 105: 751–757
41. Nouri M, Terada H, Alfonso EC et al (2001) Endophthalmitis after keratoprosthesis: incidence, bacterial causes, and risk factors. Arch Ophthalmol 119:484–489
42. Ohji M, Mandarino L, SundarRaj N et al (1993) Corneal epithelial cell attachment with endogenous laminin and fibronectin. Invest Ophthalmol Vis Sci 34:2487–2492
43. Pellier de Quengsy G (1789) Precis ou cours d'operations sur la chirurgie des yeux. Didot, Paris
44. Pettit DK, Horbett TA, Hoffman AS et al (1990) Quantitation of rabbit corneal epithelial cell outgrowth on polymeric substrates in vitro. Invest Ophthalmol Vis Sci 31: 2269–2277
45. Pintucci S, Pintucci F, Caiazza S et al (1996) The Dacron felt colonizable keratoprosthesis: after 15 years. Eur J Ophthalmol 6:125–130
46. Sayegh RR, Ang LP, Foster CP et al (2008) The Boston Keratoprosthesis in Stevens-Johnson Syndrome. Am J Ophthalmol 145:438–444
47. Strampelli B (1963) Keratoprosthesis with osteodontal tissue. Am J Ophthalmol 89:1029–1039
48. Sweeney DF, Xie RZ, Evans MD et al (2003) A comparison of biological coatings for the promotion of corneal epithelialization of synthetic surface in vivo. Invest Ophthalmol Vis Sci 44:3301–3309
49. Tan D, Tay A, Theng J et al (2008) Keratoprosthesis surgery for end-stage corneal blindness in Asian eyes. Ophthalmology 115:503–510
50. Temprano J (1993) Keratoprosthesis with tibial autograft. Refract Corneal Surg 9:192
51. Thompson RW, Price MO, Boweers PJ et al (2003) Long term graft survival after penetrating keratoplasty. Ophthalmology 110:1396–1402
52. Tugal-Tutkun I, Akova YA, Foster CS (1995) Penetrating keratoplasty in cicatrizing conjunctival diseases. Ophthalmology 102:576–585
53. Whitcher JP, Srinivasan M, Upadhyay MP (2001) Corneal blindness: a global perspective. Bull World Health Organ 279(3):214–221
54. Williams KA, Muehlberg SM, Lewis RF et al (1995) How successful is corneal transplantation? A report from the Australian corneal graft register. Eye 9:219–227
55. World Health Organization (2004) Magnitude and causes of visual impairment. Fact sheet No. 282. http://www.who.int/mediacentre/factsheets/fs282/en/. Accessed on 5 Nov2009
56. Yaghouti F, Nouri M, Abad JC et al (2001) Keratoprosthesis: preoperative prognostic categories. Cornea 20:19–23
57. Yakimenko S (1993) Results of a PMMA/titanium keratoprosthesis in 502 eyes. Refract Corneal Surg 9:197–198
58. Yamagami S, Suzuki Y, Tsuru T (1996) Risk factors for graft failure in penetrating keratoplasty. Acta Ophthalmol Scand 74:584–588
59. Zerbe BL, Belin MW, Ciolino JB et al (2006) Boston keratoprosthesis study group: results from the multicenter Boston type I keratoprosthesis study. Ophthalmology 113:1779–1784

Chapter 11

Posterior Lamellar Keratoplasty in Perspective

Arnalich-Montiel F and Dart JKG

Core Messages

- Posterior lamellar keratoplasty (PLK) offers many substantial benefits compared to penetrating keratoplasty (PK) including: closed eye surgery, elimination of both regular and irregular postoperative astigmatism leading to full visual rehabilitation with spectacles within 3-6 months, elimination of postoperative corneal anaesthesia, and a reduced risk of postoperative globe rupture.
- Disadvantages of PLK compared to PK include: corneal stromal scarring is untreatable by PLK, complex anterior segment reconstruction is more difficult with PLK, PLK often fails in patients with aphakia and/or an incomplete lens iris diaphragm, early donor dislocation in PLK remains a problem.
- PLK techniques, and the indications for it, are still evolving.
- PLK is rapidly replacing PK as the procedure of choice for patients with otherwise uncomplicated endothelial cell loss such as pseudophakic bullous keratopathy and Fuchs' endothelial dystrophy.

11.1 Introduction

Endothelial dysfunction is a leading indication for corneal grafting. Although selective replacement of the dysfunctional endothelium is the logical approach, the procedure of choice, for over 100 years, has been penetrating (full thickness) keratoplasty. However penetrating keratoplasty leads to a variety of postoperative complications that burden the outcome, including high and/or irregular astigmatism, a long rehabilitation time, suture related complications, graft rejection and late wound dehiscence following trauma.

Posterior lamellar keratoplasty (PLK) as a selective replacement of posterior stroma and endothelium, was performed for the first time in humans by Tillett in 1956 [1]. Decades later, Melles described a sutureless corneal surgical technique for PLK, having done the first human case in 1998 [2, 3]. Terry and Ousley later modified this procedure and popularised it as deep lamellar endothelial keratoplasty (DLEK) performing their first case in 2000 [4]. Further modification of the technique, called small-incision DLEK, enabled the surgeon to introduce the donor material through an opening as small as 5 mm [5].

Since then the technique has been simplified by Melles with the elimination of the deep lamellar dissection, required by DLEK, being replaced by the scoring and stripping of the host Descemet's membrane and endothelium [6, 7] known as Descemet-stripping endothelial keratoplasy (DSEK). The combination of DSEK with the use of the automated microkeratome for donor preparation [8], instead of manual deep lamellar dissection, has resulted in the technique of Descemet-stripping automated endothelial keratoplasty (DSAEK). The ease of use of DSEK and DSAEK, which eliminate many of the disadvantages of penetrating keratoplasty, are responsible for the increasing use of PLK by corneal surgeons. In the United States alone, more than 14,000 corneas were provided by US eye banks for PLK in 2007, as compared with 1,400 corneas in 2005 (Eye Bank Association of America 2007 Eye Banking Statistical Report).

Descemet's membrane endothelial keratoplasty (DMEK) in which Descemet's membrane alone, without any supporting stromal tissue, is transplanted is currently experimental [9, 10].

In our practice endothelial keratoplasty has become one of the most commonly performed transplant procedures, accounting for around 40% of cases; including Fuchs' dystrophy, bullous keratopathy, and corneal graft failure.

11.2 Choosing Endothelial Keratoplasty Procedures

11.2.1 Indications

Endothelial dysfunction is one of the most frequent indications for corneal transplant surgery, varying from 12 to 60% of all transplant procedures in different series [11–14]. Table 11.1 summarises the most common causes of endothelial dysfunction, dividing them into primary endothelial dysfunctions, in which there is no established extrinsic precipitating cause as in the dystrophies, or endothelial dysfunctions secondary to extrinsic insults such as trauma, glaucoma, previous surgery or intraocular inflammation.

The recent update from the The Australian Corneal Graft Registry (ACGR), which covers all registry data from 1985–2006, reveals that out of more than 17,000 corneal grafts, bullous keratopathy (26%) follows keratoconus (32%) as a leading indication of keratoplasty. Other causes of endothelial dysfunction such as Fuchs' dystrophy (6%), or decompensated corneal transplants (14%) also account for a substantial proportion of cases needing keratoplasty [15].

11.2.2 Preoperative Considerations

All corneal transplant surgery demands the preoperative assessment of the underlying cause of the corneal opacity, any comorbidity including the visual potential and the presence of cataract or lens implant function. For posterior keratoplasty additional considerations, that are less relevant to penetrating keratoplasty, are the degree of stromal scarring, any requirement for anterior segment reconstruction, and the integrity of the lens iris diaphragm which will influence the success of the current air bubble techniques for facilitating the attachment of posterior lamellar grafts.

11.2.2.1 Confirming the Extent of Endothelial Dysfunction

There are several approaches for the evaluation of endothelial function:

- *Visual symptoms*. Blurred vision on waking that improves during the course of the day suggests endothelial failure.
- *Morphological evaluation:*
  - Slit lamp: Gross or microcystic epithelial oedema is often present except in very early cases. Bilateral corneal guttata indicate Fuchs' dystrophy as the cause of the disease.
  - Specular microscopy: endothelial imaging with a range of specular microscopes can assess the morphology, size and density of the endothelial cells as well as identify guttata. However when the epithelium and stroma are opaque (due to oedema or scarring) the images are often too poor for meaningful analysis. This is also the case when there are dense guttata as these mask the underlying endothelial cells.
  - Confocal microscopy: this permits easier imaging in the presence of corneal opacity. Guttata appear as hyporeflective images with occasional central bright images. Neither specular nor confocal microscopy assess endothelial cell pump function or the integrity of the intercellular tight junctions.

Table 11.1 Causes of corneal endothelial dysfunction

Primary[a]	Fuchs' dystrophy
	Posterior polymorphous dystrophy.
	Iridoconeal endothelial syndromes (ICE).
	Congenital hereditary endothelial dystrophy (CHED)
	Primary endotheliitis
Secondary[b]	Surgical trauma including aphakic and PBK, retinal and glaucoma surgery
	Glaucoma: angle closure, open angle and congenital
	Failed corneal transplants
	Chemical injuries
	Chronic uveitis
	HSV keratitis
	Ocular trauma

[a]No established extrinsic precipitating cause for endothelial dysfunction
[b]Endothelial dysfunctions secondary to extrinsic insults

However normal endothelial cell morphology appears to be closely associated with normal pump function.

- *Functional evaluation:*
  - Ultrasound or optical pachymetry: Corneal thickness is an indirect measurement of endothelial function and is used as an index of severity of endothelial dysfunction. Some authors have used a pachymetry measurement of greater than 640 μm [16] to indicate that the risk of corneal decompensation is too high to carry out cataract surgery without combined corneal transplant surgery. However this presupposes that the risk of endothelial cell loss with cataract surgery has remained constant with the introduction of newer techniques, and that there is minimal individual variation in normal corneal pachymetry. However corneal pachymetry varies widely with sex, age and ethnic group [17–19] such that a corneal thickness of 640 μm does not indicate the same degree of endothelial cell dysfunction for a patient who had a normal baseline pachymetry of 600 μm compared to another with a normal baseline pachymetry of 490 μm. As a result we use serial pachymetry to assess progression of disease in an individual and only recommend combined cataract and keratoplasty in patients who have clearly developed corneal epithelial oedema.
  - Recovery after occlusion test: The ability of the cornea to de-swell after overnight eye closure also reveals the quality of the endothelial function. It is not uncommon to see patients who describe early morning blurring of vision which does not correlate with reduced acuity, signs of corneal decompensation or abnormal pachymetry. In this situation the patient can apply a patch the evening before a clinic visit; removing the patch in clinic mimics the early morning situation and shows both increased corneal thickness by pachymetry and clinical signs of corneal decompensation in patients with clinically significant endothelial dysfunction.

11.2.2.2 Corneal Scarring

Advanced corneal decompensation may lead to corneal epithelial hypertrophy and subepithelial, stromal or pre-Descemet's corneal scarring. Corneal epithelial hypertrophic membranes can be peeled off to reveal whether or not there is significant subepithelial fibrosis. The extent of stromal and pre-Descemet's scarring can be assessed with anterior segment ocular coherence tomography (OCT). Stromal scarring is a relative contraindication to endothelial keratoplasty in which the benefits of the procedure may be outweighed by the potential reduction in acuity.

11.2.2.3 Cataract and Intraocular Lens Status

Cataract status in phakic patients can be difficult to assess in the presence of corneal decompensation. Because of the loss of endothelial cells associated with cataract surgery post keratoplasty, the predictability of the biometry with posterior lamellar grafts, the delay of 3 months to ensure posterior graft stability that is recommended before carrying out cataract surgery after endothelial keratoplasty, and the relative difficulty of phakic posterior keratoplasty, cataract surgery is commonly combined with PLK in post presbyopic patients and when there is a preexisting history of cataract [20].

For patients having combined cataract surgery and PLK the intraocular lens power chosen should take into account the hypermetropic shift of about +1 diopter [21, 22]. This is thought to be due to the curved configuration of the donor cornea when attached to the posterior host cornea, functioning as a negative lens, inducing 1D of myopia. As a result, for postoperative emmetropia, we use an estimated postoperative refraction of −1D when carrying out combined cataract surgery and endothelial keratoplasty [23].

The centration and condition of any intraocular lens must be assessed before PLK. Lens exchange is technically more difficult through a small incision than open sky in penetrating keratoplasty and the requirement for this may be a contraindication to PLK. An anterior chamber (AC) IOL is a relative contraindication to a PLK because of endothelial trauma during insertion, intermittent postoperative IOL touch, reduced depth of the AC and the difficulty of maintaining an air bubble in front of the IOL during DSEK/DSAEK [24]. To overcome this problem, it is possible to remove AC IOL's at the time of PLK and replace these 3 months after a successful PLK or combine, in a single procedure, the replacement of the AC IOL with a scleral-fixated posterior chamber IOL [25].

11.2.2.4 Lens/Iris Diaphragm Status

The current technique for donor attachment in DSEK/DSAEK utilises an air bubble, usually under pressure, in the AC at the end of surgery.

In patients with aniridia, aphakia, iris defects, peripheral iris adhesions, and AC intraocular lenses, this is more difficult to achieve. In aphakic patients or those with a large iridotomy an AC air bubble may be difficult to achieve at all, or move into the posterior segment, as soon as the, patient lifts their head, eliminating support for the posterior graft. Success rates can be improved at the time of PLK surgery by closing those defects that can be closed and by implanting a posterior chamber lens. The surgeon and the patient needs to be aware that failure in these situations is more likely; an air bubble retention test, before cutting the donor for PLK can eb helpful before makin a final decision about whether to proceed with a PK or PLK. Some surgeons advocate performing DLEK in such cases, as it is less dependent on the maintenance of a postoperative air bubble for graft adherence [26]; we have no experience with this technique.

11.2.2.5 Intraocular Pressure

Failure to control intraocular pressure (IOP) after surgery reduces the survival of all types of corneal graft including PLK [27]. Normalising the IOP preoperatively is essential and we rarely proceed with graft surgery in patients requiring more than one topical hypotensive medication for good pressure control. In those with more severe glaucoma drainage surgery, usually with a tube, is carried out 3 months before graft surgery. Even in patients with advanced glaucoma an intraoperative pressure of 30 mmHg for 8 min is not anticipated to prejudice optic nerve function. Penetrating keratoplasty is known to have a detrimental effect on IOP [28], possibly because of altered post operative AC angle configuration which may be eliminated in PLK; it remains to be seen whether PLK has the anticipated neutral effect on IOP, although a small series of 44 patients with DLEK has shown that glaucoma may occur de novo in 7% of the patients [29] although some of these may be steroid related.

11.2.2.6 Retinal Function

An estimate of postoperative acuity must be made before graft surgery. In patients with opaque media we find the previous history and clinical techniques, such as the assessment of pupil responses and ability to project light of more value than electrodiagnostic tests.

11.3 PLK Surgical Technique

Currently Descemet stripping techniques by DSEK or DSAEK, rather than DLEK or DMEK, are the most widely used and this perspective will focus on these techniques. Surgery may be performed under all types of anaesthesia; we prefer the use of local anaesthesia, such as a subtenons anaesthetic injection, to ensure that the patient can cooperate with face up posturing to maintain the air bubble in contact with the transplant in the immediate postoperative period.

11.3.1 Donor Preparation

Donor dissection can be done manually (DSEK) or with a microkeratome (DSAEK). Microkeratome preparation causes a relatively small loss of endothelial cells, a more reproducible donor thickness and a smoother interface, decreasing visual recovery time and a decreased incidence of interface haze [8].

- *Manual dissection of the donor* is done using an artificial chamber such as Barron´s artificial chamber (Katena, Denville, NJ). Using an AC air bubble to estimate the depth of the dissection as described by Melles [30] is useful but not mandatory to achieve the appropriate depth and many do not use it. We aim for a two thirds depth donor dissection. Once dissection is complete the donor is punched on a block with the desired size trephine.
- *Automated donor dissection* is usually performed using the Moria automated anterior lamellar keratoplasty (ALTK) system (Moria, Antony, France). When intraoperative pachymetry is available we use the 350 μm head in donors measuring >570 μm and the 300 μm head for thinner donors. When pachymetry is not available we use the 350 μm head for cold stored material and the 300 μm head for deturgesced organ cultured donors. For the Amadeus II microkeratome (Ziemer Ophthalmic Systems AG, Switzerland) the recommendation is to use the 400 μm head [31]. Automated dissection has also been effectively performed using femtosecond laser (IntraLase Corp, Irvine, CA) with no detrimental effect on endothelial cell density in eye bank eyes. Femtosecond laser lamellar dissection seemed to be less deep and less smooth [32]. Preliminary results of femtosecond laser-assisted descemet stripping endothelial keratoplasty in 20 patients showed limited improvement of BSCVA, with higher endothelial cell loss, hyperopic shift and dislocation rate than expected for ALTK dissection [33].

11.3.2 Host Dissection for DSEK/DSAEK

Our current technique is as follows:

- Lightly mark the epithelium with gentian violet using a 7.5 mm circular marker touched onto a gentian violet pad, we aim for a descemethorrexis of about 7.5 mm

that is 0.5–1.0 mm less in diameter than the size of the donor to avoid removing host Descemet's outside the donor graft site.
- Create a 5 mm temporal corneal OR scleral tunnel.
- Either use a peripherally placed self retaining infusion (Lewicky cannula) to maintain the AC or a cohesive viscoelastic while removing Descemet's. We prefer to use a cannula as it also helps to maintain the AC during the insertion of the graft (see below). If the cannula is used it is important to keep bottle height low to reduce the risk of iris prolapse which tends to recur thereafter. Persistent iris prolapse can be managed by the insertion of an IOL glide.
- Perform one or two small vertical peripheral paracenteses (outside the zone of graft) to permit air injection after graft insertion.
- Delineate the area of Descemetorhexis with a reverse (upturned) Sinskey hook (Moria, Antony, France) and use this, a Paufique knife or a Descemet's stripper (Moria, Antony, France) to remove Descemets. "Roughing up" the peripheral stroma with the reverse Sinskey, or a Terry Scraper (Bausch and Lomb, St. Louis, MO) may help adhesion [34].

11.3.3 Donor Insertion

There are several current methods in use for the introduction of the donor including forceps insertion ("taco" technique) [35], pull through [36] and glide techniques [37]. The forceps technique (Fig. 11.1a) was the first described of these, and may be the most widely used, however there have been concerns about the effect of forceps induced endothelial crush injury, as well as handling difficulties, especially when the donor lenticule is thin, which the pull through and glide techniques were introduced to address.

- *Suture guided pull through technique* (Fig. 11.1c, d): A 10-0 polypropylene suture (Prolene; Ethicon, San Angelo, Texas, USA) on a long straight needle (STC-6, Ethicon) is passed partial thickness through the edge of the cornea and tied with an overhand knot to create a loop. The length of the loop is made large enough to allow it to be cut after the donor is placed. The straight needle is passed through the incision and across the anterior chamber and out again through the cornea at 180° opposite the incision. It is important to ensure that the needle does not pass through tissue at the incision site which will prevent the graft passing into the eye. The donor, after coating the endothelium with cohesive viscoelastic, is placed in the wound entrance either folded, or unfolded with the endothelium side down. The donor is then drawn into the AC by drawing on the suture or is held there if the technique is forceps assisted. An AC maintainer is used to maintain the AC during insertion. We prefer not to use forceps assisted insertion as the cornea may be difficult to grasp, causing trauma, and can unfold endothelium uppermost which is unlikely to occur when the donor is pulled through endothelial side down.
- *Busin glide* (ref. 19,098, Moria SA, Anthony, Francia) *guided pull through technique* (Fig. 11.1b): The donor tissue is placed on the glide with the endothelium facing upward. The glide is then turned over and pushed against the entrance of the incision or into the AC. The cornea is pulled from one edge into the AC using crocodile vitreoretinal forceps that is inserted through a paracentesis opposite the main wound.
- *Other glides/injectors*: these have been reported but are not yet commercially available.

11.3.4 Techniques for Graft Centration

Once the donor cornea is in the AC and correctly oriented, the pull through suture is removed, any infusion removed and all wounds closed to be both air and watertight. An air bubble is injected under the corneal donor to hold it against the host posterior stroma. There are several techniques that can be used to position the donor. These work best at normal levels of IOP.

- Corneal "balloting" (Fig. 11.2a): in which the surface of the host cornea overlying the edge of the graft away from the desired direction of movement is firmly indented and swept towards the desired position with a blunt instrument such as a squint hook or the angled surface of a 20 gauge angled cannula [38].
- Corneal centration using a hook (Fig. 11.2b): the tip of an insulin syringe can be bent like a reverse capsulotomy needle and introduced through side port to engage the edge of the endothelial surface of the donor and pull the graft into position [38]. This results in loss of the AC air and fluid and is more traumatic than the transcorneal needle technique.
- Corneal centration using a transcorneal needle (Fig. 11.2c): a long fine needle such as the 10–0 polypropylene suture needle used for the pull through technique (Prolene, Ethicon, San Angelo, Texas, USA). The fine needle is pushed at an angle through the periphery of the host cornea to engage the stromal surface of the donor and push it into position. We use this when the cornea does not respond to "balloting".

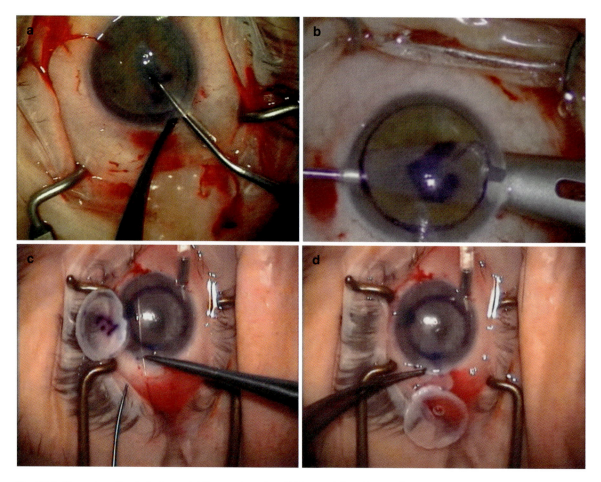

Fig. 11.1 Donor insertion techniques. (**a**) Forceps insertion. (**b**) Busin glide technique for insertion. (**c**) Suture pull through technique showing introduction of needle (here the donor lamellar has been placed on the donor anterior lamellar disc which is being used as a carrier). (**d**) Graft being pulled into the eye with the pull through technique (the donor lamellar is in the wound)

11.3.5 Techniques for Promoting Donor Adhesion

Several strategies have been advocated to improve corneal adhesion. The most effective are:

- Peripheral roughening of the host posterior stroma immediately after performing the descemetorrhexis [39].
- Sweep and compress the cornea using a blunt instrument such as an 20 guage cannula or a roller from the centre to the periphery to "milk" any interface fluid out to the edge of the graft and into the AC to ensure stroma to stroma surface contact [7].
- Place four slightly bevelled stab incisions from the surface to the interface in the pericentral zone using a 1-mm wide diamond paracentesis knife [7]. Fill the AC completely with air ensuring that the donor is fully in contact with the host cornea. The edge of the donor is visible as a refractile ring when this is achieved. Ideally ensure the pressure is between 30–50 mmHg with a tonometer and maintain this for 8–10 min in the operating theatre; then remove enough air to soften the eye but leave a bubble in the AC. Some authors recommend an inferior ocutome iridotomy (performed at the time of the descemetorrhexis) to reduce the risk of pupil block [40].
- Posture the patient face up for a period of time immediately after surgery to use the AC air to maintain the donor in position [8]. We currently recommend this for 1 h.

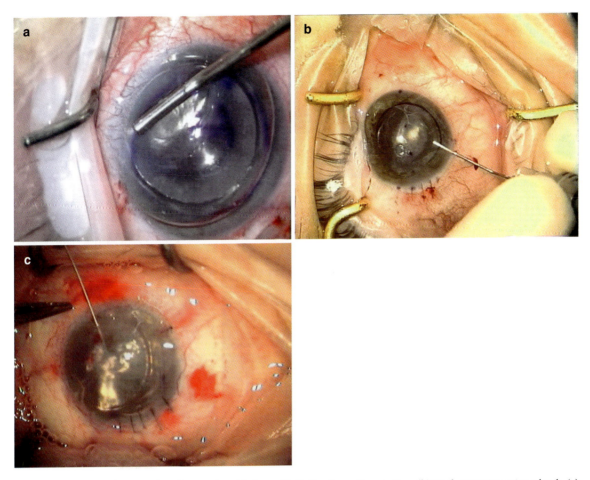

Fig. 11.2 Techniques for corneal graft centration. (**a**) Corneal balloting for graft centration. (**b**) Graft centration using a hook. (**c**) Graft centration using a transcorneal needle

11.3.6 Post-operative Care

After the period of face up posturing the patient is fully mobilised and examined to exclude the development of pupil block [8].

- If pupil block is present air can be easily removed at the slit lamp with a 30 guage cannula via a preexisting superior paracentesis.
- The patient can then be fully mobilised and instructed to take special care not to rub the eye which may dislocate the donor in the early postoperative stages. We provide a clear cartela shield to be worn at night post surgery.
- We review the patient at 24 h and 7 days to ensure that the donor is adherent. If not immediate repositioning is carried out with repeat air tamponade.
- Single sutures closing paracenteses can be removed early.
- We remove sutures closing the corneal wound at 3 months.
- We use the same postoperative topical steroid and antibiotic regimen as for penetrating keratoplasty.
- Spectacles can be changed as early as a few weeks after surgery and the vision is usually approaching the final acuity at 3–6 months.

11.3.7 Surgery for Complex Cases

11.3.7.1 Failed Grafts

Patients with previous penetrating keratoplasty that has failed can also benefit from DSAEK (Fig. 11.3c, d). In the first published series of seven consecutive patients, all cases showed successful adherence of the donor button and cleared the edema from the previous penetrating graft. Best-corrected visual acuity had improved in

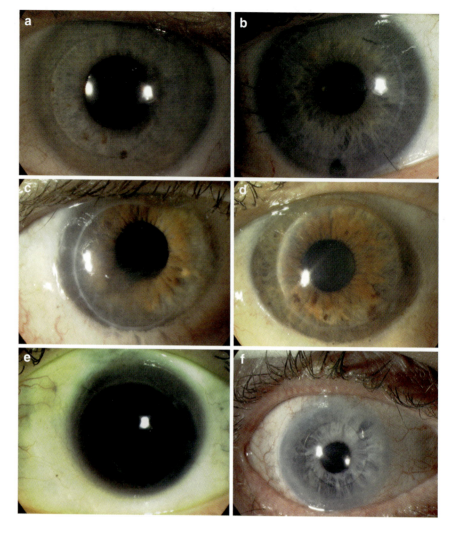

Fig. 11.3 Outcomes. (**a, b**) Pseudophakic bullous keratopathy (PBK) and Phakic bullous keratopathy after PLK. (**c, d**) Failed corneal graft before and after PLK. (**e, f**) Aphakic BK after a PLK and PBK with anterior chamber (AC) IOL after PLK

six of the seven cases compared with the preoperative vision at 3 months [41]. In another small series of seven cases with a mean follow up of 13 months, four of six eyes (67%) achieved a BCVA of 20/40 or better. One eye suffered recurrent donor graft dislocation and elected to undergo repeat PK instead of repeat DSAEK. The other six grafts remained clear at the last follow-up visit, although 2/6 needed repositioning and another 2/6 had primary iatrogenic graft failure within 1 week of DSAEK and underwent repeat DSAEK with new donor tissue with good results [42].

The technique is not much different to conventional DSAEK:

- Price et al [41], did not strip the Descemet membrane from the failed graft or recipient cornea before implanting the donor tissue in five of the seven cases where preoperative examinations determined that there were no guttata and that the Descemet membrane had been clear before corneal decompensation. The donor cornea used was 8.5–9 mm, which was probably bigger than the previous penetrating keratoplasty button although not specified.
- Covert et al [42], stripped the host endothelium and Descemet membrane corresponding to the previous 8.0-mm keratoplasty incision, and the corneal lenticule inserted was 8.5 mm which was bigger than the previous PK donor button.
- We usually remove Descemet's within the graft margins to avoid corneal dehiscence, and also make the donor larger than the previous graft by about 0.5–1 mm when possible.

11.3.7.2 Aniridics, Vitrectomised and Aphakic Eyes (Fig. 11.3e)

Maintenance of air is difficult in aphakic eyes in which there is no capsular bag to isolate the AC, increasing the risk of donor dislocation and failure after DSAEK. The main factor affecting a successful outcome in these cases is the ability to maintain air in the AC in the first postoperative hours in addition to strict face-up positioning [43]. Price and Price [44] described successful outcomes in two eyes with aphakic bullous keratopathy before DSEK with a simultaneous secondary IOL in one eye, and a secondary IOL implanted 4 months after DSEK in the other eye. A donor dislocation was successfully repositioned in one eye. Another study included three aphakic patients who underwent DSEK with varied results. Two of them had a favourable outcome using air injection in one case and longer-lasting gas (SF_6) with higher buoyancy than air to fill the AC in the other case with broad iridectomy. The last patient had donor disc displaced posteriorly leading to total RD and no perception of light [43]. The use of long-lasting, higher-buoyancy gases could be a possible solution for these patients.

Price et al [43], have modify their technique for these cases:

- Descemet's membrane was not stripped from the recipient eye.
- The stromal side of the donor tissue was stained with trypan blue to improve visualisation.
- The donor tissue was initially inserted only 80–90% of the way into the eye so that one end was held in the incision, while an anchor suture was placed in the peripheral edge of the anterior portion of the donor tissue to secure it to the overlying recipient cornea. This step can be avoided in our experience by using a pull through technique with a 10/0 prolene straight needle that secures the donor graft in the AC combined with a trailing suture, on the opposite side of the donor to hold it anteriorly, preventing dislocation posteriorly before injecting air.
- Air is not removed from the eye at the end of the case.

Some authors advocate the convenience of performing a DLEK with successful results [45] as described in 1.2.2.4 in cases where it is foreseen that the air bubble will not be retained in the AC. Placing a posterior chamber lens, closing all iris defects where possible and testing the eye for air retention before making a final decision a between PK and PLK can contribute to successful outcomes.

11.3.7.3 Anterior Chamber Lens

This is explained in Sect. 1.2.2.3. See Fig. 11.3f.

11.4 Clinical Results and Complications

The theoretical advantages and disadvantages of PLK compared to penetrating keratoplasty are summarised in Table 11.2.

11.4.1 Visual Acuity

A major concern about lamellar techniques is the creation of an interface that limits both visual acuity and quality of vision. However several studies [20, 21, 40, 46, 47] have shown that mean best corrected visual acuity in DSAEK ranges from 20/34 to 20/44 which is superior to the historical results of PK for similar indications (Fuchs', pseudophakic and aphakic bullous keratopathy) [40, 47]. In a series of 100 cases, 72/74 (97%) of the eyes with corneal decompensation and no other comorbidity achieved BSCVA of 20/40 and up to 10/74 (14%) achieved BSCVA of 20/20 after 6 months [46]. Similar levels of visual acuity have also been achieved by other posterior lamellar techniques such as DSEK [7], and DLEK [35]. The unaided and spectacle corrected visual acuity that can be achieved with PLK, which eliminates the problem of regular and irregular astigmatism that are associated with PK, are the what makes the biggest difference to the visual outcomes when comparing the results of PLK with PK.

11.4.2 Astigmatism

Induced astigmatism is not an issue after DSAEK. All the big series published so far have shown changes in mean refractive or topographic astigmatism of around 0.10 dioptres, which were not statistically significant from baseline [20, 21, 40, 46]. Similar results have been reported for DSEK [7] and DLEK techniques [35] with the exception of early cases of DLEK with a large incision of 9 mm [35]. All the endothelial keratoplasty techniques induce substantially less regular astigmatism when compared to penetrating keratoplasty [47] which also causes irregular astigmatism in some cases that requires contact lens correction for good vision [48].

11.4.3 Spherical Equivalent

Theoretically the placing of a donor corneal disc behind the host cornea posterior will steepen the posterior corneal curvature adding negative refractive power to this

Table 11.2 Advantages and disadvantages of posterior lamellar vs. penetrating keratoplasty

Advantages of PLK[a]	Closed chamber surgery: theoretically less risk of choroidal haemorrhage or endophthalmitis
	Risk of traumatic globe rupture reduced or eliminated
	More predictable visual rehabilitation; spectacle refraction stable within the first 3 months
	Few sutures resulting in:
	infrequent suture related complications (such as dehiscence, vascularisation and infections)
	minimal levels of induced astigmatism
	Predictable postoperative keratometry and refraction permits more accurate IOL power estimation for combined cataract and PLK surgery
	Less ocular surface disturbance and no disruption of corneal nerve plexus
	Probably reduced surgical time
Disadvantages of PLK	Presence of donor–host interface may reduce quality of vision and best correctable acuity
	More manipulation of donor cornea with potentially higher perioperative endothelial cell loss.
	High cost of equipment for donor preparation in Descemet-stripping automated endothelial keratoplasty (DSAEK)
	Donor dislocation relatively common
	Pupil block more common
	Scarred stroma untreatable
	Anterior segment reconstructions and IOL exchange technically more difficult
	Aniridic, aphakic and eyes with incomplete lens iris diaphragms technically more difficult
Uncertain	Routine cases probably technically more difficult
	Risks of secondary glaucoma may be less
	Risks of rejection may be less

[a]PLK, posterior lamellar keratoplasty

interface. This effect will decrease the total corneal power causing a hyperopic shift [23]. This hyperopic shift after PLK has been identified in several case series and has resulted in a change of the mean spherical equivalent from +0.50 to +1.12 D [7, 20, 21, 40]. Adjustment for the effect of this postoperative hyperopic shift, in planned cataract and PLK surgery, can be made by selecting an IOL with more power than the IOL power estimate for cataract surgery alone. We aim for a postoperative target refraction of −1D.

11.4.4 Endothelial Cell Loss

There has been continuing concern about the potential for increased endothelial cell loss in PLK compared to PK as a result of the effects of the preparation, manipulation, and insertion of the donor disc.

- Some surgeons use a larger graft diameter for PLK than PK to potentially correct for this; a 9.0 mm diameter PLK provides 26% more endothelial cells than an 8.0 mm PK graft.
- Reports of endothelial cell loss have been very variable from as high as 50% at 6 months [21], to 26% after 2 years in the Busin series [37]. Other reports suggest that there is no difference between cell loss with a 40% loss at 1 year for both PLK and PK [47] and a recent study comparing endothelial cell loss in historical PK vs. DSAEK, or other PLK techniques, showed no measurable difference [47].
- The insertion technique is likely to be an important determinant of endothelial cell loss and less traumatic techniques, such as the use of a glide, might reduce loss [49], although there are currently no definitive studies, no consensus, and techniques are still in evolution.
- The size of the wound, and its localisation (corneal vs. scleral), is also likely to have an effect with smaller corneal and scleral tunnel incisions increasing loss possibly due to compression of the donor graft during insertion [50, 51].
- A recent retrospective study showed that there was no statistical difference between forceps and pull through techniques (suture or glide guided) but that a 3 mm incision resulted in more endothelial cell loss than a 5 mm incision [52].

Further studies prospectively evaluating donor insertion protocols will establish the optimum techniques after which careful prospective comparative or randomised studies are needed to establish loss rates in PLK vs. PK.

11.4.5 Corneal Donor Dislocation (Fig. 11.4a–c)

The mechanisms of donor tissue attachment in PLK surgery are not established. Early postoperative attachment is likely to involve a combination of physical, biochemical, and physiological processes [52]. Dispersive viscoelastics like Viscoat (Alcon, Fort Worth, TX) and hydroxypropyl methylcellulose and possibly retained Descemet's membrane have been associated with dislocation [53]. However leaving host descemet's membrane intact did not cause dislocations in patients with previous PK undergoing PLK in one case series case series [41].

Evidence for the efficacy of different techniques to aid attachment is based on the reports of success rates in case series and not on experimental or prospective evaluation of different techniques. Section 1.3.5 summarises the methods most frequently described: using corneal massage, stab incisions, peripheral recipient bed roughening and high pressure with air tamponade in the AC (>30 mmHg) for 8–10 min. Donor dislocation is the most common complication of DSAEK surgery with reported rates varying from the lowest reported figure of 3/200 (1.5%) consecutive cases in which peripheral recipient bed scraping and sweeping of the corneal surface was used routinely [34] to 9/26 (35%) when the donor graft was positioned using a temporary air bubble that was partially evacuated after 7 min [40].

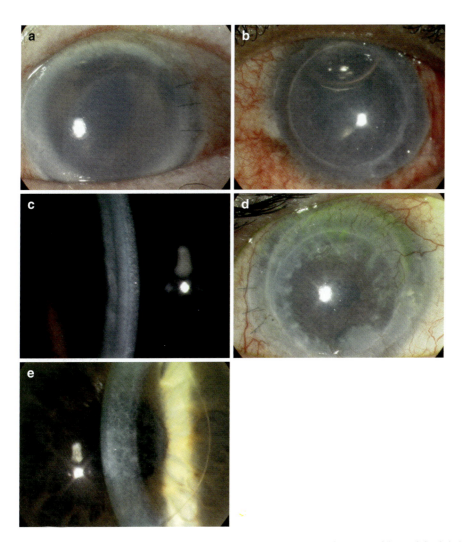

Fig. 11.4 Complications. (**a**) Total dislocation anterior view. (**b**) Dislocation without displacement of the graft for failed penetrating keratoplasty – anterior view. (**c**) Dislocation shown in 4b by slit view. (**d**) Primary graft failure in a patient with multiple previous PKs and inferior iridectomy. (**e**) Interface opacity

11.4.6 Pupillary Block

This complication is caused by the AC air bubble which can occlude the pupil and cause angle closure resulting in acute glaucoma, a flat AC, peripheral iris synechiae, iridocorneal adhesions, or a induced branch vein occlusion [40] and Urrets-Zavalia syndrome. Preventive measures are:

- To review the patient 1–2 h after the surgery to exclude this and remove any excess air if necessary [40]. We do this for all cases.
- Make an inferior iridectomy (a superior iridectomy is more easily blocked by air) [40]. This is easily carried out at the start of the procedure with an ocutome cutter. We use this procedure for phakic cases in whom we miose the pupil with pilocarpine to reduce the risk of crystalline lens damage during donor insertion.
- Dilate the pupil with topical cyclopentolate 1% and phenylephrine 2.5% at the end of surgery.
- In pseudophakic patients AC volume is greater. Some surgeons recommend removing most of the air at the end of surgery, leaving enough to cover the edges of the donor, and ensuring that the bubble is mobile in the AC by moving the patients head from side to side to assess mobility [34]. We prefer to leave the AC full of air but with a soft eye and remove any excess 1–2 h after surgery via a paracentesis.

11.4.7 Primary Graft Failure

Primary graft failure is uncommon after PK occurring at a rate of about 1:400 [34], but has been reported frequently after PLK particularly in surgeons early cases. Surgeons initial consecutive case series have reported primary failure as high as 3/34 (9%) [21] and 21/118 (18%) [54]; these high rates are likely to result from the surgeon learning curve with ten surgeons doing the 118 cases in the latter series. On the other hand some single surgeon series have reported no primary graft failures in his 200 DSAEK's [34] and only 1/100 in the first 100 DSEK and DSAEK cases. The decreased incidence of primary graft failure with increased DSAEK surgeon experience suggests that primary graft failure in DSAEK is more likely to be related to endothelial trauma during the operative procedure rather than to problems with eye bank selection and storage. In addition primary graft failure is 5 times more common in grafts that needed a second surgical intervention to treat early dislocation [55] which is in turn related to case selection being more common in patients with preoperative lens/iris diaphragm deficiency and aphakia in whom the donor dislocation rate is double [55] (Fig. 11.4d).

However the similar rates of endothelial cell loss that have been reported for PK and PLK suggest that with good currently available techniques cell loss may be no greater in PLK than PK. It is likely that as insertion and attachment protocols, and surgeon training, are improved overall endothelial cell loss and primary graft failures will be no more for PLK than PK.

11.4.8 Rejection

One series of 199 eyes, having had DSAEK or DLEK, and a follow up of 2 years had a rejection rate of 15/199 (7.5%) compared to a rate of 92/708(13%) in a historical case series of PK's carried out for similar indications [56]. In addition the morbidity following rejection was less severe in the PLK series with only 6.7% proceeding to graft failure compared to 28.3% of the PK's. However 80% of the PLK patients were still taking topical steroid medication 2 years after surgery whereas this had been stopped 1 year after surgery in the PK patients and this may have accounted for the difference rather than any potential reduction in antigenicity due to the reduced bulk of the PLK. That steroid may well have been a confounding factor in this study is suggested by the findings of a recent randomised controlled trial of topical steroid vs. no topical steroid after PK in which the topical steroid was discontinued 6 months post op in one group and continued for 12 months in the second group resulting in a 50% reduction in the rate of rejection (19/202 (9.1%) in the no steroid group vs. 10/204 (4.9%) in the topical steroid group) [57]. PLK rejection rates reported from other studies are 7/118 (6%) DSAEK's [54] in which the mean follow up was uncertain. In the largest published study by Price et al, graft rejection occurred in 54/598 (9%) eyes after Descemet stripping with endothelial keratoplasty [58]. Thirty-five per cent of the eyes were asymptomatic and were diagnosed during routine examination. Signs of immunological rejection at the initial diagnosis included keratic precipitates (69%), diffuse corneal oedema (11%) or both (20%); no endothelial rejection lines were observed [58].

11.4.9 Other Complications

Other complications of DSAEK are cystoid macular edema [54], interface opacities [54] (Fig. 11.4e), retinal detachment [54], suprachoroidal haemorrhage [54], donor dislocation into the posterior segment [54] and dislocation of an intraocular lens into the vitreous cavity as a consequence of the increase in AC volume during air tamponade [59].

11.5 Conclusion

This perspective shows that an experienced surgeon, operating on patients with corneal endothelial disease, such as Fuchs' dystrophy or pseudophakic bullous keratopathy (PBK), can expect to obtain more predictable results, much more quickly, with PLK than with PK and with fewer postoperative complications, particularly those relating to astigmatism, sutures and resistance to trauma. Following PLK using DSAEK or DSEK most patients can expect to achieve vision that is adequate for them to meet the driving standard within 3 months, using spectacles. Combined cataract and PLK surgery works well also. We believe that PLK will rapidly supersede PK for this patient group in the same way that phacoemulsification has replaced large incision extracapsular cataract extraction for most cataract patients.

However there remain many areas where the role of this technique is uncertain. It can provide excellent results for restoration of corneal clarity in patients with failed PK. It can also succeed in patients with AC lenses although success is uncertain in this situation. It can be difficult, or impossible, to do DSAEK or DSEK when an air bubble cannot be retained in the AC as can happen in some patients with a deficiency in the lens iris diaphragm. In patients with some stromal opacity PLK may still be a better option than PK, with less risk, even though the visual outcome may be compromised by corneal stromal opacification and in whom residual superficial stromal opacity can be treated with an excimer laser phototherapeutic keratectomy. Because of the difficulty of access to lens and iris structures through a small incision patients requiring lens exchange and/or pupilloplasty may be better having a conventional PK. Prospectively collected data on the use of PLK for complex and high risk cases will answer many of the questions raised in this perspective and the risks and benefits of the technique will be clarified in the next few years.

PLK is also an evolving technique with regard to the success of protocols for ensuring donor graft adhesion in DSEK and DSAEK. Prospective case series can be expected to clarify the optimal techniques for this and, like all new surgical procedures, a stable and effective solution will be developed in time. Meanwhile refinements to the procedure, including the development of DMEK, can be expected to improve the already remarkable visual results available using DSAEK and DSEK.

Lamellar corneal procedures promise to replace PK as the procedure of choice for corneal replacement surgery except for corneal disease involving both stroma and endothelium and for therapeutic procedures.

References

1. Tillett CW (1956) Posterior lamellar keratoplasty. Am J Ophthalmol 41(3):530–533
2. Melles GR, Lander F, Beekhuis WH, Remeijer L, Binder PS (1999) Posterior lamellar keratoplasty for a case of pseudophakic bullous keratopathy. Am J Ophthalmol 127(3): 340–341
3. Melles GR, Eggink FA, Lander F et al (1998) A surgical technique for posterior lamellar keratoplasty. Cornea 17(6):618–626
4. Terry MA, Ousley PJ (2001) Deep lamellar endothelial keratoplasty in the first United States patients: early clinical results. Cornea 20(3):239–243
5. Terry MA, Ousley PJ (2005) Small-incision deep lamellar endothelial keratoplasty (DLEK): six-month results in the first prospective clinical study. Cornea 24(1):59–65
6. Melles GR, Wijdh RH, Nieuwendaal CP (2004) A technique to excise the descemet membrane from a recipient cornea (descemetorhexis). Cornea 23(3):286–288
7. Price FW Jr, Price MO (2005) Descemet's stripping with endothelial keratoplasty in 50 eyes: a refractive neutral corneal transplant. J Refract Surg 21(4):339–345
8. Gorovoy MS (2006) Descemet-stripping automated endothelial keratoplasty. Cornea 25(8):886–889
9. Ham L, Dapena I, van Luijk C, van der Wees J, Melles GR (2009 Jan 30) Descemet membrane endothelial keratoplasty (DMEK) for Fuchs endothelial dystrophy: review of the first 50 consecutive cases. Eye [Epub ahead of print]
10. Melles GR, Ong TS, Ververs B, van der Wees J (2006) Descemet membrane endothelial keratoplasty (DMEK). Cornea 25(8):987–990
11. Sony P, Sharma N, Sen S, Vajpayee RB (2005) Indications of penetrating keratoplasty in northern India. Cornea 24(8):989–991
12. Al-Towerki AE, Gonnah el S, Al-Rajhi A, Wagoner MD (2004) Changing indications for corneal transplantation at the King Khaled eye specialist hospital (1983–2002). Cornea 23(6):584–588
13. Al-Yousuf N, Mavrikakis I, Mavrikakis E, Daya SM (2004) Penetrating keratoplasty: indications over a 10 year period. Br J Ophthalmol 88(8):998–1001
14. Kang PC, Klintworth GK, Kim T et al (2005) Trends in the indications for penetrating keratoplasty, 1980–2001. Cornea 24(7):801–803
15. The Australian Corneal Graft Registry (ACGR) (2007) Department of Ophthalmology FMC. 2007 Report. Bedford Park, SA 5042. Flinders University: Australia
16. Seitzman GD, Gottsch JD, Stark WJ (2005) Cataract surgery in patients with Fuchs' corneal dystrophy: expanding recommendations for cataract surgery without simultaneous keratoplasty. Ophthalmology 112(3):441–446
17. Ti SE, Chee SP (2006) Cataract surgery in patients with Fuchs'. Ophthalmology 113(10):1883–1884
18. Shimmyo M, Ross AJ, Moy A, Mostafavi R (2003) Intraocular pressure, Goldmann applanation tension, corneal thickness, and corneal curvature in Caucasians, Asians, Hispanics, and African Americans. Am J Ophthalmol 136(4):603–613
19. Foster PJ, Baasanhu J, Alsbirk PH, Munkhbayar D, Uranchimeg D, Johnson GJ (1998) Central corneal

thickness and intraocular pressure in a Mongolian population. Ophthalmology 105(6):969–973
20. Covert DJ, Koenig SB (2007) New triple procedure: Descemet's stripping and automated endothelial keratoplasty combined with phacoemulsification and intraocular lens implantation. Ophthalmology 114(7):1272–1277
21. Koenig SB, Covert DJ, Dupps WJ Jr, Meisler DM (2007) Visual acuity, refractive error, and endothelial cell density six months after Descemet stripping and automated endothelial keratoplasty (DSAEK). Cornea 26(6):670–674
22. Price MO, Baig KM, Brubaker JW, Price FW Jr (2008) Randomized, prospective comparison of precut vs surgeon-dissected grafts for descemet stripping automated endothelial keratoplasty. Am J Ophthalmol 146(1):36–41
23. Rao SK, Leung CK, Cheung CY et al (2008) Descemet stripping endothelial keratoplasty: effect of the surgical procedure on corneal optics. Am J Ophthalmol 145(6): 991–996
24. Chen ES, Terry MA, Shamie N, Phillips PM, Friend DJ (2009) Retention of an anterior chamber IOL versus IOL exchange in endothelial keratoplasty. J Cataract Refract Surg 35(4):613; author reply 614
25. Wylegala E, Tarnawska D (2008) Management of pseudophakic bullous keratopathy by combined Descemet-stripping endothelial keratoplasty and intraocular lens exchange. J Cataract Refract Surg 34(10):1708–1714
26. Chen E, Shamie N, Terry MA (2007) Deep lamellar endothelial keratoplasty. In: Fontana L, Tassinari G (eds) Atlas of lamellar keratoplaty. Fabiano Editore, 185–192
27. Al-Mohaimeed M, Al-Shahwan S, Al-Torbak A, Wagoner MD (2007) Escalation of glaucoma therapy after penetrating keratoplasty. Ophthalmology 114(12):2281–2286
28. Rahman I, Carley F, Hillarby C, Brahma A, Tullo AB (2009) Penetrating keratoplasty: indications, outcomes, and complications. Eye 23(6):1288–1294
29. Hyams M, Segev F, Yepes N, Slomovic AR, Rootman DS (2007) Early postoperative complications of deep lamellar endothelial keratoplasty. Cornea 26(6):650–653
30. Melles GR, Lander F, Rietveld FJ, Remeijer L, Beekhuis WH, Binder PS (1999) A new surgical technique for deep stromal, anterior lamellar keratoplasty. Br J Ophthalmol 83(3): 327–333
31. Mendicute J, Villarubia A, Irigoyen C, Arnalich-Montiel F (2008) Distrofia de Fuchs y DSAEK. In Cirugia de Cristalino. Lorente R, Mendicute C eds. Sociedad Española de Oftalmología
32. Jones YJ, Goins KM, Sutphin JE, Mullins R, Skeie JM (2008) Comparison of the femtosecond laser (IntraLase) versus manual microkeratome (Moria ALTK) in dissection of the donor in endothelial keratoplasty: initial study in eye bank eyes. Cornea 27(1):88–93
33. Cheng YY, Hendrikse F, Pels E et al (2008) Preliminary results of femtosecond laser-assisted descemet stripping endothelial keratoplasty. Arch Ophthalmol 126(10): 1351–1356
34. Terry MA, Shamie N, Chen ES, Hoar KL, Friend DJ (2008) Endothelial keratoplasty a simplified technique to minimize graft dislocation, iatrogenic graft failure, and pupillary block. Ophthalmology 115(7):1179–1186
35. Terry MA, Ousley PJ (2005) Deep lamellar endothelial keratoplasty visual acuity, astigmatism, and endothelial survival in a large prospective series. Ophthalmology 112(9): 1541–1548
36. Bradley JC, McCartney DL (2007) Descemet's stripping automated endothelial keratoplasty in intraoperative floppy-iris syndrome: suture-drag technique. J Cataract Refract Surg 33(7):1149–1150
37. Busin M, Bhatt PR, Scorcia V (2008) A modified technique for descemet membrane stripping automated endothelial keratoplasty to minimize endothelial cell loss. Arch Ophthalmol 126(8):1133–1137
38. Koenig SB, Meisler DM, Dupps WJ, Rubenstein JB, Kumar R (2008) External refinement of the donor lenticule position during descemet's stripping and automated endothelial keratoplasty. Ophthalmic Surg Lasers Imaging 39(6):522–523
39. Terry MA, Hoar KL, Wall J, Ousley P (2006) Histology of dislocations in endothelial keratoplasty (DSEK and DLEK): a laboratory-based, surgical solution to dislocation in 100 consecutive DSEK cases. Cornea 25(8):926–932
40. Koenig SB, Covert DJ (2007) Early results of small-incision Descemet's stripping and automated endothelial keratoplasty. Ophthalmology 114(2):221–226
41. Price FW Jr, Price MO (2006) Endothelial keratoplasty to restore clarity to a failed penetrating graft. Cornea 25(8):895–899
42. Covert DJ, Koenig SB (2007) Descemet stripping and automated endothelial keratoplasty (DSAEK) in eyes with failed penetrating keratoplasty. Cornea 26(6):692–696
43. Suh LH, Kymionis GD, Culbertson WW, O'Brien TP, Yoo SH (2008) Descemet stripping with endothelial keratoplasty in aphakic eyes. Arch Ophthalmol 126(2):268–270
44. Price FW Jr, Price MO (2006) Descemet's stripping with endothelial keratoplasty in 200 eyes: Early challenges and techniques to enhance donor adherence. J Cataract Refract Surg 32(3):411–418
45. Huang T, Wang Y, Gao N, Wang T, Ji J, Chen J (2009) Complex deep lamellar endothelial keratoplasty for complex bullous keratopathy with severe vision loss. Cornea 28(2):157–162
46. Chen ES, Terry MA, Shamie N, Hoar KL, Friend DJ (2008) Descemet-stripping automated endothelial keratoplasty: six-month results in a prospective study of 100 eyes. Cornea 27(5):514–520
47. Bahar I, Kaiserman I, McAllum P, Slomovic A, Rootman D (2008) Comparison of posterior lamellar keratoplasty techniques to penetrating keratoplasty. Ophthalmology 115(9): 1525–1533
48. Geerards AJ, Vreugdenhil W, Khazen A (2006) Incidence of rigid gas-permeable contact lens wear after keratoplasty for keratoconus. Eye Contact Lens 32(4):207–210
49. Bahar I, Kaiserman I, Sansanayudh W, Levinger E, Rootman DS (2009) Busin guide vs forceps for the insertion of the donor lenticule in Descemet stripping automated endothelial keratoplasty. Am J Ophthalmol 147(2):220–226.e1
50. Price MO, Price FW Jr (2008) Endothelial cell loss after descemet stripping with endothelial keratoplasty influencing factors and 2-year trend. Ophthalmology 115(5): 857–865
51. Terry MA, Wall JM, Hoar KL, Ousley PJ (2007) A prospective study of endothelial cell loss during the 2 years after deep lamellar endothelial keratoplasty. Ophthalmology 114(4):631–639

52. Terry MA, Saad HA, Shamie N et al (2009) Endothelial keratoplasty: the influence of insertion techniques and incision size on donor endothelial survival. Cornea 28(1):24–31
53. Kymionis GD, Suh LH, Dubovy SR, Yoo SH (2007) Diagnosis of residual Descemet's membrane after Descemet's stripping endothelial keratoplasty with anterior segment optical coherence tomography. J Cataract Refract Surg 33(7): 1322–1324
54. Suh LH, Yoo SH, Deobhakta A et al (2008) Complications of Descemet's stripping with automated endothelial keratoplasty: survey of 118 eyes at one institute. Ophthalmology 115(9):1517–1524
55. O'Brien PD, Lake DB, Saw VP, Rostron CK, Dart JK, Allan BD (2008) Endothelial keratoplasty: case selection in the learning curve. Cornea 27(10):1114–1118
56. Allan BD, Terry MA, Price FW Jr, Price MO, Griffin NB, Claesson M (2007) Corneal transplant rejection rate and severity after endothelial keratoplasty. Cornea 26(9): 1039–1042
57. Nguyen NX, Seitz B, Martus P, Langenbucher A, Cursiefen C (2007) Long-term topical steroid treatment improves graft survival following normal-risk penetrating keratoplasty. Am J Ophthalmol 144(2):318–319
58. Jordan CS, Price MO, Trespalacios R, Price FW Jr (2009) Graft rejection episodes after Descemet stripping with endothelial keratoplasty: part one: clinical signs and symptoms. Br J Ophthalmol 93(3):387–390
59. Tay E, Rajan MS, Saw VP, Dart JK (2008) Dislocated intraocular lens into the vitreous cavity after DSAEK. J Cataract Refract Surg 34(3):525–526

Index

A

ABO antigens, 6
ACAID. *See* Anterior chamber-associated immune deviation
Acute allograft rejection, 38
Acute rejection, 19, 25, 26
Allergic asthma, 5
Allergic conjunctivitis, 5
Allergic disease, 97–116
Allergic inflammation, 106
Allergic keratoconjunctivitis, 108–110
Allergic process, 105–106
Allogeneic tissue, 62
Allograft response, 17
Allografts, 1
AlphaCor Kpro, 139–140
Alpha-melanocyte-stimulating hormone, 46
Anirida, 56
Anterior chamber-associated immune deviation (ACAID), 8, 9, 37
Anterior chamber fluid, 14
Antibiotics, 130–132
Antibodies, 4
Antigen presentation, 15–17
Antigen presenting cells (APC), 5, 7, 8, 15
Antigen processing, 15, 16
Antigen uptake, 15–16
Antihistamine/mast cell stabilizers, 112
Apical clearance method, 90
Aqueous humor, 37–49
Atopic dermatitis, 28
Atopic keratoconjunctivitis (AKC), 97, 99–101
Autoimmune polyglandular syndrome, 56
Autologous stem cells, 62

B

Barrier function, 70
Basiliximab and Daclizumab, 31–32
B-cell activation, 38
Bcl-xL, 22
Biologic agents, 31
Biologic scaffolds, 142
Blood vessels, 14
B lymphocytes, 9
Boston type 1 Kpro, 138–139
Boston type 2 Kpro, 140–141
Bullous keratopathy, 70

C

Calcitonin gene-realted peptide, 46
Calcitonin gene-related peptide (CGRP), 10, 37
CD4+ T lymphocytes, 3, 9
CD8+ T lymphocytes, 3–4, 9
Cell cycle control, 69–83
CGRP. *See* Calcitonin gene-related peptide
Chlamydia trachomatis, 121
   infection, 126–127
Chronic bullous keratopathy, 56
Chronic limbitis, 56
Chronic rejection, 26
Cicatricial pemphigoid, 56
Class II expression, 14
Complement regulatory proteins (CRP), 10
Confocal microscopy, 108–109
Conjunctival limbal autograft (CLAU), 58
Contact blepharoconjunctivitis, 101
Contact dermatitis of the eyelid, 99
Contact inhibition, 69
Contact lenses (CL), 87–94
   fitting, 87
Contact lens-induced keratopathy, 56
Corneal allograft, 13–22
Corneal contour, 89
Corneal endothelium, 69–83
Corneal infection, 110
Corneal opacification (CO), 121, 122
Corneal privilege, 14–15
Corneal transplant, 110–111
Corneal transplantation, 1
Corticosteroids, 2, 28, 112, 114
Cross linking, 90
Cyclosporin A, 18
Cyclosporine, 25, 115
Cyclosporine A, 28–29
Cytokines, 37–49
Cytology, 105
Cytotoxic lymphocyte antigen 4-Ig fusion protein (CTLA4-Ig), 21

D

Deep vascularization, 28
Delayed-type hypersensitivity (DTH), 8
Dendritic cells, 14
Diabetes, 32
Diagnostic tests for ocular allergy, 105

Direct pathway of allorecognition, 26
DNA damage, 69
DNA duplication, 74
Draining lymph node, 8
Drug induced conjunctivitis, 99, 101–102

E
Endostatin-kringle 5 fusion protein (EK5), 21
Engineered antibodies, 19–20
Entropion, 122
Epithelium, 3, 8, 53
Ex vivo expansion, 60

F
Fas ligand (FasL), 8, 10, 44–45
Fitting CLs, 88
Fitting techniques, 89–90, 93–94
FK506, 18
FK788, 31
FTY 720, 31

G
Gene therapy, 20
Giant papillary conjunctivitis (GPC), 99, 101
G1-phase, 74
    inhibition, 79
    inhibitors, 69

H
Hemangiogenesis, 6
High-risk transplantation, 27
High-risk transplants, 25
HLA matching, 2, 13, 18
Human corneal endothelial cells (HCEC), 69
Hydroxyapatite biologic haptics, 141

I
IFN-γ, 37
IgE production, 38
IgG production, 38
IL2, 19, 25
IL-4, 37
IL-5, 37
IL-10, 17, 37
IL-12, 37
IL2 receptor (IL2R), 19
Immune privilege, 1, 18, 38
Immune reactions, 92
Immune rejection, 2
Immune response in trachoma, 128–129
Immunologic rejection, 25
Immunomodulatory cytokines, 14
Indirect pathway of allorecognition, 26
Indoleamine 2,3-dioxygenase (IDO), 21
Indoleamine dioxygenase (IDO), 10
Inflammation, 2
Innate immunity, 104–105
Interferon gamma (IFN-γ), 42
Interleukin 2, 37, 40
Interleukin 4 (IL4), 21, 46
Interleukin 5, 46
Interleukin 6, 37, 41

Interleukin 8, 46
Interleukin 10 (IL10), 21, 41–42
Interleukin 12, 46
Interleukin 1b, 40
Interleukin1 receptor antagonist, 45

K
Keratoconjunctivitis, 101–102
Keratoconus (KC), 88–91
Keratoconus and allergic conjunctivitis, 109
Keratoglobus, 109–110
Keratolimbal allograft transplant, 59–60
Keratoprosthesis, 137–142
Kpro, 138–140

L
Langerhans cells (LC), 7, 14
LESC niche, 55
Limbal stem cell deficiency (LSCD), 28, 55
Limbal stem cell transplantation, 53–63
Limbus, 53–55
Living-related conjunctival limbal allograft transplant, 58–59
Loss of endothelial cells, 70
Low compliance, 32
LUCIDA, 33
Lymphangiogenesis, 6
Lymphatics, 14
    vessels, 8
Lymph node, 15

M
Macrophages, 4–5, 14
Major histocompatibility complex (MHC), 6, 8, 14, 26
    class II, 15
MHC. *See* Major histocompatibility complex
Migration inhibitory factor (MIF), 10
α-MSH, 10, 37
Mycophenolate mofetil (MMF), 25, 29–30

N
Natural killer (NK) cells, 4–5
Neovascularization, 2
Nerve growth factor (NGF), 21
Neurotrophic keratopathy, 56
NKT cells, 8, 9
Normal-risk transplantation, 27

O
Ocular immunity, 104–106
Osteo-odonto keratoprosthesis (OOKP), 140
Oxidative DNA damage, 81–82

P
Partial LSCD, 58
Patch test, 105
p21Cip1, 69
Pediatric application of Boston type 1 Kpro, 139
Penetrating keratoplasty, 37, 91–94
Perennial allergic conjunctivitis (PAC), 98
Peripheral ulcerative keratitis, 56

Pimecrolimus, 31
p16INK4a, 69
Pintucci Kpro, 141
p27Kip1, 69
Previous graft rejections, 28
Programmed death ligand-1 (PD-L1), 8
Proliferative capacity, 71–72
p40 subunit of interleukin 12 (p40-IL12), 21
Pterygium, 56

R
RAD (Everolimus), 30
Rapamycin (Sirolimus), 30
Regulation of G1-phase, 73–74
Reshape and splint method, 89
Risk factors for active trachoma, 126–127

S
SAFE strategy, 121, 130
Scarring in trachoma, 127–128
Scleral fitting method, 90
Seasonal allergic conjunctivitis (SAC), 98
Seoul-type Kpro, 141
Serum specific IgE, 105
sFasL, 37
Short telomeres, 81
Skin prick test, 105
Soft lenses, 89
Soluble fas ligand, 44–45
SOM. See Somatostatin
Somatostatin (SOM), 10, 37, 46
Steroids, 25
Stevens–Johnson syndrome, 56
Stimulus for inflammation, 127–128
Surgical treatment of keratoconjunctivitis, 116
Suture removal, 93–94
Systemic immunomodulation, 28
Systemic immunosuppression, 13, 18, 25, 27

T
Tacrolimus (fk506), 29
T cell, 25
    activation, 17
    receptor (TCR), 5, 16
Tear IgE, 105
Tear instability and corneal involvement, 107
TGF-β, 10
TGF-β2, 37, 38
Thermal burn, 56

Three-point touch method, 89–90
Th1 responses, 38
Th2 responses, 38
Thrombospondin, 37, 46
Th1/Th2 paradigm, 39
Tissue matching, 62
T lymphocytes, 9
Topical and systemic immunomodulation, 25–33
Topical immunomodulation, 27–28
Topical immunosuppression, 25
Topical steroids, 28
Total LSCD, 58
Trachoma, 121–132
    control, 130–132
Transforming growth factor-beta2 (TGF-beta2), 69, 75
Transforming growth factor beta (TGF-β), 43–44
Transgenes, 20
Treatment
    of AKC, 115–116
    of allergic conjunctivitis, 112–114
    of GPC, 114
    of ocular allergy, 111–116
    of vernal keratoconjunctivitis (VKC), 114–115
Trichiasis, 121, 122
Tumor necrosis factor alpha (TNF-α), 37
    levels, 42–43
Tumor necrosis factor-related apoptosis-inducing ligand (TRAIL), 8

U
Ultraviolet B (UVB), 8
Urban allergy, 99
Urban eye allergy syndrome, 102

V
Vasoactive intestinal peptide (VIP), 10
Vasoconstrictor, 112
Vectors for gene therapy, 20
Vernal keratoconjunctivitis (VKC), 97–100
Viral macrophage inflammatory protein II (vMIP II), 22

W
WHO system for the assessment of trachoma, 123
Worst-Singh Kpro, 141

X
XYZ hypothesis, 54

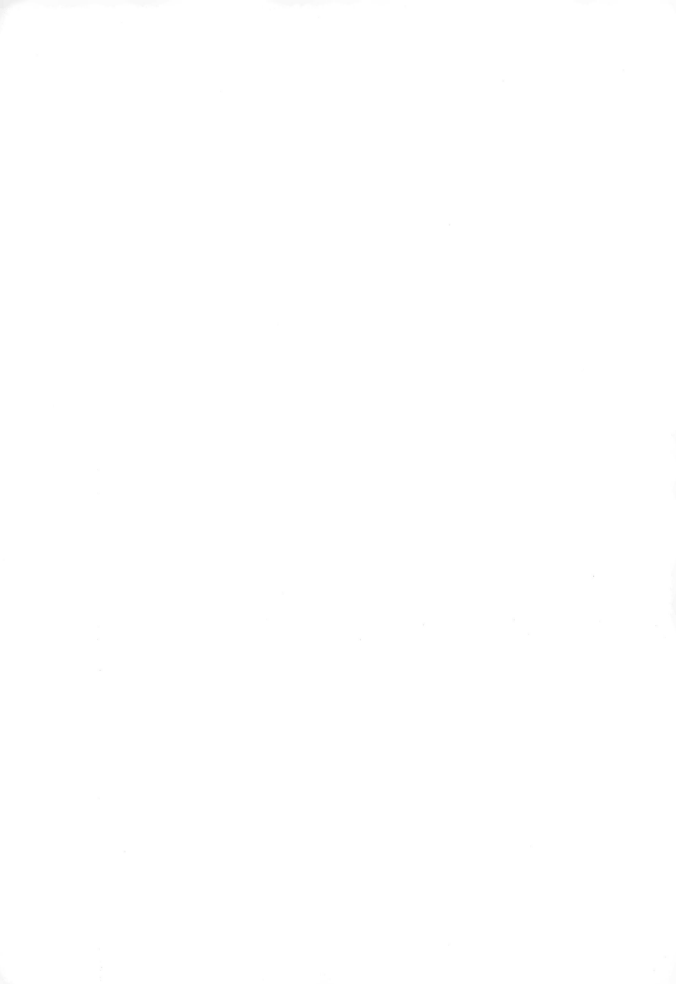

Printing and Binding: Stürtz GmbH, Würzburg